The
History of
Massage

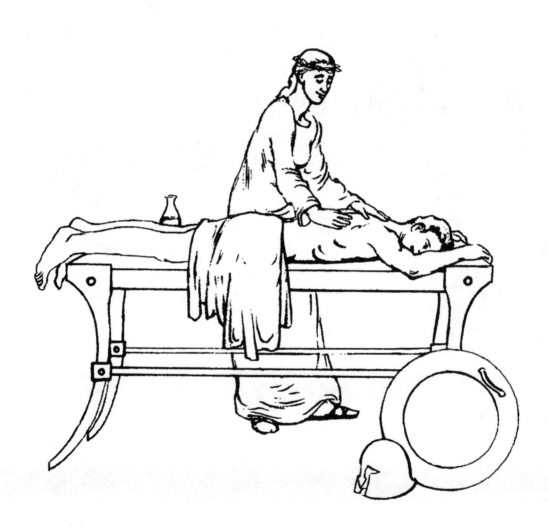

The
History of
Massage

AN ILLUSTRATED SURVEY

FROM AROUND THE WORLD

Robert Noah Calvert

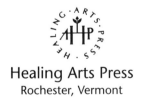

Healing Arts Press
Rochester, Vermont

Healing Arts Press
One Park Street
Rochester, Vermont 05767
www.InnerTraditions.com
Healing Arts Press is a division of Inner Traditions International

Library of Congress Cataloging-in-Publication Data

Calvert, Robert Noah.
    The history of massage : an illustrated survey from around the world / by Robert Noah Calvert.
        p. ; cm.
Includes bibliographical references and index.
    ISBN 0-89281-881-6 (pbk.)
 1. Massage—History. 2. Massage therapy—History.
    [DNLM: 1. Massage—history. WB 537 C167h 2002] I. Title.
    RM721 .C345 2002
    615.8'22'09—dc21

                           2002000056

Printed and bound in the United States at Edwards Brothers

10 9 8 7 6 5 4 3 2 1

Text design by Cindy Sutherland; layout by Priscilla Baker

This book was typeset in Garamond, with Futura, Stone Sans, and Berkeley as the display typefaces

Frontispiece: Polykaste Anoints Telemachos, *The Odyssey,* Book III. Reprinted with permission from *Anoint Yourself with Oil for Radiant Health* (Vital Health Publishing, 1997).

Grateful acknowledgment to the American Massage Therapy Association for permission to reprint excerpts from *Massage Therapy Journal* vol. 25, no. 3 (summer 1986), vol. 26, no. 1 (winter 1987), and vol. 32, no. 4 (fall 1993).

Contents

Foreword

How appropriate that, at the dawn of the twenty-first century, we consider the significant contribution massage has made to the health and well-being of humanity throughout the ages. Soft-tissue manipulation is no doubt one of the oldest forms of therapy, practiced for its health benefits and fulfilling the essential human need for contact with others. As this informative and enlightening book shows, massage is a universal practice crossing all borders and boundaries; it does not belong exclusively to any one profession, or even to one tradition. Massage is a shared human experience.

The History of Massage brings massage as a healing practice out of the shadows and offers an understanding of the place of massage in the evolution of medicine and natural healing. The stuff of history—people, places, things, events, everyday life—comes alive in quotations and in vintage drawings, photographs, and advertisements. But this project has a value that transcends curiosity about old things and nostalgia for days gone by. Background material for discussion of current isssues in the field is also presented. These issues include the association of massage with prostitution, accusations of quackery, unethical behavior of practitioners, and the connection of massage with the New Age phenomena of the 1970s and 1980s. Attempts to regulate massage are examined. Context is given to issues raised by the professionalization of a field considered holistic and alternative, and one that draws from many traditions.

For professionals who use massage in their work, and especially for developing their leadership, historical literacy is imperative. It offers perspective to see the big picture, deepens understanding of current events, and helps today's leaders make better decisions for the future. Robert Calvert captures the breadth of massage as a world phenomena and offers a sense of its pervasiveness in the human experience throughout time. In many places massage was (and still is) a health practice as common as eating the right foods and getting enough sleep and exercise. Among indigenous people in places such as Africa, Australia, and Hawaii, and in ancient civilizations such as Egypt, China, and India, massage was part of the fabric of life. In an unbroken chain from ancient Greece and Rome, Western civilization has enjoyed the benefits of massage at the gymnasium, at Roman and Turkish baths, at hot springs and health resorts, and now at destination and day spas and health clubs.

Of particular interest in this book are explorations on the history of massage in specific occupations. Massage has been a main feature in treatments offered historically by barbers, cosmetologists, physicians, nurses, midwives, physical therapists, and athletic trainers, as well as massage specialists. Massage practitioners and students will especially enjoy discovering the roots of their specialty and appreciate the antiquity of their chosen work.

An awareness of the past defends against a provincialism of time as well as place. *The History of Massage* explores the theory behind the practice of massage in different cultures and time periods, including the association of massage with traditional healing practices also involving magic and ritual, the empirical development of knowledge and skill in massage, and the assumptions underlying early scientific research. Such an exposé broadens our understanding of massage theory, inviting us to explore perspectives other than Western science and encouraging us to think about the validity of different approaches to knowledge and the impact of culture on how we think and act.

The universality of the simple yet profound benefits of skilled and caring touch is evident in the many guises massage has taken throughout world history. Any attempts to pin massage to one paradigm—be it Western biomedicine or esoteric systems such as Chinese medicine and Ayurveda—fail as massage's universal nature is unveiled. We are blessed with the challenge of a global consciousness; that is, to see the underlying truth in it all.

Massage practitioners who read *The History of Massage* will enjoy a sense of identity with those who came before. Current practitioners are the latest in a long line of those who answered the calling to help humankind through the practice of massage. It is true that we today "stand on the shoulders of giants," as well as on the shoulders of all the ordinary people throughout the ages whose livelihood has been massage. An unbroken chain from teacher to student to practitioner and round again brings us to today. We see that chain in our history.

I have known Robert Calvert for more than ten years as a fellow activist in the massage profession. His dedication to massage and its traditions is undeniable and shows through clearly in this panoramic view of massage history. Robert brings the same enthusiasm and love of massage to this work as he did to founding *Massage Magazine* in the 1980s and establishing the World of Massage Museum in the year 2000. I am pleased to watch the development of WOMM and its collections and to serve on its first advisory council.

The History of Massage is a great reference book. My appreciation and congratulations go out to Robert on this sterling contribution to understanding our past.

Patricia J. Benjamin, Ph.D.
Executive Director, Chicago School of Massage Therapy
February 2002

Acknowledgments

My mother started me on the way to healthy touch by having me rub her feet when I was ten years old. My upbringing was a very touchy one, too. Each morning and upon returning home from school all us kids would kiss and hug Mom and Dad. Even today at family gatherings we continue to give and receive hugs. So thanks, Mom, for getting me started rubbing the right way.

My formal education in the touching arts and sciences was initiated by my dear friend Sherry Lauer, a midwife extraordinaire. At the time I was a journeyman ironworker—you know, one of those guys who works on bridges, dams, and nuclear plants. Sherry recommended that I read a book called *Your Healing Hands.* This book and the experiences Sherry provided in giving me the honor of practicing polarity therapy on her pregnant patients were the catalysts that moved me formally into healing touch.

The everyday experience of being touched with the great love and care of my wife, Judi, a professional massage therapist of almost two decades, has also contributed to my appreciation for this kind of caregiving. Since 1984 Judi and I have shared the joys and mystery of touch with each other and with many other people around the world during our travels as self-proclaimed ambassadors of touch and as representatives of *Massage Magazine.*

Ashley Montagu's seminal book, *Touching: The Human Significance of the Skin,* has had a powerful influence on my studies in the tactile arts and sciences. His book, one of the cornerstones of my inquiry, provides an exciting springboard of possibilities. I hope others will follow his lead.

My own career in massage began in 1979 when I first experienced and later trained in polarity therapy. Pierre Pannetier, M.D., Cambodian physician and successor to osteopath, chiropractor, and naturopathic doctor Randolph Stone, the founder of polarity therapy, was my first teacher of this comprehensive healing art system. I attended the ALIVE Polarity Institute on Orcas Island and later studied at the Calistoga and Murrieta Hot Springs locations as well. Through my polarity therapy training and through reading and working with clients in my counseling practice, I realized that the body needed accessing, not just the mind, for bringing to light the many struggles we humans undergo.

Writing a book is an adventure. To begin with, it is a toy and an amusement. Then it becomes a mistress, then it becomes a master, then it becomes a tyrant. . . . Just as you are about to be reconciled to your servitude, you kill the monster and fling it to the public.

—Winston Churchill

I enrolled in the East West College of Massage and then studied Pfrimmer deep-muscle technique with George Siegfried, D.C.

Finally I was ready to open my own massage therapy practice. Then in 1984 my clinic and school—The Bodyworks School of Muscle Therapy in Spokane, Washington—burned to the ground, leaving me without a home or a business.

Judi says I moved in with her then and never left. The truth is she was overjoyed to marry a massage therapist because, and rightly so, she figured she'd have her personal in-house therapist. In January of 1985 we moved to Hawaii, where I conceived of and started *Massage Magazine* with a group of dedicated and intrepid friends. Since those fateful days of our inception, when we were working with a lot of energy and little publishing experience, *Massage Magazine* has become the leading publication of its kind in the world.

Massage Magazine has afforded Judi and me many wonderful opportunities to explore and learn about touch therapies around the world, and about myself and my relationships in the process. I extend my deeply felt appreciation to the staff of *Massage Magazine,* past and present, for their unending support and enhancement of my vision for the magazine, a vision that is now theirs as well. I have enjoyed their support of numerous other projects, which on occasion have not succeeded. Our shared vision of bringing touch to the world continues to drive all of us in our everyday endeavors.

Specifically, I extend my gratitude to Lori Bertis for her excellent help during the initial research phase that manifested in the world's first display on the history of massage. Our research began in 1994, and in 1995 we created a display of the history of massage in the United States, from its ancient roots to modern times, which stood 9 feet tall and spanned 54 feet in length. That display has since been dismantled, and its contents are now a part of this book. I'm pleased to announce that all that research has resulted in the establishment of the world's first museum dedicated to the history of massage. The World of Massage Museum, created in 2000 by Judi and me, is now housed in the *Massage Magazine* facilities in Spokane, Washington.

My appreciation goes, too, to Patricia Benjamin, Ph.D., for her work delving into massage's past, and for her courage in clarifying some of the lingering myths about massage. I especially appreciate the accuracy and integrity of her reporting over the years. I am thankful to Richard van Why for his extensive research of the formal literature on massage and for categorizing that which he discovered. Thank you to Frances Tappan for her early work in the field of massage technique and her indomitable spirit. Thank you to Emil Kleen, M.D., for his provocative pursuit of the best of massage in the midst of major changes in medicine, and to Douglas Graham, M.D., for his considerable historical research and candid writing. The work of John Harvey Kellogg, M.D., has been instrumental in the development of massage therapy in the United States and abroad.

Thank you, John V. Basmajian, for your research into the historical traditions of massage and for providing such rich reports of those findings; to Herman L. Kamenetz, my deep appreciation is extended for providing a look at the foreign language materials regarding massage and its historical development and his extensive compilation of reference materials; and to the distinguished Albert Schatz, Ph.D., no less than the discoverer of streptomycin, the cure for tuberculosis. Thank you, "Al," for your unbridled and valuable assistance.

Thank you to Tiffany Field, Ph.D., for assistance in organizing and leading contemporary research on touch. Thank you, Corey Bippes, for your help in bringing me to consider that one book was really two, and for your expertise in bringing the graphics in this work to light. Through the help of the editors at Healing Arts Press, a somewhat ragged manuscript has been turned into an actual book. A special thank-you to project editor Susan Davidson for spearheading the Healing Arts Press effort to publish this book.

To the publishers, authors, and artists who kindly gave their permission to reprint portions of their work in this book, thank you very much. And finally a posthumous thank-you to the "encyclopedists" who labored to reproduce, protect, and retrieve the teachings of the ancients for the benefit of their own time and for unknown future generations.

Human touch as rendered by healing massage is an inherent need. The roots of massage lie solidly in the touch of a caring hand. The art of massage is its female side, while the science of massage is its complementary opposite, the male side. And with the flow of energy created by the contact of two human beings, the yin and the yang move in a dance of life. Healing can and often does ocurr under such circumstances. In the end it is the reaching that serves our need, making contact is the rich reward. Finally, how does one thank the almighty Creator? Words of appreciation to my fellow humans seem inadequate as they are, and yet I wish to acknowledge the benevolent gift of the Lord's grace in my life and in this work. The creation of this material and all that has preceeded it is only a process toward which His light and grace is becoming known to me.

Namaste,
Robert Noah Calvert

Introduction

Describing the application of massage as a design of "the Creator," as Dr. Graham does, might seem a bit overzealous, but most massage practitioners I've met in more than twenty years in the field *do* feel as if their chosen work is something akin to a sacred mission. My own work has very often been motivated by ideals beyond those of profit or career satisfaction. During the years I was a massage practitioner I witnessed how thousands of people were helped not so much by the technique I was administering, but by being touched with care and compassion. I began to understand the power of touch and how it is needed by people everywhere. I expanded my reading in the subject area and discovered that what I had been observing in my clients was the profound and dynamic human need to be touched.

No history of massage had given me this perspective, or detailed how massage was a part of other human activities that included touch of some kind. Aside from prefatory chapters contained in books about massage, my research uncovered only one other text primarily dedicated to a history of massage—Walter Johnson's 1866 book, *The Anatriptic Art, A History of the Art*. The rest of the title reads, *"Termed Anatripsis by Hippocrates, Tripsis by Galen, Friction by Celsus, Manipulation by Beveridge, and Medical Rubbing in ordinary language, from the earliest times to the present day."* Although that is the title, much of the book consists of case histories of massage treatments. Johnson's book is no longer available and can only be found in university libraries and museums, but his work was significant because he pioneered a trail of discovery for those who came after him.

Massage schools seldom offer more than a few hours of historical background to educate those entering the field. Just like any other aspect of the healing arts, massage has a long and informative history, but it has been mostly forgotten and is rarely discussed. There is too little knowledge and a lot of misinformation about the past of this important and incredible field. *The History of Massage* was written to begin to fill that gap and to stimulate a new dialogue about where we've come from, so that we might be better prepared for where we are going. It is a text filled with information, but it is much more than that, and I hope that my readers will find it inspirational as well as educational. It is my hope that it will provide the foundation for the development of massage-history coursework in schools around the world.

A careful study of the structure of the human body, its contours and conformations, together with the most agreeable and efficacious manner of applying massage to it, results in proving that the Creator made the body to be manipulated and that He put it into the heart of man to devise massage as a means of arousing under-action of nerve, muscle, and circulation.

—Douglas Graham, M.D.,
a Massachusetts practitioner
writing in 1884

The history of massage is the history of touch, both intertwined with human history. Since prehistoric time, touch has been an integral part of the primate social system, initially as an element of grooming behaviors. During the long transition from primate grooming behaviors to human contact systems, touch took on other social characteristics. As human beings evolved to develop organized civilizations, touch was transformed into a variety of behavioral modes. The study of prehistoric touch is outside the scope of this work; I am currently writing a book on the subject entitled *Evolution of Human Touch*. This book begins where that one will end—with the advent of formal touching methods that eventually developed into massage therapy as we know it today.

Manual treatment as a remedy for disease is believed to be as old as humankind. The most common proof offered as evidence for this claim is a very simple one— humans instinctively respond to pain by touching where it hurts. In all ages and all places, in all cultures, human beings reach for the spot that hurts and rub it, usually making it feel better. This reflexive response to pain serves as the validation that massage is as old as humanity.

"Even in the remotest times massage was in use. . . . It was regarded as a universal remedy, a panacea, to which uncivilized man had recourse in all his difficulties. This ought not to astonish us so much, as 'uncivilized' man has few remedies, and no instrument but the hand, which he instinctively uses for relieving his pain. We ourselves, when we feel pain from some cause or other—a blow, cut, fall, etc.—instinctively put our hand to the part affected, for the purpose of rubbing or pressing it—in other words, to massage it."[1]

Since the time when human beings inherited socially laden grooming behaviors from their primate ancestors and evolved them into more complex and structured manual arts, massage has always been a part of a larger picture. It has been an integral part of several aspects of human life, including religious and healing rituals; healing arts such as midwifery, medicine, and hydrotherapy; exercise and movement; and the pleasurable pursuits of sensuality.

Massage was not advocated nor practiced as a singular therapeutic tool until modern times. The shaman rubbing evil spirits out of the body, the deaconess laying on her hands to inspire the healing power of the Holy Spirit, the midwife soothing a mother from the pains of childbirth, the trainer preparing for and administering after athletic pursuits, the nurse applying a healing balm in battle or the bath, the doctor treating an injury with a liniment or mechanical treatment, the woman applying healing and soothing creams to her skin for beauty and health, a couple rubbing as a part of the rituals of sexual behavior, and any person touching another simply for feeling good and getting relaxed—massage was a part of the repertoire of each of these activities before it broke free in the nineteenth century. It remains a complement to them all even though it is now recognized as a stand-alone therapeutic tool.

The commingling of massage with a broad range of human activities makes writing about its history challenging and sometimes a bit confusing. But this *is* its past, a legacy primarily based on association with better-known aspects of human life. In each of these massage has found a place—sometimes thriving, sometimes faltering, but always surviving. Massage has survived because it is the most fundamental means of giving care, affection, and aid between human beings. Its healing qualities differ from those of other healing modalities because massage confers its benefits through the character and healing intention of those who give and receive it. The true value of massage comes from the inherent need of humans to have contact with one another.

This work offers a new direction in the exploration of massage history. Most previous writers on the subject have limited themselves to the medical literature, thus missing the broader cultural perspectives pertinent to the story of massage. Evidence contributing to a more comprehensive picture of the role of human touch comes from everyday life and from cultural phenomena, such as religious rite and ritual, exercise and movement programs, baths, spas, and sanitariums. Massage has played a significant role in the history of medicine, midwifery, nursing, and sports. It is also evident in the advertising and use of a variety of products, from mechanical inventions to liniments and tonics, as well as in the professional practices of barbers and beauticians. Although each of these areas is a part of the history of massage, most have been forgotten or misunderstood in other writings about massage's history.

It may be surprising to some readers, but this book also includes discussion of what has been called the world's oldest profession—prostitution—in order to clarify the long-standing connection between prostitution and massage. The link between them has its roots in ancient cultures and, in more recent times, prostitution has often operated under the guise of massage parlors in the United States and other countries. As a result, virtually all of the state massage regulations and city or county ordinances that are now aimed at practitioners were originally intended to control prostitution. However, this book will make the distinction between massage and prostitution very clear, a distinction that fortunately became widely evident by the end of the twentieth century.

A Japanese midwife massaging a pregnant woman's belly. Drawing adapted from an 1827 woodcut by Japanese artist Ohta. Courtesy of *Massage Magazine.*

This work differs from previous models of written history about massage. I have chosen not to cover every event and personality. It does provide an interesting and entertaining survey of massage's historical place in our world—a history of massage never before written. It is my hope that it will foster further efforts to put readers of our time and future generations more in touch with this unique and fascinating hands-on healing art. This book will be invaluable for massage practitioners, as well as fascinating for anyone who wishes to learn more about massage. My primary purpose in writing this book is to continue to spread the good word about massage—its great value in relieving human suffering and fostering beneficial human relationships.

While I feel compelled to apologize for any errors I may have made in this book, they have been unintentional. If they do exist, I hope that I will learn about them so that the same mistakes will not be passed down in successive works. This is a wide territory, and exploring it is an ongoing project. Like those who have come before me, I have had to rely on the translations of ancient texts. In order to glean a completely accurate and full perspective on the subject, it will be necessary to read the ancient texts in their original form. I hope this challenge will be met someday.

This book is organized around one central theme—exploring the world for evidence of massage. It begins with a revealing look at history from the point of view of definitions of massage, from their first appearance to current usage. The book then explores the role of massage in the shamanic/priestly tradition, source of the most ancient healing practices. This tradition, found in ancient human civilizations around the globe, developed differently in different areas, so I then present an exploration of the use of massage in different regions of the ancient world. Although the practice of massage dwindled during the Middle Ages and the Renaissance, massage continued as part of other traditions until the nineteenth century, when it enjoyed increasing use and popularity as a part of medicine, gymnastics, and the movement cure, and in a variety of health institutions, such as spas and sanitariums. Along with a detailed exploration of all those developments, particular attention is given to the evolution and use of various tools and techniques of massage.

During the last few decades of the twentieth century massage at last began to stand on its own as a healing art. Massage attained growing acceptance and legitimacy as a healing method and witnessed increasing mainstream use. Because the field of massage experienced something akin to the incredible growth of the industrial and electronic revolutions in the twentieth century, there is arguably as much to write about in the twentieth century as in the ten thousand years that preceded it. In the attempt to provide a firm historical perspective, I have chosen to cover the entire span, rather than providing an exhaustive study of all the developments of the twentieth century. However, I have included an overview of the extensive recent history of massage. The book concludes with some comments about the destiny of massage in the new millennium.

I invite you to join me on this journey through time and world cultures to discover the place of massage in human history. It is a journey I believe you will find informative, pleasurable, and enlightening.

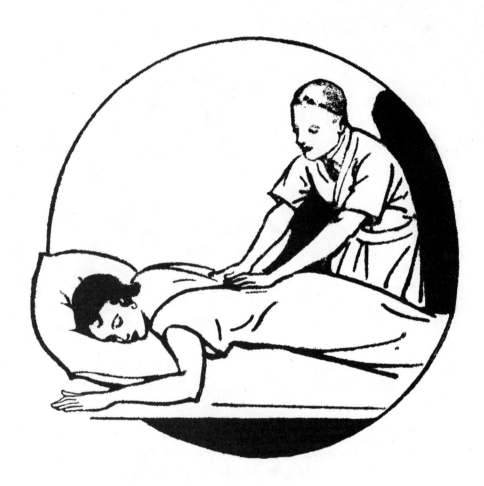

The cover graphic from *Massage: Its History, Technique and Therapeutic Uses,* Dr. Richard Haehl's 1898 introductory text of massage for medical students.

1 What Is Massage?

Many definitions of *massage* can be found in the literature and regulatory texts of modern times, but there is no known definition of *massage* from the ancient world. Gertrude Beard and Elizabeth Wood, professors of physical medicine at Northwestern University Medical School and authors of the well-known book *Massage: Principles and Techniques* (1964), assert that "the early medical literature is devoid of any comprehensive definition of massage." They also claim that "there is little description of massage movements in the early literature."[1] However, Hippocrates (460–377 B.C.E.), widely regarded as the Father of Medicine and a renowned advocate of massage, wrote about the use of friction in the treatment of many ailments, as well as about its physiological effects: "Rubbing has the effect of relaxing, constricting, thickening, and thinning; hard rubbing constricts, soft relaxes, much rubbing thins, and moderate thickens."[2] The ancient Greeks used techniques that they called *anatripsis* and *frictio*. The word *anatripsis*—meaning "to rub up"—represents a transitional period in the history of massage. Prior to Hippocrates the shamanic/priestly healing traditions directed rubbings downward, out the extremities. But Hippocrates' rubbings were performed by rubbing up, from the extremities toward the body's center.

Greek physicians performed anatripsis on patients suffering from intestinal ailments and on athletes suffering from waste buildup in their muscles. Today we use anatripsis in much the same way, even though we have our own word for it and have developed more techniques and better rationale to describe its effects. The ancient physician Claudius Galenus, commonly known as Galen (131–201 C.E.), was a strong proponent of the Hippocratic method. In his extensive writings about massage he did not provide a definition; however, in his *De Sanitate Tuenda (Hygiene)* he did give descriptions of massage from which we might draw elements of a definition. He wrote that the objective is "to soften the body" before exercise. "And the rubbings should be of many sorts, with strokes and circuits [*sic*] of the hands, carrying them not only from above down and from below up, but also subvertically, obliquely, transversely, and subtransversely."[3] He goes on to give more details about how the hands should move "from every direction."

From these instructions we can conclude that massage as practiced by the Greeks was a manual treatment of the body utilizing a variety of techniques. The descriptions

Massage . . . is a very ancient form of treatment, so ancient that one may consider its history to be as old as that of mankind, and its beginning prehistoric.

—Emil A. G. Kleen, M.D., *Massage and Medical Gymnastics*, 1921 of massage have changed between the time of the ancient physician and the modern practitioner, but the essence of massage has remained unchanged—the application of human hands or another object to the superficial skin of a recipient for the purposes of rendering remedial or palliative aid.

Although positive references to the healing power of touch can be found in historical documents in many fields, the first lucid descriptions of the movements of massage, such as friction and rubbing, were given by the French physician Joseph-Clement Tissot, acknowledged as one of the leading figures in the history of massage. Writing in his 1770 classic text on exercise, Tissot devotes more than twenty pages to the subject of "friction, rubbing, kneading and alternate compressions." He does not use the word *massage* because the word had not yet been created. Even so, Tissot expounds on the ancient virtues and modern benefits of the movements that make up, in large part, what we now know as massage.

Even though there has been no consistent definition of massage through the ages that could provide us with a historic reference point for comparing what the ancients did and what we do today, it seems clear the tradition is seamless—the one thread that has passed through time is the act of human contact with the intent to give relief from suffering.

Where did the word *massage* come from?

Herman L. Kamenetz, M.D., provides a useful description of the etymology of *massage*. He writes: "The controversy about its etymology deals mainly with two possible derivations, one Semitic, the other Greek.

"To the first belongs the Arabic verb *mass*, to touch. This origin was proposed by Savary as early as 1785 in his report on Egypt, where he observed massage. The Greek origin from the word *massein*, to knead, was suggested in 1819 by Piorry. Littre, in 1873, held the Arabic origin more likely than the Greek, because of the widespread use of massage in the East. However, most lexicographers today favor the Greek etymology."[4]

Gunilla Knutson, in her 1972 book *Gunilla Knutson's Book of Massage*, provides another look at the origins of the word. "Scholars differ on the origin of the word *massage*. Some say it derives from the Greek word *massein*, meaning to knead, and was originally applied to the act of washing hair," as practiced first by the people of India and called by them *tshampua* (shampooing). "Others," Knutson continues, "trace the word to the Arabic *mass*, which specifically describes the act of massage as 'the pressing of the muscular parts of the body in order to give suppleness and stimulate vitality.'" She claims that historians consider the Arabs to be the inventors of massage because of the precision of their description of it.[5]

Adding a little humor to an otherwise very dry subject, Dr. Graham provides the following comment in a footnote to his *Treatise on Massage* (1902): Arabic, *mas'h*, "Those who inadvertently or through ignorance call *masseurs* 'mashers' are oftentimes not so far out of the way after all."[6] In Sanskrit we find *makch*, meaning "to strike" or "to press." Derivatives of the word *massage* can be found in a number of other languages, such as Hebrew (*mashesh*), Latin (*massa*), Japanese (*anma*), and Chinese (*amma or anmo*).

Kamenetz clarifies the French derivatives with the following. "Any of these roots [Greek or Arabic] may have evolved into the French words: *masser* (verb), *massage* (action), *masseur and masseuse* (operator)."[7] According to Kamenetz, "the first use of the word seems to come from French colonists in India. Guillaume Joseph Le Gentil, who went to India in 1761 and 1769, wrote: 'I mention here the art of massaging, which is practiced by women as well as by men. . . . Here, along the Coromandel Coast, they call it *macer* or *masser* (having oneself massaged), and there are *masseurs* and *masseuses*.' He reports that *massement* 'renders the limbs more supple and more agile.'"[8]

Kamenetz claims the first appearance of the word *massage* as a noun was "possibly for the first time in print, in a French-German Dictionary, in 1812." However, the word or phrase he refers to in the dictionary is *massage a' friction*. This French phrase does not mean "massage"; rather, it means "to use friction." He cites the second appearance of the word *massage* as coming seven years later. In 1819 it appeared in volume 31 of the sixty-volume French Dictionary of Medical Sciences, with an eight page article entitled "Massage."[9]

English physician William Murrell, in his 1886 book *Massage as a Mode of Treatment,* reports he found the word *massage* used in an 1839 French-language edition of *Lancet,* an English hospital gazette. According to the 1993 edition of the *Oxford English Dictionary,* the word *massage* was first found in the English language in 1876.[10] Although the first appearance of the word *massage* in the English language in the United States has traditionally been reported as being in 1876 in an English medical dictionary, Richard P. Van Why claims that the word first came into the American medical lexicon in 1874, when it appeared in articles published in the *New York Medical Record* (William Fischer) and the *Philadelphia Medical and Surgical Reporter* (Douglas Graham).[11]

However, I have found one piece of evidence that the word *massage* was used in the United States as early as the 1830s. A poster dated 1837 depicts a Dr. Swift purportedly giving a massage at home. Historical record leaves us uncertain whether Dr. Swift was a practitioner of massage, a physician offering gynecological exams at home to make them less threatening, or a male midwife using massage—then considered more acceptable—as a ruse for his services. In any case, his poster is a clear indication that the word *massage* was in use in America much earlier than previously thought. Three other Dr. Swift posters have been discovered in New York and California, giving further proof to their reliability as authentic documents from the year 1837.

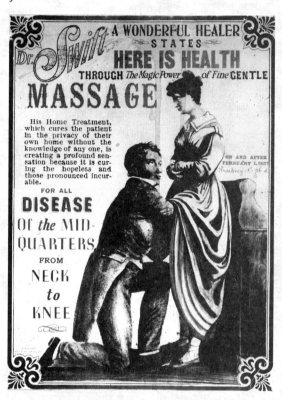

This advertisement from 1837 provides one piece of evidence that the word *massage* was used in the English language prior to the conventionally accepted date of 1876. This poster also suggests that massage was in common usage as an in-home therapy during this time. Courtesy of World of Massage Museum.

Early Medical Definitions of Massage

An examination of early definitions of *massage* in dated progression in itself provides an important perspective on the history of massage. As we will explore in detail in chapter 6, massage was an integral part of movement therapy and gymnastics before it was adopted by the medical profession. It was gradually incorporated into the practice of allopathic medicine in the nineteenth century, as demonstrated by numerous references to massage found in medical textbooks and dictionaries.

During the latter half of the nineteenth century medical doctors in Europe and America began writing about the benefits of massage. As more physicians were introduced to the domain of manual therapeutics the terminology of the practice began to change, reflecting the physicians' disdain for common massage; the commonly used terms were gradually replaced by more medically oriented terms. For example, *rubbing,* a term used in 1866 by Walter Johnson, became *medical rubbing* by the 1880s. By the turn of the century *medical rubbing* was replaced by *Massage* with a capital M. The distinction between *massage* with a little m and *Massage* with a big M reflects the physicians' dislike of gymnasts, or "common rubbers" as they were called. The doctors argued that the massage done by gymnasts did not have the credibility of the Massage used medically.

Thomas's Medical Dictionary of 1886 defines *massage* in this terse way: "Massage, from the Greek, meaning to knead. Signifying the act of shampooing."[12] There is evidence in other historical texts that *shampooing* initially meant massaging or rubbing; only later did it come to mean cleaning the hair with special products.

George H. Taylor, M.D., in his 1887 book, *Massage: Principles and Practice of Remedial Treatment by Imparted Motion,* writes: "The word *massage* denotes any process of conjoint motion and pressure applied to parts of the living body, for remedial purposes. Massage implies some source from which the pressure-motion is derived and involves the production of physiological consequences adapted to remedy defects arising from insufficient muscular action of the usual forms."[13] Dr. Taylor was very concerned in his book with what he called "motor-energy," derived from "nutrition" and responsible for all motion or power of the body. "The motor power of the human hand," he affirms, "easily lends itself to this generous purpose; and it thus, almost by instinct, but in strict conformity with scientific principles and purposes, reinforces the vital needs and waning energies of the suffering."[14]

Douglas Graham, M.D., American Medical Association member and author of *Manual Therapeutics, A Treatise on Massage* (1890), defines *massage* in this way: "Massage . . . is a term now generally accepted by European and American physicians to signify a group of procedures which are best done with the hands, such as friction, kneading, manipulating, rolling, and percussion of the external tissues of the body in a variety of ways, either with a curative, palliative or hygienic object in view."[15]

Although not specified in most definitions, these early authors also limited massage movements to those performed solely by the hands, often as an adjunct to other therapies in the treatment of disease. In his 1895 book, *The Art of Massage,* John Harvey Kellogg, M.D., of the Battle Creek Sanitarium states, "Massage, or systematic rubbing and manipulation of the tissues of the body, is probably one of the oldest of all means used for the relief of bodily infirmities."[16] He also provides several terms related to the word *massage,* as well as their "right and proper" pronunciations:

> *Massage* is a noun, the literal meaning of which is kneading, as a baker kneads bread. This word, like many other terms relating to massage, is derived directly from the French. It retains its French pronunciation, and is pronounced as though spelled *mas-sahzh,* and not as though spelled *massaj* or *massaje,* which is so frequently heard.

Masser is a verb, meaning the act of applying massage.

Pe'trissage is pronounced as though spelled *pa-tris-sahzh.* It is a French term applied to deep kneading, as distinguished from superficial kneading.

Tapotement is pronounced nearly as though spelled *tah-pote-mont,* and indicates the act of percussion.

Effleurage is pronounced as though spelled *ef-flur-ahzh.* It means light friction.[17]

Noah Webster's 1899 *An American Dictionary of the English Language* does not contain the word *massage.* It does define *friction* first as the act of rubbing two objects together to produce heat; second, as the scientific meaning of mechanical rubbing of two moving objects; and third, "In medicine, the rubbing of the body with the hand, or with a brush, flannel, etc., or the rubbing of a diseased part with oil, unguent, or other medicament." *Rub* is also referred to as "the act of rubbing, friction."

Axel V. Grafstrom, M.D., in his 1904 book, *A Text-book of Mechano-Therapy,* writes, "By **massage** we understand a series of passive movements on the patient's body, performed by the operator for the purpose of aiding nature to restore health. These passive movements are friction, kneading, percussion, stretching, pressure, vibration, and stroking."[18] Dr. Grafstrom used bold text in his book to assist students in finding key words for their studies.

Emil G. Kleen, M.D., of Sweden, a contemporary of Dr. Graham, defines *massage* in his 1921 edition of *Massage and Medical Gymnastics* as "a manipulation or handling of the soft tissues by movable pressure in the form of stroking, rubbing, pinching, kneading or beating performed with a therapeutic aim. This is generally applied by hand, but can, of course, also be given by means of instruments and apparatus of different kinds."[19]

Dr. Thomas Stedman's 1936 edition of *A Practical Medical Dictionary* defines massage as "a scientific method of manipulation of the body by rubbing, pinching, kneading, tapping, etc.; it is employed in therapeutics to increase metabolism, promote absorption, stretch adhesions, etc."[20]

Contemporary Definitions of Massage

By the middle of the twentieth century the definitions of *massage* began to show evidence of a growing disassociation between the medical profession and the practice of massage that was slowly establishing itself as a separate vocation. The definitions, primarily appearing in nonmedical sources, became more descriptive in terms of technique as they moved away from association with general body systems or movement theory.

In 1947 Rodale Press published a book called *The Word Finder* that lists verbs, adverbs, and adjectives for the word *massage.* Among the adjectives are "invigorating;

stimulating; scientific; frictional; and healing." Under the adverbs they recommend also looking under "rub and knead."

Gertrude Beard, in her 1952 classic textbook, *Massage: Principles and Techniques,* defines *massage* as a "term used to designate certain manipulations of the soft tissues of the body; these manipulations are most effectively performed with the hands, and are administered for the purpose of producing effects on the nervous, muscular and respiratory systems and the local and general circulation of the blood and lymph."[21] This definition became a standard for several decades within the massage trade.

In 1972, during the peak of the human potential movement, George Downing, teacher of massage and body awareness classes at the Esalen Institute at Big Sur, California, published *The Massage Book.* An international classic that continues to be sold in bookstores around the world, it has introduced hundreds of thousands of people to the art of massage. Although Downing doesn't define *massage,* he provides a humanistic description: "In its essence massage is something simple. It makes us more whole, more fully ourselves. Your hands have the power to give this to others. Learn to trust that power and you will quickly find out better than anyone can tell you what massage is all about."[22]

In 1977 Ruth E. Williams wrote in her book, *The Road to Radiant Health,* "Massage is a manual manipulation of the soft tissue by methodical pressure, stroking, friction, kneading, compressive movement, vibration, tapotement (percussion) and active and passive joint movement, usually applied upon the bare skin."[23] Her book, a standard-bearer in the trade for more than a decade, was used as a text in many schools throughout the country.

Evidence of the growing separation between massage and medicine can be found in a variety of publications. For example, in 1936 Dr. Stedman's *A Practical Medical Dictionary* classified massage as a "scientific method" and included it among "therapeutics," but his twenty-fifth edition—with its title changed to *Stedman's Medical Dictionary*—dropped all reference to "scientific" or "therapeutic." His 1980 definition of *massage* was, "A method of manipulations of the body by rubbing, pinching, kneading, tapping, etc." Perhaps the change in title of his own dictionary may be the reason for the changes in the definition of *massage.*

Few health care professionals today define *massage* as having value for easing stress or relieving simple aches and pains, nor do they mention its role in providing the benefits of human contact. However, these are perhaps its most important healing attributes because it is touch—not a specific massage technique—that is inherently needed by humans and yet is practically nonexistent in much of today's allopathic health care.

By the 1980s the breach between massage and medicine had become so significant that it was professionally risky for Frances M. Tappan, a physical therapist by training, to explore the world of massage. However, her pioneering work in the field of massage therapy led to the establishment of one of the country's first substantive massage courses in a college physical therapy program. Her 1980 book, *Healing Massage Techniques,* now in its third edition, continues to be used as a reference text in many massage schools. In it she defines *massage* as "the systematic and scientific manipulation of the soft tissues of the body."[24]

For their part, many practitioners of massage were eager to establish a nonmedical status for their profession. From the 1980s we find numerous terms from the human potential movement describing massage. Albert Schatz, Ph.D., gives this exposé of a few terms from this period and their meanings. "During the 1980s I found 20 or more names for massage, such as planetary massage, psychic massage, universal massage, healing massage, stellar massage, individualized massage, personalized massage, spiritual massage, vital massage, etc., in various local magazines. They were usually ads—all trying to be different. When I [telephoned] the people involved, most were self-taught or had very little 'training.' The names were designed to get more clients by creating the impression that what was offered was something unique and not available elsewhere. If I recall correctly, the individual who did spiritual massage said that she mentally massaged the person's spirit while she massaged his or her body."[25]

In their 1987 consumer-oriented book, *Massage: Total Relaxation,* Time-Life Books defines *massage* as "the systematic manipulation of the body's soft tissues, primarily the muscles, to benefit the nervous, muscular and circulatory systems. Usually this manipulation is performed with the hands, although some forms of massage also use the forearms, elbows, knees, and even the feet."[26]

The best-selling massage textbook available today is *Mosby's Fundamentals of Therapeutic Massage* by Sandy Fritz. In it the author accurately writes that the massage field has yet to agree on one comprehensive definition of *massage,* and offers her own definition of *therapeutic massage.* "The scientific art and system of the assessment of and the manual application to the superficial soft tissue of the skin, muscles, tendons, ligaments, fascia, and the structures that lie within the superficial tissue by using the hand, foot, knee, arm, elbow, and forearm through the systematic external application of touch, stroking (effleurage), friction, vibration, percussion, kneading (petrissage), stretching, compression, or passive and active joint movements within the normal physiologic range of motion. Also included are adjunctive external applications of water, heat, and cold for the purposes of establishing and maintaining good physical condition and health through normalizing and improving muscle tone, promoting relaxation, stimulating circulation, and producing therapeutic effects on the respiratory and nervous systems, and the subtle interactions between all body systems. These intended effects are accomplished through the energetic and mind/body connections in a safe, nonsexual environment that respects the client's self-determined outcome for the session."[27]

Note that these definitions rarely mention the whole person; they seldom use terms such as *holistic, energetic systems,* or *energy;* and they usually do not include the mind, soul, or spirit as part of the person or healing process. Albert Schatz, Ph.D., a distinguished professor emeritus from Temple University and massage practitioner, criticizes these kinds of definitions as "describing massage only in terms of technique."[28]

The Impact of Massage Regulation and Medical Dominance

The qualification of massage as "therapeutic" in the current most popular textbook on massage is evidence that massage practitioners yearn for their field to find its place once again in medical practice. However, in the face of substantial opposition, the massage profession has not done its work to establish itself along the lines of its medical roots despite ample historical evidence of the role of massage as a therapeutic modality within the medical profession.

The American Massage Therapy Association, established in 1943 and now the largest national organization of its kind, gives its own definition of *massage*. "Massage is manual soft tissue manipulations, and includes holding, causing movement, and/or applying pressure to the body. Manual means by use of hand or body."[29] This definition certainly leaves plenty of room for interpretation and is clearly calculated to step on no one's toes. It reflects the massage profession's fear of reprisal for infringing on the medical profession's legal scope of practice bolstered by law and political clout.

Beginning in the 1970s and continuing through today, there has been a dynamic movement to establish massage as a viable stress management, health enhancing, and health maintenance modality outside medical practice, but this has yet to be reflected in the legal definitions found in most states. Current regulation is careful about mentioning diagnosis and typically denies that massage is a medical practice. A little more than half of the states in the United States have such regulations. In those states where there is no statewide regulation, municipal or county ordinances exist in wide variety. The definitions given here represent a geographic cross section of the country and are also some of the most established laws in the nation.

Connecticut's state law is somewhat contradictory in its definition, first stating: "'Massage therapy' means the systematic and scientific manipulation and treatment of the soft tissues of the body, by use of pressure, friction, stroking, percussion, kneading, vibration by manual or mechanical means, range of motion and nonspecific stretching. Massage therapy may include the use of oil, ice, hot and cold packs, tub, shower, steam, dry heat, or cabinet baths, for the purpose of, but not limited to, maintaining good health and establishing and maintaining good physical and mental condition." It then adds the following qualifications: "Massage therapy does not encompass diagnosis, the prescribing of drugs or medicines, spinal or other joint manipulations, nor any service or procedure for which a license to practice medicine, chiropractic, naturopathy, physical therapy, or podiatry is required by law."[30] How you can provide "treatment of the soft tissues of the body" without some form of diagnosis is questionable, although the term *assess* is often used to skirt this issue.

The 1997 laws of the state of Florida define *massage* as "the manipulation of the superficial tissues of the human body with the hand, foot, arm, or elbow, whether or not such manipulation is aided by hydrotherapy, including colonic irrigation, or thermal therapy, and electrical or mechanical device, or the application to the human body of a chemical or herbal preparation."[31] Considering that the state of Florida has been at the leading edge of massage regulation and development during the past fifteen years, this definition is surprising. It would appear that any technique that works below the "superficial tissues of the human body" is off limits to massage therapists in Florida. Currently the Florida Board of Massage is engaged in a controversy to determine whether Reiki, an energy-healing technique, should be considered massage or not. Their inquiry stems from the fact that Reiki practitioners lay their hands on the person receiving treatment; therefore, by the state of Florida's definition, this constitutes massage. However, any definition of *massage* includes strong elements of manipulation with the hands, which Reiki does not provide. Several other states, including Utah, have exempted Reiki from the massage statutes after similar appeals from the Reiki community.

Oregon provides another example of ambiguity and open interpretation in its massage law. "'Massage' or 'massage therapy' means the use on the body of pressure, friction, stroking, tapping or kneading, vibration or stretching by manual or mechanical means or gymnastics, with or without appliances such as vibrators, infrared heat, sun lamps and external baths, and with or without lubricants such as salts, powders, liquids or creams for the purpose of, but not limited to, maintaining good health and establishing and maintaining good physical condition."[32] I wonder why "maintaining good health and physical condition" are mentioned at all, because the practitioner is "not limited to" these purposes?

Iowa, a middle-America state, attempts to provide a definition of *massage* that would apply to just about any form of body-oriented therapy. "'Massage therapy' means performance for compensation of massage, myotherapy, massotherapy, bodywork, bodywork therapy, or therapeutic massage including hydrotherapy, superficial hot and cold applications, vibration and topical applications, or other therapy which involves manipulation of the muscle and connective tissue of the body, excluding osseous tissue, to treat the muscle tonus system for the purpose of enhancing health, muscle relaxation, increasing range of motion, reducing stress, relieving pain, or improving circulation. 'Massage therapy' does not include diagnosis or service which requires a license to practice medicine or surgery, osteopathic medicine or surgery, osteopathy, chiropractic, or podiatry, and does not include service performed by athletic trainers, technicians, nurses, occupational therapists, or physical therapists who act under a professional license, certificate, or registration or under the prescription or supervision of a person licensed to practice medicine or surgery or osteopathic medicine or surgery."[33] It seems very difficult to find any service *not* provided by one or more of these medical professions left available for massage therapists. Yet physical therapy, osteopathy, naturopathy, podiatry, and chiropractic are all relatively new professional practices compared to massage, which historically predates them all as a part of the medical profession.

Calvert's Definition of *Massage*

In the professional world of massage there is no method or technique simply called *massage*. Rather, *massage* is a broad term under which specific methods or techniques are categorized. There is Swedish massage, Esalen-style massage, connective tissue massage, medical and sports massage, and so on. There is a plethora of historic and contemporary words that mean *massage,* some discussed in this work. Synonyms for the word *massage* include stroking, rubbing, unction, inunction, anatripsis, tripsis, apotherapeai, flagellation, frolement, fustigation, pressures, touch therapy, tactile application, effrayante, slapping, shaking, hacking, beating, rolling, handling, mechanotherapy, medical gymnastics, physical treatment, bathing, friction, effleurage, petrissage, tapotement, vibration, kneading, compression, cutaneous stimulation, Swedish gymnastics, smoothing, pressing, and flexing.

Defining the term *massage* is a difficult task because massage is more than all of its specific techniques. Many modern definitions of *massage* provide for the physical and therapeutic aspects but fail to include the range of methods or the effects of human contact. The inclusion of a list of tools and devices in a contemporary and comprehensive definition of *massage* will also provide a historic context missing from most other definitions. As I will demonstrate, the history of massage is the story of changing attitudes toward massage and how those attitudes have either sustained or altered the methods, applications, and usefulness of massage. A definition of *massage* must therefore be inclusive, not exclusive to any particular type of technique or approach. Massage is more than all the purposes for which it is used, and it is more than all the changing modes by which it is applied.

The human element of connecting for the betterment of another is deeply ingrained in the practice of massage in all its forms. The virtue of human contact through the medium of massage is that its benefits are automatically given. This is not to say that massage is an unconscious act. Quite the contrary—giving massage is a very conscious act that almost always includes the intent to help and heal. But the help and healing come not so much because of that intent, but because those benefits are intrinsic to the act of human contact. For that reason, evidence of massage can be found in all cultures and ages.

Massage can console, nurture, support, feed the spirit, create bonds, and establish and maintain friendships; it is often given and received simply because it is pleasurable and feels good. We can say that massage therapy is "the formal application of a variety of manual or mechanical methods to the body of a recipient for the purposes of promoting and maintaining health and well-being, used in conjunction with other healing arts modalities," but that leaves out some of what massage is. A proper definition of *massage* must include not only its therapeutic role and historic development, but also its capacity to nurture and support—to feed the spirit, bind relationships, and please the senses. Massage is about relationships and it is about healing. Massage is the highest order of touch.

Taking all of these factors into consideration, I offer Calvert's definition of *massage:*

> *Massage:* From the Greek word *massein* (to knead). The manipulation of the body by kneading, stroking, friction, percussion, vibration, and other methods applied with the hands, feet, elbows, forearms, or with tools such as stone, wood, ceramic, ivory, metal, bone, or devices that operate by hand-crank, steam, battery, or electric power, and the use of water, herbs, salts and muds, any or all of which may produce directly or indirectly various therapeutic effects, feelings of pleasure or pain, a sense of being nurtured and supported, an uplift of the spirit, and general well-being . . . are often used adjunctively with massage.

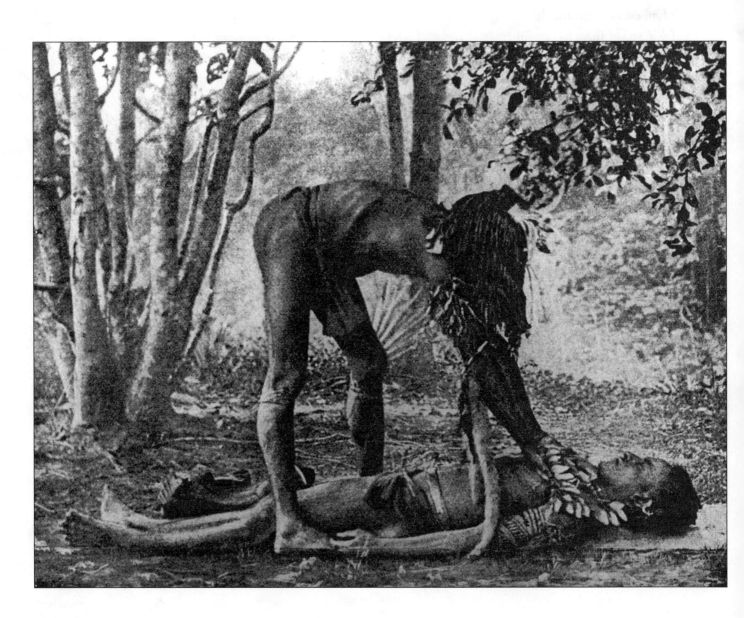

A Papuan shaman uses leaves believed to have curative qualities to gently massage the evil spirits of illness from his patient. From *Manners and Customs of Mankind* (vol. I), edited by J. Alexander Hammerton (London, 1923).

2 Shamanic and Priestly Origins of Massage

Medical lore was passed down from generation to generation long before human beings settled in mud huts or crude villages between the Tigris and Euphrates Rivers nearly ten thousand years ago. In this and subsequent civilizations members of the priestly classes were the keepers of most knowledge, especially that related to the healing arts—spiritual and physical. They were the overseers of the welfare of the people, and healing practices were intricately tied to their religious rituals.

The shaman was the first identifiable priest-physician. Today most people think of the shaman as a medicine man, sorcerer, or witch doctor, dancing amid beating drums, chants, and the rattling of beads and charms. The image of the shaman is that of a primitive, archaic, outdated, strangely bizarre, and mysterious man. But the true picture of the shaman is far from this myopic and masculine view. The shaman is a noble figure in history, and both men and women have served their people in this venerable role. The shaman was the first undisputed champion of magico-religious life in society. It is from the ritualized healing practices of the shaman that civilized societies have inherited nearly all their healing arts.

Two important facts must be remembered when considering the shamanic lineage of healing. First, the shaman's practice included both medicine and magic ritual. And second, the keepers of the tradition in the earliest civilizations were both physicians and priests. The earliest written records of medical practices—carved on stone and clay or written on papyrus—reveal a combination of incantations, spells, exorcisms, prescriptions, and clinical observations.

In *The Epic of Medicine*, medical historian Felix Marti-Ibanez, M.D., writes: "Magic represented man's earliest attempts to use his own strength to solve the problems of health and disease."[1] He refers to the incantations, spells, amulets, and other magico-religious rituals used in ancient healing practices. Then he adds, "Also used in therapy were fruit, cereals, spices, flowers (garlic, roses, oats, laurel, and tamarind), mineral and animal substances, massage, plasters, and baths."[2] His conclusions are based on archaeological evidence such as fauna, artifacts used for containers, and domestic remains.

The medicine man first rubs his hands several times as if washing them, then stretches his fingers quickly one after another so that the joints crack. This he does to imitate the crackling of fire. He next breathes on his hands and, holding them together, spits on them. He then holds them out towards the south, north, west and east, and also towards the ground. . . . Making a kind of gargling noise, he sucks out the disease in the form of a grain of corn or small stone, afterwards coughing. . . . He then breathes on the affected part, making passes as if to sweep the disease away.

—John Hammerton, *Huichol Indians of Mexico* (1938)

13

In ancient times disease was believed to be caused by demons, spirits, or the sinful acts of the patient. This concept of disease was based on something magically put into the body or magically taken from it. Despite the use of herbal remedies, ritual was the significant aspect of treatment—the superior power of one magic over another was regarded as the curing factor. Massage was used in these rituals as a part of the overall treatment for a disease. It was a form of coaxing or intimate and personal coercion by use of the skilled hands of the practitioner to cleanse or chase demons from the body.

The fundamental remnants of an archaic past remain evident in the practices of contemporary shamanic ritual healing. Modern shamans, according to the world's leading expert on the subject, Mircea Eliade, retain many of the same attributes and methods used by their ancient counterparts. There is ample evidence linking the shaman's healing ways found today with those of their ancient predecessors. We can thus examine contemporary shamanic practices for insight into the role played by massage in the healing ways of the first human civilizations.

Australia

The most ancient people of Australia are the Aborigines. Although the arrival of immigrants from Great Britain and other countries in the eighteenth century had a devastating impact on Aboriginal peoples and their cultural traditions, currently there is a resurgence of Aboriginal culture and a growing respect for traditional Aboriginal knowledge among both Aborigines and non-Aborigines.

The common belief as reported by white men (because the Australian Aborigines developed no written language except pictographs) is that the Aborigines attribute illness and death to magical practices and the activities of spirits. The shaman is the one trained and able to free the spirits of the departed who haunt the living or clear the cause when a person has broken a taboo. Massage's role in their considerable arsenal of healing arts usually consisted in pushing the demon or evil spirit from the abdomen out through the top of the head with vigorous massaging. In his book *Aboriginal Men of High Degree,* Adolphus Elkin claims that body aches and pains are treated with herbs or healing waters rather than massage.[3] But in an interview the author conducted with twentieth-century Aboriginal medicine man Kakkib li'Dthia Warrawee'a, massage is a common remedy used for a variety of ailments, including muscle aches and pains. The medicine man told me, "Touch is vital to my people and is called *yabung.*" It is used for physical ailments but is a component of social binding as well. "Kids learn massage from the elders by doing it on them." It is one of the many daily activities that provide Kakkib's people with the opportunity to share knowledge while building relationships between the generations.

Kakkib illustrated the daily use of massage with the following story. "An elder is sitting around at the end of the day. He looks about and calls a young boy over to him. The elder points to a place on his shoulders and tells the boy 'press here.' The elder then gives the boy instructions on how long to hold the pressure, to increase or lessen the pressure, and when to move to another spot. He explains to the boy why he's pressing that particular spot and how it is useful. This isn't an apprenticeship but a way of life like so many other activities—like using herbs for headaches or sinus congestion. Everyone knows the way of healing to a certain degree because we lived primarily in small bands of twelve to twenty-four people and had to be able to take care of ourselves out there in the middle of the Bush."

Kakkib relayed that massage among the Australian Aborigines is also used in their tribal hospitals. These are circular stone buildings about twenty feet in diameter and "staffed" by young people who take care of the elders who can no longer keep up with the nomadic life of their people.

An ancient game of football has been played by Kakkib's people for thousands of years and includes the use of massage. "The body is looked after" during the long game, one that continues for several days. There is "lots of massage used on the key players during the time they take breaks, because my people know how valuable it is to rejuvenate and heal tired and sore muscles and keep the main players in the game."

Kakkib also told me that "several women massage the expectant mother during the birth," but this is not the same massage given at other times, because of the special needs of the pregnant woman. He said that young boys learn massage from their mothers so they can massage their pregnant wives in the months before birth.

Africa

Massage in Africa has been a part of folk medicine, or "the way of the people," for centuries. Massage in ancient times was associated with the bath, a practice probably exported by travelers through Africa to Mesopotamia, Egypt, and the Greek empires. Abdominal massage—the kind of massage most often written about by those who have traveled through Africa—has been used as part of the medicine of the village shaman to help push out evil spirits and to aid poor digestion. The African midwife also used a type of abdominal massage during pregnancy to correct malpresentation of the fetus. A modern form of African massage focuses on the center of the abdomen, or what the Asians call the "hara."[4] Also a part of this modern massage from Africa are elements of tribal dance, giving balance, rhythm, and style to the artistic performance of massage.

Central and South America

When the Spanish marched into Tenochtitlán, what is today Mexico City, in November 1519, they compared what they saw to the city of Venice, Italy. There were bridges, temples, huge palaces, and streets bustling with commerce. Tenochtitlán had been built on an island in the middle of a large lake; it was surrounded by a city with a population of more than one hundred thousand people. At that time London was only a city of about fifty thousand and Paris seventy thousand.

Fertile fields of corn and other crops marched in rows up to the foothills of distant mountains, punctuated by villages here and there. Hernando Cortés and his Spanish conquistadors had entered the capital city of the Aztec nation, a city surpassing anything found in all of Europe. Sanitation was very advanced, with garbage collection, clean public toilets, and paved streets of mud bricks that were swept clean regularly. Cortés wrote in his journal, "Houses were found in which they kept pharmacies where remedies ready to drink, ointments, and plaster can be bought. You see barber shops where you can bathe and have your hair cut."[5] The Aztec physicians treated every kind of disorder with their healing arts, crowned by the use of medicinal plants and drugs. The maize goddess, Chicomecoatl, was thought to both give and cure disease, disease believed to be a consequence of sins against the gods. Although this belief was common in most ancient civilizations, it was uniquely resolved by the ancient peoples in this part of the world through human sacrifice.

The Olmecs had been the first people to erect a great civilization in the region. Around 600 B.C.E. the Olmecs, like the Egyptians, transported huge stones from inland volcanoes to sites in and around what is now Mexico City, to be carved into gigantic stone statues and used as building material. They were followed by the Toltecs and then the Chichimecs, who were conquered by the Aztecs. Each civilization had a tradition of baths, both public and private, and healing arts of a magico-religious character. The Aztecs had entered the region about four hundred years prior to the Spanish, conquering its inhabitants in the course of a century. The Spanish conquered the Aztec nation in just a few years, destroying their magnificent city and, with smallpox, most of its people. The massive ritualistic killings by the Aztecs to feed their god Huitzilopochtli provided the Spaniards with ample incentive to destroy all the Aztec's temples, statues, and traditions, and nearly all their writings.

Not long after, the Spaniards also conquered the Mayan peoples of the Yucatan region who had lived there perhaps thousands of years before the Christian era.[6] Like the Aztecs, they had vast city complexes with baths to rival even those of Rome and Greece. The Incas of Peru had baths as well, as attested to by historian Garcilaso Inca de la Vega in his book, *Commentarios Reales de los Incas* (1609). The author provides a firsthand account: "The buildings consisting of houses, temples, gardens, and baths of the Incas were marvelously hewn from stone, highly polished, and with the rocks so well fitted together that they seemed to leave no room for cement."[7]

Throughout the area, tremendous steam baths, or *temazcalli,* with hot and cold rooms and exercise areas have been discovered. The steam rooms were used for treating exhaustion, rheumatic disorders, and neuralgia; for women who had just given birth; and for the relief of tired and aching muscles. The steam rooms were shaped like beehives and made of brick or stone. Medical treatment was given inside by burning a combination of remedies in the fire or releasing them directly into the steam.

Reports from most historians on the steam bath practices of the Aztecs, Olmecs, Incas, and Mayans refer to the use of massage. In fact, several medical histories refer to

SHAMANIC AND PRIESTLY

ORIGINS OF MASSAGE

massage as "one of their favorite methods" of treatment in the steam bath. Lashing or flagellation was practiced as well, using the leaves of the maize plant. Pinewood ointments were rubbed on the chest for lung ailments and elsewhere for muscular aches and pains.[8] Other ointments made from herbs, animal fats, or oils and a variety of special leaves were used in the application of massage during the steam. Temazcalli were found in nearly every village. It seems reasonable to infer that massage was applied by either slaves or adepts in the baths, because slavery was widely practiced by these peoples, and specialization was a common part of medical practice, even in the steam bath.[9]

When the Spanish arrived, conquering each civilization, they outlawed the practice of bathing and steam rooms because they thought frequent bathing was enervating to the body and could lead to disease, even though the hot springs were often frequented by the Spanish themselves. Most of the temazcalli in Mexico disappeared, except in obscure locations. However, the tradition of massage continued. In the epigraph at the beginning of this chapter John Hammerton alludes to an ancient Mexican healing tradition. I have been told by Delores, a Tarahumara Indian living in the Sierra Madre Mountains of north central Mexico, of a similar ceremony used to initiate her into the manual healing arts. Before she was allowed to begin her training in massage she was first rubbed with a masticated mixture of aromatic herbs. Her teacher, like the ancient shamans, first prepared herself by concentration, by expressing words of power, and then by rubbing, sucking, brushing, and performing other activities that are all a part of the sacramental forms of healing. Delores, the Tarahumara Indian I talked with, performs a prayer ritual prior to each massage treatment she delivers. And like those who came before her, she works from the core of the body out to the extremities so as to remove the spirits of illness, to press and rub them out of the body.

Elisabeth Brooke, an herbalist and author, tells about a woman living in Sante Fe, New Mexico, in the 1990s who worked as both a midwife (curandera) and massage therapist (sobadora). Gregorita "was taught by her aunt and practiced on her seventeen children. She claims that 'curanderas cure with their minds, with their experience, and with herbs.' She feels energy flowing from her hands as she begins to massage the abdomen. Sometimes she examines patients at their hospital bedside, and on one occasion took a very ill patient home with her. This patient was described as having a spleen that 'jumped.' Gregorita massaged the patient throughout the night and put towels soaked in cold water on her abdomen. Next morning she had recovered. Gregorita returned to the woman's doctor, angry that he had diagnosed heart trouble when all she needed corrected was her loose spleen."[10] Constipation and other intestinal difficulties are also treated by massage in the sobador tradition. Brooke writes: "Constipation or intestinal blockage responds brilliantly to Gregorita's strong massage. She locates the hard area and, with kneading, pushing, and shoving, manages to soften it and cause the symptoms to disappear. Often she prays for strength to carry on her healing work and offers up petitions for her sick patients."[11]

North America

Some early writers from England and other parts of Europe who traveled to North America remarked in their journals about the healing arts of the Native Americans. Elisabeth Brooke reports that colonial settlers in the New World "learned much of their medicine from the Native Americans."[12] Her reference is to herbs and medicinal plants found within the local areas familiar to the Native Americans and unfamiliar to new inhabitants. Although massage was rarely mentioned as a part of native therapeutic arts, two types of massage were noted as being used in Native American healing practices: percussions, such as beating, thumping, and slapping; and a kind of vigorous kneading and pushing. Some observers claim a kind of general massage was given to villagers by the medicine man.[13] Whether this was therapeutic massage or a shamanistic ritual healing method is not clear. It was most likely a ritualized method of exorcising spirit demons from inside the patient. Often the medicine man or woman would actually take the spirit within his or her own body and then release it from themselves, or have another shaman do so. The massage that was a part of these healing rituals is ancient and typical of the shamanistic traditions around the world.

In his 1902 book, *Manual Therapeutics, A Treatise on Massage,* Douglas Graham provides a fascinating look at how massage was used by the Navajo Indians during the nineteenth century. This is a classic example of how massage was intertwined with the mystic and ritual practices of the native shaman.

A method of curing the sick among the Navajo Indians of Arizona is given by James Stevenson in the "Ceremonial of Hasjelti Dailjis," in the eighth annual report of the Bureau of Ethnology, Washington, 1891, from which the following abstract is made. For a prehistoric, antediluvian performance in modern times it surpasses anything I have yet found:

> "During his visit to the Southwest in the summer of 1885 it was Mr. Stevenson's good fortune to arrive at the Navajo healing ceremonial. The ceremony was to continue nine days and nights. The occasion drew to the place about twelve hundred Navajoes, on an extensive plateau near Keane's Canyon, Arizona. A variety of interesting occurrences attended the great event, such as mythologic rites, gambling, horse- and foot-racing, general merriment, and curing the sick, the last being the prime cause of the gathering.
>
> "A man of distinction in the tribe was threatened with loss of vision from inflammation of the eyes, which was supposed to have arisen from his looking upon certain sacred masks with an irreligious heart. He was rich and had many wealthy relatives, so they 'soaked it to him.' A celebrated theurgist was solicited to interfere. He arrived October 11, 1885.
>
> "A bright light burned in the lodge, and shortly after dark the invalid appeared and sat upon a blanket in front of a song-priest. Three men personated the gods, Hasjelti, Hostjoghon, Hostjokobon, and one the goddess, Hostjoboard. They left the lodge and put on their masks.

"On the second day, after singing and chanting and pouring medicine from a gourd on heated stones, Hasjelti lifted the coverings from the entrance to the sweat-house, and the patient, having donned his breech-cloth, came out and sat on a blanket. Hasjelti then rubbed the invalid with the horn of a mountain sheep held in the left hand and in the right a piece of hide from between the horns of the sheep. The hide was held flatly against the palm of the hand, and in this way the god rubbed the breast of the invalid while he rubbed the back with the horn, occasionally alternating his hands. After this Hostjoghon put the invalid through the same 'course of sprouts.' The gods then gave him drink four times from the gourd containing medicine-water, composed of finely chopped herbs and water, from which they had first taken a draught themselves.

"On the third day the same procedures, with variations, took place. This time Hasjelti began with the limbs, and as he rubbed down each limb he threw his arms towards the eastern sky and cried 'Yo, Yo!' He also rubbed the head and body, holding the hands on opposite sides. After this the sick man again drank from the bowl of medicine-water.

"On the fourth day, after the invalid had drunk of pine-needle water and been bathed with the same, Hasjelti manipulated the right leg with the sheep's horn and hide, rubbing the upper part of the leg with the right hand and the lower part with the left; then the sides of the leg in the same manner, each time giving a hoot. The arms, chest, face, and head were similarly manipulated, and every time he changed the position of his hands he gave a shout.

"On the eighth day the hands were placed to the soles of the feet, varied with hooting, then 'the heart of the invalid was touched' with the palm of the right hand, the left being placed upon the back. The body was pressed in this way four times amid loud cries. After touching each figure of a sand-painting, the right hand was placed to the forehead of the invalid and the left hand to the back of his head and the head pressed this way on all sides."

"Many other details are given, but quite enough has been said. Whether the invalid was killed or cured does not appear. At any rate his pocket must have been touched, seeing that he had to pay for all this racket, including the entertainment of the twelve hundred Navajos."[14]

As in South and Central America, the steam room was popular with the Apache, the Cheyenne, the Klickitat, the Shoshone, the Pueblo, the Delaware, and many other tribes. Hot springs, where they existed, provided the most sacred of healing waters. Some sweat lodges were built into the earth with a tunnel for access. The sweat lodge continues to play an important part in Native American traditional rites, primarily for cleansing and purification as preparation for contacting one's animistic spirits or for initiation rites of passage. Massage has survived only in a few Native American nations, usually employed during childbearing and used along with herbs in the treatment of abdominal pains.

The Pacific Islands

In Hawaii, massage—called *lomi-lomi*—was an integral part of the native healing arts system for centuries. Passed down through family traditions, the *kahuna,* a rough equivalent to the shaman, was taught by the grandfather or grandmother over a period of years, oftentimes secretly, until the apprentice proved him- or herself to be worthy and truly sincere in wanting to be a kahuna healer. Several categories of kahuna exist, some for purely spiritual purposes and others for a variety of healing purposes. Not all kahuna learned the art of lomi-lomi, and not all learned about herbs or incantations. Today we find lomi-lomi being practiced with and without prayer as a part of the session.

The word *lomi-lomi* comes from the Hawaiian word *roromed,* which may be translated to mean "a pressing of the hand when tired." *Roromed* was the term used by Archibald Campbell when he reported his experiences with the technique in 1810. But another source of the same time, Thomas G. Thrum, defined *lomi-lomi* as "to rub or chafe the body."[15] This massage style resembles what is today called Esalen-style massage from California, with long flowing strokes, rhythmic patterns, and use of the forearms.

In ancient Hawaii, lomi-lomi was performed on the king and queen after they had eaten in order to allow them to eat even more. Apparently the massage helped their digestion. Otto von Kotzeblu relates that, during a visit he made to the islands in 1824, "it seems that the Queen Nomahana, after feasting heartily, turned on her back whereupon a tall fellow sprang upon her body and kneaded her as unmercifully with his knees and fists as if she had been the dough of bread. Digestion was so assisted that the queen resumed her feasting."[16] N. B. Emerson, M.D., as told by Douglas Gra-

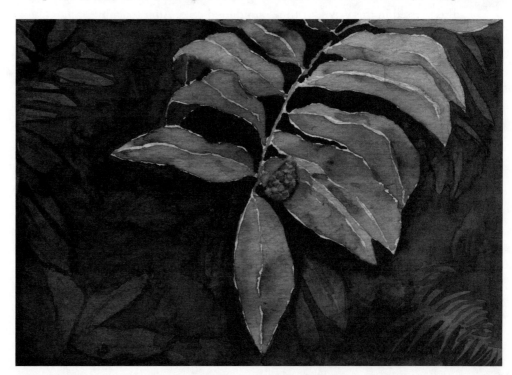

The Polynesian wild ginger plant *(Zingiber zerumbet)* of Hawaii. The flowers exude an abundance of perfumed liquid that was used as a massage lubricant and shampoo before the arrival of Europeans. From *Maui's Hana Highway* by Angela Kepler (Honolulu, 1987).

SHAMANIC AND PRIESTLY

ORIGINS OF MASSAGE

ham, relates his experiences from the year 1870 receiving massage in Hawaii. Douglas Graham writes:

> He [Dr. Emerson] describes it as a luxurious and healthful form of passive motion which the Hawaiians bestow upon one another as an act of kindness and which constitutes their crowning act of generous hospitality to a well-behaved stranger. When foot-sore and weary in every muscle, so that no position affords rest and sleep cannot be obtained, it relieves the stiffness, lameness, and soreness and soothes to sleep, so that unpleasant effects of excessive exercise are not felt the next day, but in their stead a suppleness of muscle and an ease of joint entirely unwonted. . . . They have various ways of administering the *lomi-lomi*. When one is about to receive it he lies down upon a mat; and he is immediately taken in hand by the artist [as Dr. Emerson calls the person who lomi-lomies], generally an elderly and experienced man or woman. The process is spoken of as being neither that of kneading, squeezing, nor rubbing, but now like one, and now like the other. Those skilled in the art come to acquire a kind of tact that enables them to graduate the touch and force to the wants of different cases. . . . The Hawaiians are a famous race of swimmers, and to a foreigner they seem amphibious. When wrecked they sometimes swim long distances, and if one of their number becomes exhausted they sustain him in the water and *lomi-lomi* him at the same time.[17]

Charles Nordhoff, in his 1874 book, *Northern California, Oregon and the Sandwich Islands,* provides a description of Hawaiian massage.

> Wherever you stop for lunch or for the night, if there are native people near, you will be greatly refreshed by the application of lomi-lomi. Almost everywhere you will find some one skilled in this peculiar and, to tired muscles, delightful and refreshing treatment. To be lomi-lomied you lie down upon a mat or undress for the night. The less clothing you have on, the more perfectly the operation can be performed. To you thereupon comes a stout native with soft, fleshy hands, but a strong grip, who, beginning with your head and working down slowly over the whole body, seizes and squeezes with a quite peculiar art every tired muscle, working and kneading with indefatigable patience, until in half an hour, whereas you were weary and worn out, you find yourself fresh, all soreness and weariness absolutely and entirely gone, and mind and body soothed to a healthful and refreshing sleep.[18]

Today lomi-lomi is being practiced and taught in Hawaii along with other aspects of ancient Hawaiian healing arts, which include herbs, saltwater plunges, and a steam hut called an *imu loa,* where the steam bath was given.[19]

———— ✺ ————

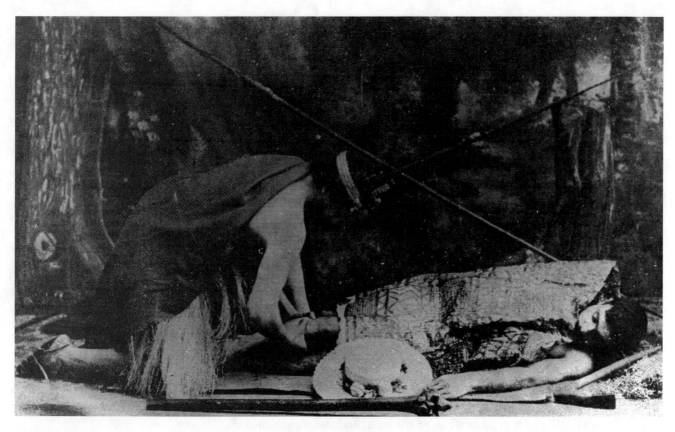

A Polynesian administering massage. Completely apart from any outside influences, the Tongans developed massage techniques and a nomenclature similar to the European Swedish massage: *toogi-toogi* (tapotement), *mili* (effleurage and friction), and *fsota* (petrissage). From *The Art of Massage* by John Harvey Kellogg, M.D. (Battle Creek, Mich., 1895).

Emil Kleen, M.D., reports in 1892 that "among the . . . Pacific Ocean . . . tribes it [massage] is employed both as general-massage (chiefly as a restorative), and for local purposes. Its technique seems to have attained a considerable degree of development, the different manipulations being classified by the Tongas, quite after the method of the modern Mezger school."[20]

A hospital gazette from the year 1839 tells its French readers about massage in Tonga and provides further insight into their techniques. "Toogi-Toogi or tapotement consists of continuous soft striking with the closed fist. Mili or effleurage and friction is done by rubbing with the palm of the hand. And petrissage or Fsota presses and squeezes the muscles between the fingers and the thumb. Usually these techniques are performed by females among the Tongans, but sometimes children will walk all over the person if the condition dictate [*sic*] this type of treatment."[21]

Captain Cook—the purported first European visitor to Hawaii—also landed in Tahiti. The local native chief, being a friendly sort of guy, offered to help Captain Cook with his severe rheumatism. The chief gathered up a few of his women relatives and other female practitioners in the village. Captain Cook is reported to have had no less than twelve large women pounce upon his body while he was spread out on mats and blankets laid on the ground. After only a few minutes of being pummeled and squeezed and beaten with fists and hands and elbows and knees and feet, and nearly every joint in his body cracked, the captain stood up astonished that he was relieved of pain. The women asked him if he wanted more and he immediately laid back down and called out, "Indeed." With three additional sessions his pain was alleviated.[22]

SHAMANIC AND PRIESTLY

ORIGINS OF MASSAGE

In the Fiji Islands massage is also performed on the naked skin using coconut oil. It has been a family tradition for as long as anyone can remember. In Fiji a kind of foot massage is used where the practitioner doesn't stand on the recipient but instead uses his or her feet while standing at the side of the recipient. The practitioner also sits and lies on the floor and uses his or her feet, especially the heel, to work the recipient's body from head to toe.

In New Guinea, the wide variety of village tribes have little traces of any therapeutic rubbing within their highly ritualized and magical healing arts. The rubbing that is practiced is done to extricate evil demons or disease from the body, using pushing or raking motions nearly always performed toward the head in a technique very similar to some of the South American tribal customs. In Malaysia and Indonesia massage is called *pidjet-ten,* or *urut.* Its historical roots and uses have been primarily as part of folk remedies and midwifery practice. Like the healing arts systems from other countries of the region—Thailand's *nuat bo'rarn,* Burma's *hneit chin,* Cambodia's *chap sosai,* and Korea's *hanpang*—it is also practiced by village doctors, found in hospital clinics and urban healing centers, and available to tourists on the beach, on a park bench, or in the privacy of their hotel rooms.

The Philippines

Missionaries stationed in the countryside of the Philippines reported massage being used as a medical treatment. Sometimes called "Oriental rubbers" and occasionally referred to by the English equivalent, "masseur," these practitioners also utilize herbs and magic in their remedies.[23] But the true Filipino healing art of therapeutic massage is called *hilot* (pronounced **hee**-lote). From the shamanic tradition of their ancestors, Filipino healers derived their calling from visions or from having been born breech. The first of these healers were midwives who followed their destiny into the birthing rooms of their neighbors and relatives, usually getting payment in the form of livestock, vegetables, or services. The hilot system of massage was born from these traditions and continues to thrive even today.

According to the authors of the book *The Healing Hands of Hilot: Filipino Therapeutic Massage,* hilot is very similar in technique to massage practices found in Indonesia, particularly the island of Bali, "such as strokes which move away from the heart, sideways rubbing or going across the muscle fibers, and the principles and function of the channels."[24] Coconut oil is used, as it has been since ancient times. Before the massage begins, range-of-motion exercises are conducted on the "patient." These are also common in Thai massage and other Asian systems of manual healing arts.

The system of hilot has a correspondence with the Chinese system of six internal organs—heart, liver, spleen, kidney, lungs, and pericardium. The first stage of hilot massage helps soften the musculature, increases circulation, and prepares the body for deeper pressure. "In Hilot, an experienced [practitioner] would . . . check for blockages or stiffness in areas that directly or indirectly correspond to the injured body part. . . . By opening up these blockages, the blood and energy flow is unimpeded and healing takes place faster."[25] A lot of pressure techniques are used in hilot, and it is sometimes described as being painful, yet the pressure is usually varied depending upon the condition being treated.

Russia and the Ukraine

There is very little English literature available on the rich and long history of massage in Russia and the Ukraine, but it can be safely assumed that it was a part of ancient folk remedies, practiced within the mystical, magical, and often superstitious practices of religious cults and rituals before it rose to the attention of the medical community. According to Zhenya Kurashova Wine, a Russian immigrant now living and teaching in the United States, massage was not scientifically studied in Russia until 1860; prior to that it was considered "part of folk remedy." Wine claims that the ancient Slovaks did something called "twigging." Using the softened leaves of a birch tree twig, a practitioner in the sauna "would hit the body . . . and follow by rubbing the body with the branches. After this the masseur would pour water (hot first, followed by cold) on the body. . . . That process was repeated several times during the bathing, and was finished with a bather going for a dip in the snow. This severe amount of friction prevented the body from serious over-cooling, and helped the bather to better adapt to the cold temperatures of Winter Russia."[26]

Experts who study the healing arts and ritual practices of shamans living in the world today find many remnants of their ancient past. This is certainly true in the realm of massage. Ancient and contemporary shamans utilize rubbing in some form during their highly ritualized healing sessions. In almost every case the shaman rubs from the core of the body out the extremities. The purpose is to remove the bad deed or evil spirit that occupies the body and brings on sickness or injury to the one suffering. Whether they use compressions, shaking, rolling, stroking, or brushing techniques, they all remove the sickening spirit from within. All of these are, according to experts, evidence of the ancient ways of healing that can best be described as "rubbing down."

As we will see in the following chapters, modern massage also has its roots in ancient practices, but not from the same source nor from as far back in the history of humankind. Most every modern system of massage in the world today that derives from the Western model moves from the extremities toward the core of the body. This method began with the great physician Hippocrates, approximately 450 years before the birth of Christ. His method of doing massage—or anatripsis or frictions, as it was called then—was to rub up, not down.

Hippocrates' medicine was a natural medicine, based strongly on observation of the patient's body and utilizing natural methods of treatment, such as rest, hydration, and diet. Neither Hippocrates nor his contemporaries knew much about human anatomy and physiology; the circulatory system of the human body wasn't recognized and known for many centuries after he lived. (Human dissection was not allowed during Hippocrates' time, and so much of what was known about the internal systems of the body was derived from animal dissection.) Even so, with little hard data and a lot of observation and experience, Hippocrates altered the course of anatripsis forever when he ordained that rubbings should be conducted from the extremities inward to the center of the body, so waste materials—which would contain disease—could be removed through the alimentary tract with vibration and friction, assisted by proper diet, rest, and plenty of water.

And so today we find in our world the practice of the ancient shaman still rubbing down alongside the modern practitioner rubbing up. Both practices have similar intentions, to help heal the infirm, but utilize different methods to achieve their goals.

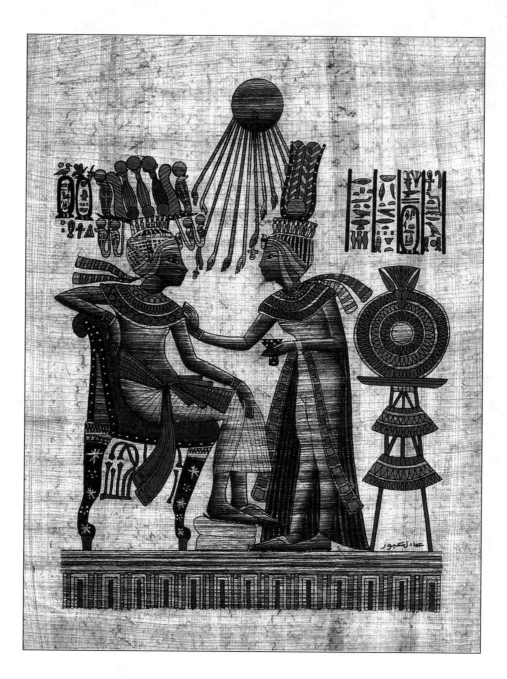

King Tutankhamun sits on a cushioned throne
as his wife, the queen, anoints her husband
with perfumed oil. Contemporary rendering of
a painting on a throne chair in King
Tutankhamun's tomb.

3 Massage in the Ancient World: Babylonia, Egypt, China, and India

The first recognized civilizations were well established about eight thousand years ago. However, written records were not made until the Babylonians, living in the Mesopotamian region of the Near East (in today's Iraq), circa 2350 B.C.E. created a way to express themselves in what is called cuneiform writing. Cuneiform text is made up of wedged or arrowhead-shaped lines inscribed on wet clay tablets. Cuneiform writing predates Egyptian hieroglyphs.

In *The Epic of Medicine* (1959) medical historian Felix Marti-Ibanez, M.D., writes that evidence of massage was first found in the Code of Hammurabi, carved upon a pillar of black diorite stone. His claim is not based on an actual mention of massage in the Code, but on inferential evidence. Law number 221 of the Code (there are a total of 282 laws) states, "If a physician heal the broken bone or diseased soft part of a man, the patient shall pay the physician five shekels in money."[1] The inference of massage is based on the reference to a "diseased soft part"—apparently meaning soft tissues such as muscles, tendons, and ligaments—the healing of which would indicate massage.

Babylonia

Massage historian Herman Kamenetz discusses massage in ancient Babylonia in his writing on the history of massage. Citing an article in the 1917 issue of the *Annals of Medical History* by M. Jastrow, Kamenetz writes, "The evolution of medicine from magic to religion to empiricism to science is recognized in the history of massage. The phases are often difficult to distinguish, notably in ancient cultures. Characteristic is the following reference to Babylonian-Assyrian medicine: 'If a man has cramps . . . place his head downwards and his feet [under him?], manipulate his back with the thumb, saying 'be good,' manipulate his arms 14 times, manipulate his head 14 times, rolling him on the ground.'"[2] Jastrow, as reported by Kamenetz, comments further.

The human organization, so delicate and so varied, is like a musical instrument of complicated and exquisite workmanship, and easily loses its harmony. Thus it is with much reason that the poets unite in Apollo the arts of music and of medicine, perceiving that the genius of the two arts is almost identical, and that the proper office of the physician consists in tuning and touching in such a manner the lyre of the human body as that it shall give forth only sweet and harmonious sounds.

—Francis Bacon, English philosopher (1561–1626)

Massage must have been recognized as beneficial in certain cases, but the point of view necessarily was that what was good for the patient was bad for the demon. The drugs, the poultices, the hot and cold douches and the massage all were supposed to act not on the patient but on the demon who was in this way to be forced out or to be coaxed out."[3]

Jastrow's description sounds quite similar to the shamanic exorcism of evil spirits using incantations, magic, massage, and other mystical methods. It thus provides not so much direct proof of massage being used within the first human civilized cities, but a confirmation of the continuation of the archaic ways of healing associated with superstition, magic, and the conception of disease as being primarily the result of an evil possession.

In *The History of Medicine* (1922) by Walter Libby, M.D., we find reference to the use of massage in Mesopotamia. After presenting several examples of cures administered by the ancient Babylonian physicians and their considerable pharmacopoeia of drugs, Dr. Libby expounds upon "the therapeutic agents relied on by the Babylonian priest-physician" as "purgatives, diaphoretics, enemata, compresses, salves, poultices, liniments, fumigations, diet, and rest." Next he mentions the use of "salves, poultices, liniments" from which we can reasonably suppose the use of some kind of rubbing.[4] These salves, poultices, and liniments were smeared on the patient's skin and rubbed in in order to obtain their therapeutic effect. Dr. Libby does not address the issue of whether their use implied rubbing them on or massaging them in.

A modern-day rendering of a circa 2330 B.C.E. wall painting in the tomb of Akhmahor (Ankh-mahor) at Saqqara, known as the physician's tomb. The wall painting has been used as evidence of reflexology dating back to ancient times.

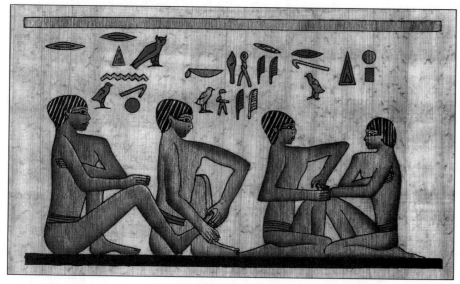

Egypt

The graphic at the opening of this chapter is a contemporary rendering of a painting found on the back of a throne chair in King Tutankhamun's tomb. Scholars have interpreted this scene as clearly showing Tutankhamun's wife, Ankhesenamon, applying perfumed oil to her husband. Is this a scene demonstrating massage? Regrettably not; however, although this graphic merely illustrates a ceremonial act of anointing, there is other pictorial evidence of Egyptian massage.

The painting on the tomb of Akhmahor is an example of Egyptian pictographs providing evidence of massage in Egypt more than four thousand years ago. This painting of Akhmahor, an Egyptian priest, was made circa 2200 B.C.E. The hieroglyphs in the painting have been translated to read "Don't hurt me," leading to the certain

MASSAGE IN THE ANCIENT
WORLD: BABYLONIA, EGYPT,
CHINA, AND INDIA

Reconstructing history from ancient records

The use of circumstantial evidence and inference is a respected technique in archaeological and anthropological studies, especially in examining prehistoric civilizations, for which written records and hard physical evidence are often lacking. For example, it is generally agreed that agriculture was the predominant activity for most of the common people of the world for thousands of years before the first historical records were kept. Even so, scientists tell us that scenes of agriculture are rare on vases, drawings, carvings, and other such physical remains of the most ancient developed civilizations, such as Mesopotamia, Sumeria, and Babylon. The Egyptians had highly evolved agricultural techniques and irrigation systems, yet little record remains of this aspect of their lives; thus we must make certain assumptions about their lives based on evidence that is indirectly derived. This is also true in our search and reporting about the history of massage. According to massage historian Herman L. Kamenetz, massage was "at times not named at all but understood when therapeutic manipulations . . . or . . . simply external measures were mentioned."[5]

This is an important point because it is not always from formal literature that we learn about massage. Not all history is written in the texts of the past. It seems a small leap to conclude that just because proof isn't found in an ancient text, it doesn't mean a particular practice wasn't being carried out at the time. This is especially true when it comes to massage—the basic and fundamental practice of rubbing people to help them feel better and aid in their healing process, a practice known to have been a part of almost every culture in the world throughout human history.

Even after writing was invented, much of history was not preserved as written documents. Very few of the world's ancient writings have survived in their original form. The decline and fall of civilizations often brought with it the burning of manuscripts and the destruction of libraries and temples where records were kept. Fortunately, some knowledge was saved by oral traditions—teachers verbally passing on their work to eager students—as well as by encyclopedists, who copied what was left after wars had subsided. Scholars of some civilizations, such as the Arabs, were insightful enough to compile these worthy treasures in their own languages. At times the manuscripts of a culture that were captured by an invading force were saved from destruction, becoming a part of the invader's literary heritage. For example, Greek and Roman medicine was influenced by the cultures they conquered, such as Egypt and Persia.

From 500–400 B.C.E. the Greeks compiled the records of those who came before them, adding to them information from their own medical practices. This compilation has come to be known as the Corpus Hippocraticum. The Corpus preserved a significant body of the Egyptian medical practices that had been recorded on papyri. Much of our knowledge of Egyptian therapeutic practices, and many other insights into the extremely well-developed culture of ancient Egypt, come from the Corpus Hippocraticum.

The Corpus comprises seventy-two volumes, including the teachings of the Greek physician Hippocrates (460–380 B.C.E.), and thus contains quotes of his many references to massage. Although the Corpus is attributed to Hippocrates, scholars have determined that the vast majority of the text—and perhaps all of it—was written hundreds of years after Hippocrates' death by Alexandrian scholars. It is not uncommon in history for the knowledge and deeds of a person to be immortalized by writers and myth-makers long after that person has passed on. For example, it is believed that the famous Yellow Emperor's Classic of Internal Medicine, a considerable medical text, was not actually written by the emperor but was instead written much after his time, to give his name historical honor.

Even when ancient texts do exist, modern historians and writers about massage, medicine, exercise, and related subjects have had to resort to translations, sometimes through several languages, such as Greek to Latin to German to English. Fortunately we have direct translations from the ancient Greek to English for the works of Hippocrates, and for some of Galen's work as well.

conclusion that some form of bodywork is being performed. The fact that two different techniques or applications are pictured suggests this might be the recording of an ancient system of bodywork.

The ancient Egyptians devised a form of paper made from the pith of the papyrus, a tall-water plant that grew in abundance in the Nile River Valley. Many papyrus records have been discovered, and reveal much about Egyptian medical practice. Stone carvings, reliefs, and clay tablets were copied on what are called medical papyri (medical records). Medical historians refer to eight of these papyri for accounts of medical practice by the Egyptians. These documents date from 1,900 to 1,200 years before Jesus Christ and well over a thousand years before the Roman empire rose to world power. One such document, written in cuneiform and translated into Egyptian hieroglyphic characters, is called the Ebers Papyrus. This papyrus, circa 1600 B.C.E., contains the statement, "rubbed with vinegar."[6] This may be a reference to rubbing vinegar as part of a ritual practice; or it could be a formula denoting a poultice application based on vinegar; or the word *rubbed* could infer massage. If so, this might be the earliest written record of massage.

Scholars of Egyptian medicine claim it is Imhotep, rather than Hippocrates, who should be known as the Father of Medicine. According to Sir William Osler, Imhotep is "the first figure of a physician to stand out clearly from the mists of antiquity."[7] Even Galen (131–201 C.E.), the Roman physician and follower of Hippocrates—whose works influenced medical practice for nearly fifteen hundred years after his death—wrote, "The invention of medicine was the experience of the Egyptians." Imhotep lived in the reign of the Egyptian king Djoser (2650–2631 B.C.E.), who ruled during the third dynasty. Imhotep was more than a physician; he was a priest, an architect, and an administrator. The Egyptians later deified him as the god of healing. According to James Breasted, "2500 years after his death he had become a God of Medicine, in whom the Greeks, who called him Imouthes, recognized their own Aesculapius."[8]

Imhotep is the male version of Egypt's first physician, but there is another famous personage, a female, who has laid claim to the first physician of the ancient world. Isis, the Divine Mother, was a queen of Egypt and mortal goddess who reigned circa 4000 B.C.E., long before Imhotep. In her book *Medicine Women* Elisabeth Brooke tells us that Isis was worshiped throughout Egypt and administered many temples in her name. One of these is depicted in the National Geographic collection of Egyptian artifacts as an immense multicolumned structure with myriad drawings and carvings. Brooke writes:

> Her priestesses, consecrated to purity, had to bathe daily, wore linen robes free from animal fiber, and were strict vegetarians. . . . [They] were also physicians. They used "rational" medicine, herbs, massages, baths, and so on, and combined them with the "irrational medicine" of prayer, incantations, and ritual.[9]

Selim Hassan, Ph.D., in his *Excavations at Giza I,* described the discovery in tomb writings of yet another early Egyptian physician, one with different significance. Lady Peseshet was the "overseer of the doctors." She was a female doctor overseeing all other female doctors circa 2400 B.C.E. In addition she enjoyed the title of "soul-priestess" with the responsibility of overseeing the funeral cults of private citizens. One authority on medical history claims Lady Peseshet was the world's "first female physician in Africa and in world history."[10]

The demon of consumption and the demon of liver complaint were common ailments (and spirit forces) to be reckoned with by the priest/physician four, five, and even six thousand years ago. Ritual medicine comprised the use of magico-religious methods, such as incantations, spells, and exorcisms, along with drugs, herbs, and surgical procedures. In Egypt these ancient ways still persisted, even amid the progressive approach toward rational medicine. It was not until about 1300 B.C.E., near the end of the Egyptian monarchy, that medicine and magic and religion would begin to differentiate themselves from one another, culminating with the Greeks, in a true separation of medicine from mysticism. Based on the medical papyri, Dr. Marti-Ibanez makes this comment about the study of anatomy during the time of the Egyptians: "Yet, though millions of embalmings were performed, not the slightest progress was recorded in anatomy, which was studied only in animals in the kitchen or in sacrifices at the temples."[11]

For four thousand years, starting long before Imhotep, Egyptian men and women studied medicine. Several royal schools of medicine existed where free dispensaries were open to the poor. Scholars and physicians from other empires gave and received lectures at these institutions, spreading medical knowledge and advancing its wisdom. Egyptian healing arts enjoyed a considerable reputation in the known world at that time, and many stories are told of high-status persons of other areas, even as far away as Mesopotamia, visiting Egypt to secure a cure for their illnesses. Women, like men, were trained through apprenticeships with their fathers or husbands and often carried on the practice of their deceased husbands as bonesetters and surgeons or as administrants of drug therapies. There are believed to have been more than one hundred prominent female doctors in ancient Egypt, while there were no known female physicians in the Mesopotamian cultures.

Egyptian medicine, passed down through the family, was greatly specialized. There was a doctor available for a wide variety of illnesses: diseases of the eye, the head, the teeth, the intestines, and so on. It isn't too much of a leap to suppose that there were specialists in massage as well. Not only did Egyptian physicians travel widely to learn new methods; they taught as well. And many travelers from other empires visited Egypt to learn and share their knowledge. At its peak, Alexandria, a great city at the mouth of the Nile River, offered vast educational, cultural, and commercial opportunities to the world. The existence of massage practices in Turkey, Greece, Rome, Asia, and Persia suggests that the Egyptians were or had available to them specialists in massage. Like so many other ancient cultures, massage was probably a common craft, details about which were not recorded.

In all cultures of the world with traditions of the bath, massage was a significant part. Russell T. Trall, M.D., writes about baths in Egypt: "When Alexandria was conquered by the Moslems [642 C.E.] it contained four thousand baths, constructed on the Roman plan."[12] Writing about baths in Egypt during his own time (1851), Trall says, "In Egypt and India bathing is practiced in a manner very similar to that of the Turks. In Cairo there are about seventy public baths. In addition to the manipulations of a Turkish bath, the attendant of the Egyptian bather rubs the soles of the feet with a kind of rasp, made of baked clay. . . . The three stages of the bathing process consist of sweating, rubbing, and washing."[13]

Dr. Graham relays that Alpinus (1553–1617), "a celebrated Italian botanist who occupied the chair of botany at Padua in 1593," wrote about massage in Egypt during his time.

> Friction's [sic] are so much in use amongst the Egyptians that no one retires from the bath without being rubbed. For this purpose the person is extended horizontally; then he is malaxated, manipulated, or kneaded, and pressed in divers manners upon the various parts of the body with the hands of the operator. Passive motion is then given to the different articulations. Not satisfied with masse'ing [sic], flexing and extending the articulations alone, they exercise the same pressures and friction's [sic] upon all the muscles.[14]

A quote from the hieroglyphs of an Egyptian tomb reads, "Ointment is the prescription for her body."[15] In a 1978 National Geographic Society book, *Ancient Egypt*, author Barbara Metz adds these comments, "The sage spoke well; a freshly anointed body made life more bearable in a hot, dusty land. Even the humble prized oil as a daily necessity, as vital as food."[16] With the wide popularity of oil, a natural and readily available lubricant and elixir, massage from the many slaves at one's service must have been common in Egypt considering the multitude of slaves attendant at many households and temples.

In 1785 Savary, a Frenchman, wrote about his experiences receiving massage in Egypt.

> Perfectly masseed [sic], one feels completely regenerated, a feeling of extreme comfort pervades the whole system, the chest expands, and we breathe with pleasure; the blood circulates with ease, and we have a sensation as if freed from an enormous load; we experience a suppleness and lightness till then unknown. It seems as if we truly lived for the first time. There is a lively feeling of existence which radiates to the extremities of the body, whilst the whole is given over to the most delightful sensations; the mind takes cognizance of these, and enjoys the most agreeable thoughts; the imagination wanders over the universe which it adorns, sees everywhere smiling pictures, everywhere the image of happiness. If life were only a succession of ideas, the rapidity with which memory retraces them, the vigor with which the mind runs over the extended chain of them, would make one believe that in the two hours of delicious calm which follow a great many years have passed.[17]

China

Cuneiform scholars date the beginning of Chinese culture earlier than 781 B.C.E., or, at the furthest, 1154 B.C.E.[18] If we assume that estimates can vary as much as 1,500 years, as scholars attest, then it is fairly safe to assume that Chinese and Egyptian cultures began about the same time. But most historians cite a lack of Chinese archaeological data to substantiate a cohesive culture contemporary with Egypt. They claim that Chinese culture was just beginning its rise at approximately the time Egyptian culture was beginning its decline. Even with cultural evidence lacking, human remains have been found and verified from Chinese archaeological sites that date human existence in the region at around five hundred thousand years ago, making it one of the earliest places of human inhabitancy.[19]

Much of the development of Chinese civilization, particularly its healing arts, occurred prior to the building of the Great Wall, during the Ch'in dynasty (221–206 B.C.E.).[20] Archaeological findings, especially scripts carved on bones, reveal an ancient people who worshiped many gods and demons. Before the development of rational medicine based on plants and manual therapies, Chinese healing arts were—like those of the Egyptians and Babylonians—deeply rooted in their religious beliefs. Through many years of meditation, the priests of the Shang dynasty (1766–1122 or 1523–1028 B.C.E., depending on the source) developed a conception of the spirit world, the Tao, from which all the world is made. J. J. M. de Groot explains the ancient concept of the Tao as being "composed of two souls, the Yang and the Yin; the Yang represents light, warmth, production, and life, as also the celestial sphere from which all those blessings emanate; the Yin is darkness, cold, death, and the earth, which, unless animated by the Yang or heaven, is dark, cold, dead. The Yang and the Yin are divided into an infinite number of spirits respectively good and bad, called shen and kwei; every man and every living being contains a shen and a kwei, infused at birth, and departing at death, to return to the Yang and the Yin."[21] This cosmological view is known as "animism."

Circa 1027 B.C.E. the Shang dynasty was brought to an end by a new class of rulers, the Chou dynasty (1122–221 or 1027–256 B.C.E., again depending on the source). But their rule did not do away with the Shang priests, who had created a new cosmology for their people. Instead, the Chou dynasty elevated these former priests to a scholarly class of sages who were quickly taken into the new empire as favored sons. During the eight hundred years of the Chou Empire these scholars wrote and further developed their ideas. From this tradition has come to our time some of the most ancient texts and philosophical ideas of humankind.

The primary texts were the Book of History *(Shu Ching)*, the Book of Ceremonies *(I Li)*, the Book of Odes *(Shih Ching)*, and the famous Book of Prophecies or Changes *(I Ching)*. These sages developed concepts of the five elements (fire, wood, metal, earth, and water), five directions, five planets, five seasons, five times of the day, five colors and tone, and so on. In 213 B.C.E., emperor Shih Huang Ti (Ch'in dynasty), who is responsible for having the Great Wall built, ordered all books except those on medicine, agriculture, and prophecy to be burned. A short time later the Han dynasty fell as a result of a series of disasters and internal conflicts. This period marks the end of ancient China; it would be more than five hundred years before the nation was once again unified.

The cosmological notions of health and sickness derived from the ancient priests served as a principle guide for the later development of Chinese traditional medical practice. Anatomy was not advanced in ancient China, for many of the same reasons as in other cultures, including a prohibition against human dissection. The worship of ancestors and the belief that one's soul lived within the remains of one's relatives made dissection unthinkable. This and other prohibitions led to speculation about anatomy and physiology and to the linking of disease to the cosmological elements— a concept that led to the development of what is uniquely Chinese medicine.[22]

From these religious roots Chinese medical practices were first developed in large part from what nature had to offer. Taking from plants and trees and animals and insects—from virtually all of nature's bounty—the Chinese fashioned treatments for disease and pain. Two areas are commonly thought to be the source of Chinese medical practices: the Yellow River basin and the Yangtze River region.

The Yellow River basin produced acupuncture, moxibustion, and anmo massage. There the soil is infertile, rocks and boulders abound, and the major plants are small grasses, one of which is mugwort. Over the ages Chinese people have applied dried mugwort plant to (or near) a painful area, lit it, and gained relief from pain from its heat. This practice continues to flourish worldwide today in various forms. Acupuncture developed in the Yellow River area supposedly from the very ancient practice of pricking the skin with slivers of rock to discharge suppuration (pus) in wounds. As time passed and centuries of experiments were conducted, they found that stimulation of certain specific points on the body by acupuncture, moxibustion (mugwort), or anmo gave even more relief than the stimulation of random points. These vital points, called *tsubo,* were systematized with yin and yang knowledge to form the meridian system, the basis for most Oriental healing practices.

Chinese writers tell us that anmo massage slowly developed first from a way to keep fingers and toes warm. From pressing and rubbing cold toes or fingers evolved manipulations applied around or on the tsubo. These methods, the first half of the great body of Chinese medicine developed in the northern lands, remain in use today.[23] In the southern lands of the Yangtze River region, where plants and trees were abundant, remedies made from herbs, roots, and bark were used for healing practices.

North and south China were united circa 205 B.C.E., during the Han dynasty, which also brought together the two branches of medical practice. Today this commingling of ancient medical practices is called *kampo,* or Chinese medicine.

There is some controversy today about the ancient Chinese sources, particularly regarding which texts on medical practice are the oldest, the derivation of important terms, and whether massage was a part of the ancient healing arts. Franz Hubotter, a German scholar, believes that the oldest book on Chinese medicine is entitled the *Shen Nung Pen Tsao,* or Classification of Roots and Herbs. There are no reports of massage mentioned in this work; it is fifty-two volumes pertaining only to drugs.

In 1892 Swedish physician Emil Kleen wrote: "It is in Asiatic literature of hoar antiquity that we find the first known works which touch upon mechano-therapeutics. Among them is the oft-referenced *Kong-Fu,* of great age, but uncertain date, possibly 2700 B.C. It is a description of gymnastics, and contains illustrations showing a variety of positions. Whether it contains anything about massage I cannot say; but it is certain that its importance in this connection has been greatly overrated."[24] The following quote is from Dr. John Harvey Kellogg's 1895 book, *The Art of Massage:* "There is evidence that massage was employed by the Chinese as early as 3000 B.C. . . . An ancient Chinese book entitled 'The Cong-Fou of the Tao-Tse,' of which a French translation appeared about a century ago, was probably the foundation both of our modern massage and of the manual Swedish movements so admirably elaborated and systematized by Ling."[25]

Kamenetz provides some insight into this disagreement. Kung fu was "a system of physical and religious philosophic discipline. . . . This system, together with many other observations . . . was brought to the attention of the Western world by missionaries upon their return to France from Peking [circa 1776]. Pierre Martial Cibot, the interpreter of the 'Cong-Fou,' did not translate the entire system. His 11 pages . . . including 20 figures, deal only with postures, exercises and the schooling of respiration. No mention is made of massage. Massage is, however, briefly mentioned in a later volume as having been directly observed by the reporting missionaries."[26]

Kamenetz goes on to cite several scholars of Chinese literature who assert first that Taoism, the religious philosophy of Lao-tse (600 B.C.E.), is related to kung fu and that it was common practice to append the ancient writings as time and ages passed. Material that had been added to the ancient writings was interpreted later as having been written with the original material; because of this we may be finding references to massage in certain Chinese texts because they were "super-added." It is therefore difficult to pinpoint precisely when these writings were made, although it is clear from some scholars that these practices (including massage) were indeed conducted long before being recorded in written form. Dr. Kleen's earlier comment concerning massage being a part of the Kong-Fu texts were "greatly overrated" may refer to the fact that these reports provided no written evidence but were based only on statements that the missionaries had "observed" such practices.

The Yellow Emperor's Classic of Internal Medicine, also known as the *Nei Ching* or *Neijing,* is most likely from circa 1000 B.C.E. Some authors claim it dates back to circa 2500 B.C.E., while others date it at circa 100 B.C.E. One plausible explanation for the considerable difference in these estimated dates of origin is that it was common among Chinese writers and historians to give credit for works done in later periods to a popular previous emperor as a token of honor.

On the Yellow Emperor's Classic of Internal Medicine, Kamenetz comments:

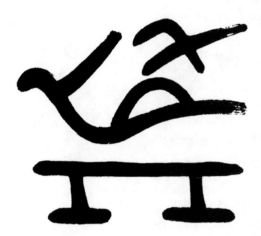

An ancient Chinese ideogram for massage. From *Amma Therapy* by Tina Sohn and Robert Sohn (Rochester, Vt., 1996).

> Possibly the oldest extant medical work is The Yellow Emperor's Classic of Internal Medicine, usually referred to as the *Nei Ching.* Attributed to Huang Ti, the Yellow Emperor, who died in 2598 B.C., the book dates probably back to about 1000 B.C. We find in Chapter 12 of Veith's book [a 1949 translation entitled *The Yellow Emperor's Classic of Internal Medicine,* published by Williams & Wilkins] mention of "complete paralysis and chills and fever . . . most fittingly treated with breathing exercises, massage of the skin and flesh [muscles], and exercises of hands and feet." The book discusses in Chapter 24 the cessation of the circulation in the arteries and the veins for which "one uses massage and medicines prepared from the lees of wine." [Lees of wine is the sediment that settles at the bottom of the bottle.] In Chapter 27 a question is posed about what to do when supplementing is insufficient [the word *supplementing* here means "excess." The question could be rephrased to read "What should be done when treatment for excess is insufficient?"]. Ch'i Po answered: "One must first feel with the hand and trace the system of the body. One should interrupt the sufficiency's [*sic*] and distribute them evenly, one should apply binding and massage."[27]

It is commonly agreed that the meridian system of energy pathways had been well developed as early as this time; this is likely the "system of the body" referred to in this passage. Binding may be meant as a medical treatment (bandaging) for support of veins and arteries, because the passage is discussing a blood condition.

The phrase "finger pressure" is also found within the Yellow Emperor's Classic of Internal Medicine. Sensei Masunaga, in his 1977 book *Zen Shiatsu, a Japanese Form of Manual Therapy*, provides the following quote: "In the spring and autumn, when food is plentiful and humans tend to become lazy and slothful, finger pressure is used to increase digestive fire, and restore vigor."[28]

No equivalent in English is provided for the word *massage* in these texts, although it is likely that word was *moshou* according to Zhang Tao, M.D., professor emeritus of the Department of Orthopedics for Guang An Men Hospital in Beijing, China. In an interview with *Massage Magazine* Dr. Tao said; "In ancient times the approach was called *moshou*, which translates into English as 'hand rubbing.' Later on, during the Han dynasty [25–220 C.E.], the name for these techniques changed from *moshou* to *anmo*, which in English means 'press and rub.' In the Ming dynasty [1368–1641] the name was finally switched to *tuina*." He goes on to say, "None of these different names conveys the complete scope of practice of what we now call tuina. In my opinion, a better name for this medical discipline would be something that translates as 'hand manipulation therapy.'"[29]

In an English translation of a Chinese text entitled *Chinese Bodywork, A Complete Manual of Chinese Therapeutic Massage* (1993), Sun Chengnan a fourth-generation practitioner on his father's side and a ninth-generation practitioner via his maternal grandfather, writes: "When China was unified during the Qin Dynasty in the 3rd century B.C., bodywork was known as Moshou (hand rubbing). During the Han Dynasty (206 B.C.– 220 A.D.), Chinese therapeutic massage became known as Anmo (press and rub). By the 5th century, it had evolved to such a level that a Doctoral Degree was created for it at the Imperial College of Medicine in Xian, the ancient capital of the Tang Dynasty. (Later, during the Ming Dynasty [1368–1644], the term Tuina [push and hold] was added."[30] These terms are consistent with Dr. Zhang Tao's.

In the book *Chinese Massage* (1988, 1990), translated into English by six Chinese professors, the Shanghai College of Traditional Chinese Medicine asserts that the term *anwu* was used to describe the ancient massage technique applied by a famous doctor during the reign of Emperor Hunag Yu Fu. They further state: "It was recorded in the unearthed oracle inscriptions on bones or tortoise shells of the Shang Dynasty that the female witch doctor Bi could treat the patients with massage."[31]

Numerous other Chinese writings of ancient origin mention the use of massage in therapeutic practice. One of these is worth noting for its substantial text about massage. Kamenetz reports that in *The Annals of Art*, the official history for the early Han dynasty (202 B.C.E.–9 C.E.) there is mention of a ten-chapter treatise on massage (*an mo* in old Chinese, literally translated as "press rub"). The treatise is entitled *Huang*

Ti Ch'I Pai An Mo. Like the *Nei Ching,* it was ascribed to Huang Ti as a matter of honoring the emperor, not as an indication of its authorship or age.[32]

Kamenetz writes that "during the T'ang dynasty (619–907 C.E.) four kinds of medical practitioners were recognized: physicians, acupuncturists, masseurs and exorcists."[33] Formal institutions and academic positions were well established around these categories, including a department of massage, professors of massage, and "masseurs," who comprised the majority of the labor force in the delivery of moshou.

According to Honora Lee Wolfe, writing in 1986, "Five major remedial schools of Chinese therapeutic massage can be identified. 1. The One Finger School concentrated on 'one finger pushing' to push points along the channels and collaterals by concentrating force through the tip of the thumb. This school originated in the Sui or Song dynasty [circa 580 B.C.] and is still an integral part of clinical Tui-Na today. 2. The Rolling School developed from the One Finger School. . . . The Rolling method covers a large area, is comfortable in its application, is mechanically easy on the practitioner's body, and can be adjusted to suit many different patients and situations. 3. Nei Kung Tui-Na is also called the Flat-Pushing Method. It is a combination of Internal Nei Kung exercise coordinated with massage treatment in which the practitioner channels Qi to the patient. 4. Pointing Method is the Chinese name for Acupressure. 5. Bonesetting is composed of eight basic types of manipulations: joining, holding, lifting, pushing, pinching, pressing, rubbing, and feeling. . . . Within Tui-na there is also a specialty of Remedial Infant Massage. This was developed during the Tang dynasty (600–900 C.E.)."[34]

India

Delhi, the current capital of India, was founded in 400 B.C.E., just after the death of Hippocrates in Greece. However, archaeological evidence around Delhi points to "a flourishing culture of city dwellers datable as early as 2500 B.C.E."[35] Earliest historic Indian society is known as the Vedic period. There were four ancient sacred Veda writings in India: the Yajur, Rig, Sama, and Atharva Vedas. These were known only to a few scholars of the higher castes. In the early Vedic period (2000 B.C.E.) knowledge was passed on through oral traditions. The Aryans from Persia invaded Indian territories over several centuries, and the earliest writings of Indian origin come from their religious practices in the form of their ancient hymns. The characters in these hymns later developed into divine gods, which eventually contributed to the Hindu religion extant.

The Aryans continued to move about in different directions to conquer and assimilate other societies around them, in the process developing the caste system. The Vedic period was followed by the Brahmanic period. The Brahmans were a powerful group of Aryan priests who asserted considerable influence during the period 800 B.C.E. to about 1000 C.E. Historian John Bowle writes: "The Brahmans secluded themselves from the rest of society, often in separate settlements, and transmitted their

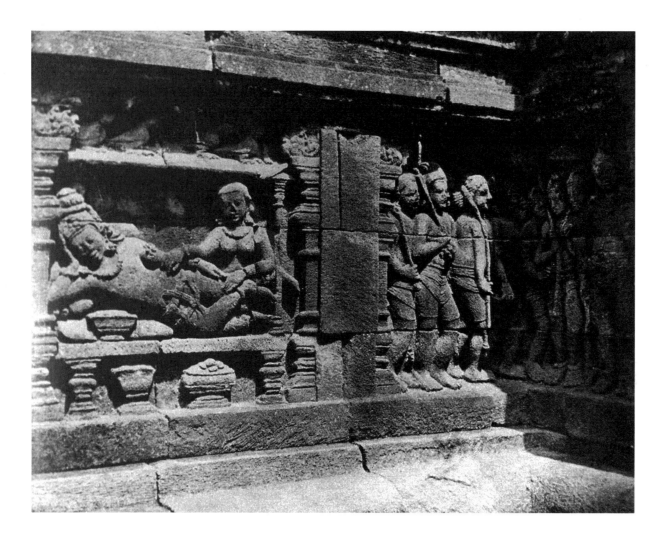

sacred learning through special schools within their own order. They performed sacrifices and other rituals for the kings and chiefs, and as their chaplains, might perform the functions of political advisers and administrators, but they remained as a class independent of royal control."[36]

The ancient Indian medical texts came from these traditions; however, during the Brahamic period (800 B.C.E.–1000 C.E.) the practice of medicine was not within the domain of the controlling priests, as it was in earlier Indian periods. According to Dr. Marti-Ibanez, the Brahman relegated the practice of medicine to a lower caste.[37] The authors of the classic medical texts, "Charaka (100 A.D.), Susruta (500 A.D.) and Vaghbhata (600 A.D.), founders of Indian medicine," based their work on the Ayur Veda (1800–1500 B.C.E.), "the supreme mystic document of Hindu medicine." According to D. Guthrie in *A History of Medicine* (1945), the Ayur Veda is an anatomy book found in the fourth volume of the *Atharva Veda*.[38]

The term *samvahana,* according to French author L. Mac-Auliffe, is an Indian word from the Ayur Veda long used to denote massage. Its translation into English means "hand rubbing," while the word *mordan,* also found in the Sanskrit literature, means "to rub."

This carved stone relief at the Buddhist temple at Borobodur, in Java, is believed to have been built circa the eighth century C.E. The caption accompanying this image in the source text states: "The Lord Buddha receives treatment at the hand of his masseuse." From *Wonders of the Past,* edited by J. Alexander Hammerton (New York, 1923).

Numerous authors claim that ancient Indian writings found in the medicine of India, called *ayurveda,* used the word *shampooing* (from the Sanskrit *tshampua*) to denote massage. Greek historians who visited India three hundred years before the birth of Christ brought back glowing accounts of the art of shampooing. "Among the Brahmins there is an order of physicians who rely chiefly upon diet and regimen . . . [and] hygienic shampooing."[39] Shampooing was a part of India's indigenous medicine when Alexander the Great passed through India in 327 B.C.E. His soldiers have been given credit for bringing the techniques to the Mediterranean region, where later it would become a part of Greek, Roman, and Turkish practices. Shampooing as practiced by the people of India can still be found today in Turkish bath houses around the world. That shampooing has a lineage more than two thousand years old is confirmed by the similarity of the descriptions of shampooing found in ancient writings of the Arabs and Romans and that given by George H. Taylor, M.D., a late-nineteenth-century physician who advocated exercise for health. In his book, *Health by Exercise,* he describes the practice as experienced by English residents living in India during his time:

> The English who reside in India frequently give accounts of the shampooing and friction, which they find a great source of delight as well as of health. The person receiving the operation is extended on a seat, while the operator manipulates his members, as he would knead dough for bread. He then strikes him lightly with the side of the hand, applies perfume and friction, and terminates by cracking the joints of the fingers, toes, and neck. After this operation, the subject experiences a sensation of ineffable happiness and energy. It is said that the Indian ladies seldom pass a day without being thus shampooed by their slaves.[40]

Although in more modern times *shampooing* implies a full-body cleaning usually done with a brush and the hands, this account leaves little doubt about the claim that Indian shampooing is massage. French scholars and historians used the term *barber-masseur* to describe the manual practices of India they discovered during their travels there in the late 1700s and early 1800s.

Wrestling was and is popular in India. Massage has been a traditional healing modality used in wrestling since ancient times, in conjunction with exercise and breath work. Harish Johari, in his book *Ayurvedic Massage* (1996), asserts that "in ancient times Ayurvedic clinics did not regularly offer massage, as everybody gave and received massage." When people did need massage they would be referred to a specialist in the tactile arts, who used oils and techniques passed down through the centuries. "Often these massage practitioners were wrestlers," says Harish Johari. He continues: "Today in India massage practitioners with this training roam public places in great numbers and give head and body massages for a few rupees."[41] Many of these practitioners work in the city parks, and some are Ayurvedic doctors as well.

Minnie Goodnow provides the following quote regarding a medical school that was also a public hospital operating in India circa 225 B.C.E.: "The nurse must be clever, devoted to the patient, and pure in body and mind; must know how to compound drugs, be competent to cook food, skilled in bathing the patients, conversant with rubbing the limbs and massage, with lifting the patient, well skilled in making and cleaning of beds, ready, patient and skilful."[42]

As we browse through the Asian continent for evidence of massage it becomes evident how the movement of manual therapies moved across the continent like a camel caravan spreading commerce with its heavy load of goods. Even without conscious effort to record the massage practices of countries, its practice is visible to us through the stories of travelers, scholars, and historians. From inferences drawn by the examination of the most ancient records made on bone, shell, and stone, kept alive through verbal traditions and finally to the venerable writings of Sanskrit scholars and historians, the evidence for massage in world cultures unfolds before us in wonderful form.

Emerging from the mists of ancient ritual practices, massage finds a place in medicine, sport, and midwifery, and becomes a little more visible and a lot more utilized. As we move into the world of the ancient Greeks and Romans, a golden period for massage, we will at the other end of these epochs learn about the first great fall of massage in the eyes of humankind and the ancient roots of its association with sexual behavior.

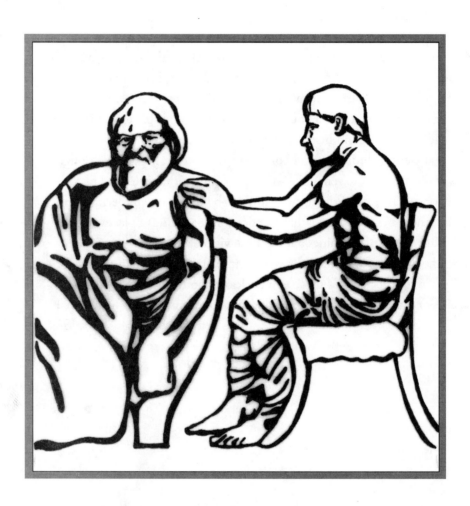

A slave *aliptae* administering massage to a Roman
gladiator. From a photograph of a stone relief fragment
believed to be from the Roman baths in Cyrene, circa
98 C.E. *From Manipulation, Traction and Massage* edited
by Joseph P. Rogoff (New Haven, 1960).

4 Massage in the Ancient World: Greece and Rome

The Hellenistic period in Greece was a time in history when the convergence of intellect, education, opportunity, and experience all came together to produce new lines of thought. A new mind emerged among the Greek people. For whatever reason—whether the builders of Greek civilization felt unburdened by the past or had achieved safe haven in the quest for survival, which allowed them greater latitude to cogitate—a turning point from the old ways to a new way of thinking took hold of humanity and spread its wings of flight to deeply influence the next two millennia.

Greek medicine represents a revolution in thinking about diagnosis and treatment. Greek physicians were well schooled in all the magico-religious cures but found them inconsistent with the emerging new philosophies of rational thought. The history of modern medicine begins with Hippocrates, who was the first to separate the physician from the historical roots of cosmological speculator and philosopher of nature. He shifted the focus of the physician away from magic, ritual, and speculation to medicine marked by keen observation, logical thought, principles of diagnosis and treatment, and a humble relationship with the patient. Beginning with Hippocrates, Greek physicians no longer approached a patient as a vessel containing evil spirits to be exhumed through rites and ritual. The Greek physician observed symptoms, related those symptoms to the patient's internal and external environment, and attempted to provide therapy that was in accord with nature's physical offerings.

Massage was a part, albeit a small part, of this medical revolution. Although there is clear evidence that massage played a significant role in ancient Greece, there is less evidence to support the claims made by some massage historians for its extensive medical use. Hippocrates' biography can be viewed as an indicator of the place of massage in ancient history because of his immense fame. More has been written about Hippocrates' philosophy and practice of medicine than about any other figure in the healing arts.[1] His was not only the first systematized medicine, but the first holistic medicine as well.[2] Yet the Hippocratic Corpus contains very few references to massage.

The excess of bodily exercises may render us wild and unmanageable, but the excess of arts, sciences, and music makes us too faddled and effeminate; only the right combination of both makes the soul circumspect and manly.

—Plato (427–347 B.C.E.)

The scant occurrence of remarks about massage in the ancient medical literature is in stark contrast to the voluminous texts on most other medical practices (diagnosis, case histories, and many other treatments) and the vast classifications of natural phenomenon. There are countless examples of Greek and Roman medical texts that provide enormous details about a wide variety of surgical methods, pharmacological formulas, and disease treatment procedures. Although references to massage do exist, the amount of material about massage is comparatively small.

The prevailing medical doctrine of Hippocrates' time was commonly known as the four humors. The theory of the four humors was central to the tenets of the Hippocratic Corpus and remained the mainstay of medicine in Europe for more than two thousand years after Hippocrates. According to this theory, the four humors—phlegm, blood, yellow bile, and black bile—had to be in balance for health to exist. Further, the humors were related to the four seasons, the wind, and to the four elements: earth, air, fire, and water. Dr. Walter Libby's medical history offers this composite view.

> Blood is hot and moist like air, phlegm is cold and moist like water, yellow bile is hot and dry like fire, and black bile is cold and dry like earth. . . . Similarly in the Hippocratic physiology, health depended on the *crasis,* or blending, of the four juices of the body. Unless they duly blend, there is a state of *dyscrasia,* or crudity, the humors, like raw food, acting as irritants. Health must be restored by a process of *coction* (or pepsis) wherein the internal heat of the body cooks the crude humors. Upon this follows a *crisis*—a separation, or elimination—of the superfluous substance. The elements may be restored to a state of harmony and equilibrium by the remedial power of Nature. It was faith in this *vis medicatrix naturae* which led Hippocrates to adopt an expectant attitude in the treatment of many of his cases, to abstain at times from surgical interference, and to prescribe drugs and cooling drinks as auxiliaries of Nature in the expulsion of the morbific matter after a fever crisis.[3]

This statement by Libby offers a good perspective on Hippocrates' belief that massage was a valuable therapeutic tool. "Nature acts without masters," wrote Hippocrates. He firmly believed that the body was capable of curing itself and that disease symptoms, particularly fever, were simply expressions of that capability.

Hippocratic Massage: Anatripsis

Although references to massage were slight in writings attributed to Hippocrates, they did occur. Hippocrates used the word *anatripsis* to "designate the process of rubbing" according to Walter Johnson (1866), whose early work was often quoted (and sometimes plagiarized) by medical historians who came after him. Douglas Graham, M.D., an American physician writing in the early 1900s, cites the following quote from

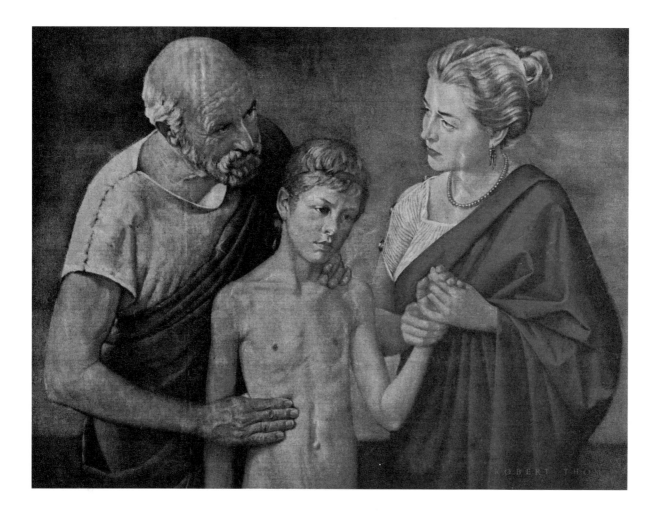

"Great Moments in Medicine—Hippocrates—Medicine Becomes Science." Oil painting by Robert Thom, commissioned by Parke-Davis & Co., the Warner-Lambert Company subsidiary. Reprinted with permission.

writings attributed to Hippocrates: "The physician must be experienced in many things, but assuredly also in rubbing (his [Hippocrates'] word, anatripsis)."[4]

The word *anatripsis,* meaning "to rub up," itself demonstrates the Greek medical revolution as it was applied to the theory and practice of massage. The antecedent priest-physician method of rubbing prior to the Greeks was to rub *down*—rub, brush, blow, or suck to move evil spirits or the invading sickness from the core of the body toward and out the extremities. "Massage, another means of inducing the evil spirit to leave the body, consisted in stroking the limbs in a centrifugal direction—that is, towards the extremities. Later, as devil possession gave place to more enlightened pathology, the direction of the massage changed and was applied in a centripetal direction."[5] The Greeks altered this tradition to move the body fluids toward the core of the body from the extremities, so to eliminate the toxic materials through the alimentary tract.

In the following extract Walter Johnson refers to anatripsis and "friction," and translates it as "rubbing."

> Hippocrates . . . frequently mentions friction as a recognized and famil-
> iar remedy; and in one pregnant aphorism he fully and tersely defines its

effects. Here and there again he takes occasion to recommend friction in terms which prove his practical acquaintance with its uses; as in the following passage, speaking of the treatment of dislocation of the shoulder-joint after reduction, he [Hippocrates] says: "Those in whom the ligaments are attacked with inflammation cannot use the shoulder, for they are prevented by the pain and inflammatory tension. It is proper to treat such patients with cerate, and to bind the part with compresses and numerous bandages; to fill up the hollow of the armpit with a ball of soft cleansed wool, as a support for the bandage and a prop to the joint. To the arm there should be given for the most part an inclination upwards; [elevation] for in this position the head of the shoulder will be most distinct from the spot into which it was dislocated. And when you have bandaged the shoulder, then it is proper to bind the arm to the side with a bandage passed round the body. *And it is necessary to rub the shoulder gently and smoothly. The physician must be experienced in many things, but assuredly also in rubbing; for things that have the same name have not the same effects. For rubbing can bind a joint which is too loose, and loosen a joint which is too hard. . . . However, a shoulder in the condition described should be rubbed with soft hands, and above all things gently; but the joint should be moved about, not violently, but so far as it can be done without producing pain.*" (Hippocrates "Peri Arthron" Littre. vol. iv., p. 100, et seq.)[6]

Hippocrates defined *anatripsis* as stroking the extremities upward (toward the heart), followed by a light stroke back, and then another upward stroke to push the venous and lymph toward the heart.[7] These strokes could be hard, soft, or moderate, depending on the condition of the tissues and the effect desired. Hippocrates was specific about the effects of each of these methods of anatripsis, saying: "Friction can relax, brace, incarnate, attenuate: hard braces, soft relaxes, much attenuates, and moderate thickens."[8] Dr. Graham comments: "The observations of Hippocrates must have been very accurate to discern that rubbing upward in the case of the limbs had a more favorable effect than rubbing downward, and doubtless in this manner he had experience in promoting the resorption of effusions; for it is now well known that upward friction on the limbs favors the return of the circulation, relieves blood stasis, and makes more room in the veins and lymphatics for the carrying away of morbid products."[9]

Hippocrates earned high praise from Dr. Graham, as from so many others: "These brief sayings of Hippocrates on anatripsis serve partly to show at the same time why he was considered a man of transcendental genius and justly styled the 'Father of Medicine,' who . . . raised the art from a system of superstitious rites practised wholly by the priests to the dignity of a learned profession."[10]

MASSAGE IN THE

ANCIENT WORLD:

GREECE AND ROME

Was anointing massage?

Anointing may be the first recorded word found in ancient writings that has links to the present-day term *massage. Anoint* comes from the Latin *inungere,* literally, "to smear on" (*in* meaning "on" and *unguere* meaning "to smear"). In practical terms this definition means "rubbing olive oil or oil essences on the body." Many historians of massage base their assumptions about how massage was employed in earlier times on the presence of the term *anoint* in ancient manuscripts. Elizabeth C. Wood and Gertrude Beard, in their classic book, *Massage: Principles and Techniques* (1964), state, "Writings of physicians, philosophers, poets, and historians show that some form of rubbing or anointing was used among both savage and civilized nations from the most ancient times."[11] In particular, Beard and Wood, Graham, and a number of other massage historians have cited Homer's *Odyssey* as containing references to massage being used in Greek times.

Homer sang songs as he wandered in the countryside and through the cities around a thousand years before Christ. His songs largely told about the heroic exploits of soldiers from various parts of the region. However, a reading of Homer's *Odyssey* reveals that the word *anatripsis,* the word commonly used in his time to denote friction massage, does not appear anywhere in those stories. However, as universally translated by modern scholars the word *anoint* appears in the *Odyssey* nineteen times, although the word does not explicitly or implicitly refer to massage. There are twelve references to a man being anointed by a slave or a family member (a daughter). Three times anointing is done by women to themselves, and there is one description of a man anointing himself. In one instance a group of women anoint each other, and there is another mention of a woman, distraught because her husband is away, saying, "Do not try and persuade me to wash and to anoint myself, for heaven robbed me of all my beauty on the day my husband sailed."[12]

Throughout most of history anointing was done after bathing, before and after exercise, and in conjunction with and in applying beauty treatments. Taking into account the dry, arid climates of these early civilizations, anointing also served as a means of moisturizing the skin. Oil gives the skin a rich look and silky feel, qualities highly prized by the ancient peoples, particularly the Egyptians. Anoint-

ing was also believed to afford curative benefits, following the application of specific kinds of oils. The oil of choice for the ancients was olive oil, often perfumed with liquid myrrh or sweetened with cinnamon, cane, or cassia. Oil is absorbed into the skin, and if of sufficient quality, can provide essential fatty acids, antioxidants, vitamins, and other nutrients. Clearly, each reference to anointing in Homer's epics is to a form of traditional practice common in Greek households as part of the cleaning and bathing ritual and as a form of beauty aid for dry, parched skin.

In ancient medical practice as well, the word *anoint* had a particular meaning. Francis Adams's translation of Hippocrates' *Treatise on Fractures* (400 B.C.E.) reveals that Hippocrates used the word *anoint* much differently than he used the word *anatripsis.* Here is an example of his use of the word *anoint:* "To the wound itself a cerate mixed with pitch is to be applied, a thin folded compress to be bound upon it, and the parts around are to be anointed with white cerate."[13] Cerate is a waxlike substance often used to help hold bandages on the body to keep them from moving, or to keep the bandage from rubbing over a wound to prevent irritation. Here Hippocrates is using the word *anoint* to denote applying an ointment (cerate) to a wound. He uses the word *anatripsis* when he is referring to massage, as in the following example taken from his *On Dislocations:* "And when you have bandaged the shoulder, then it is proper to bind the arm to the side with a bandage passed round the body. And it is necessary to rub the shoulder gently and smoothly . . . [the shoulder] should be rubbed with soft hands, and above all things gently."[14]

Walter Johnson, in his 1866 book, *The Anatriptic Art,* provides some keen insight into this subject. When you read the word *friction* here it is helpful to substitute the word *rubbing.*

The processes of Friction and Unction are broadly distinguished by Celsus, who states that the latter is advantageous in many cases in which the former is quite inadmissible. And this distinction is indeed useful for medical purposes, though it is true that there can be no unction (which is defined to be the rubbing in of greasy substances) without friction of some sort; while friction was understood by ancient medical writers to be usually performed by the aid of oil or fat. Friction, therefore, might also be termed unction. In the operation of friction, however, the greasy substance is used merely to keep the skin from chafing; but in unction no more friction is employed than is necessary to apply the oil. Friction may be extremely gentle or extremely rough—may be used for a few minutes, or for hours continuously; but the friction employed in unction is always gentle, and generally of short duration. But as I said before, this is a medical distinction—a distinction which naturally would very commonly be disregarded in ordinary language.[15]

Johnson is clearly stating that unction (anointing) is not massage but merely the application of "greasy substances," while friction (rubbing) is massage, and utilizes unction merely as a process of lubricating the skin. The clue toward solving our question lies in his last statement. It is in "ordinary language" that unction or anointing has been used to indicate massage.

The Greek Gymnasiums and Baths

If the use of massage was slight in the Greek medical context, it was highly developed in association with the gymnasiums and baths, central institutions of both Greek and Roman ancient society. Walter Johnson writes, "The rubbing practices of the Greeks and Romans may be considered under two heads, viz., as simple rubbing, and as rubbing in connection with the bath or gymnastic exercises."[16]

Six hundred years before Christ was born, Prince Anacharsis, living in self-imposed exile in Athens wrote, "In every city of the Greeks there is a designated place where they go mad daily, I mean the gymnasium."[17] The gymnasium was at first built as an institution for military and athletic training of the young Greek citizens; their education also included intellectual and artistic subjects, all taught at the public gymnasiums. The gymnasium developed into the center of Greek social activity, which included lectures on philosophy, medicine, and poetry. Cults of the traditional gods of the gymnasiums were worshiped at these facilities as well. After the Romans conquered Greece, the gymnasiums also housed libraries and provided space for civic functions; even public sacrifices of cows followed by grand feasts were conducted inside them.

The first gymnasiums were sited in open fields located on the outskirts of town, usually near a stream, river, or body of water to provide easy access for bathing after strenuous exercise and games. As gymnasiums became more popular they were developed into parklike facilities. Sporting activities were the first use of these open spaces. Ball games, wrestling, running, and jumping were the most popular sporting activities. It wasn't long before the peaceful atmosphere attracted orators and teachers and picnickers, too.

Small buildings were erected, large numbers of trees were planted, running tracks were built, and the open spaces became smaller. As the cities increased in population and territory, many of them with high walls built around them, these open spaces were encroached upon even more. Circa 400 B.C.E. there was no longer room to hold running races, and so they were contested on the streets of the city. These changes all led to the building of huge gymnasiums situated more toward the city center, or near the seashore. These buildings in turn changed the character of the Greek gymnasium.

Properly named the Esclapeion, Greek gymnasiums were everywhere, with more than three hundred in the country at one time.[18] A comparison with today's hospitals dramatizes their place in the culture of the time. Our hospitals are places of medical sterility, tile and stainless steel; buildings from which we want to leave as soon as possible. The Greek Esclapeion were built in a natural setting; the Esclapeion was an environment dedicated to healing, education, and public discourse, a place where one would want to stay. Even though there was an elite social class, the gymnasium was a public place open to all free-born citizens, even those living outside the city's boundaries. The common citizen practiced his exercises, bathed, and competed alongside the sons of noblemen and political leaders. Each shared in the spiritual, mental, and physical possibilities available at the Greek gymnasium.

Washing and bathing took place in the *loutron* of the Greek gymnasium, an open-air space used exclusively for this purpose. The loutron was nearly always a cold-water bathing room, following the "Laconian style" of bathing practiced by the Spartans (circa 750 B.C.E.), representing a frugal philosophy toward the body. After the Roman era, hot bathing became available and the Greek upper class followed the immoderate tradition of past aristocrats well described by Plato (427–347 B.C.E.), who had written at length on the subject of hot bathing as a privilege reserved for the kings and their courts.[19] The wet-steam room *(concamerata sudatio),* dry-steam room *(laconicum),* and the warm bathing room *(calda lavatio)* were specialized rooms added to the gymnasium as hot baths rose in popularity.

The buildings were palatial, with a grand central courtyard for exercising, lectures, and gatherings. Usually situated within high walls accompanied by massive columns inside, the interior held classrooms, libraries, and—when included—baths with changing rooms. There was a cold-water washing room; sweating rooms; a room for oiling the body and storing the oils; and the *ephebeum,* "the young men's hall in the middle." It was here that athletes and citizens discussed the politics and games of the day, rested, and massaged each other.[20]

At the height of their success the Greek gymnasiums were primarily devoted to exercise, massage, and baths. The exercises included wrestling, jumping, boxing, running, throwing, and games played with balls. Massage was a common service at these facilities, yet little is written about it by modern historians of medicine, architecture, or literature, perhaps because of its commonness. The earlier baths contained "tubs," which were a few feet deep, with steps leading out of the water or ledges along their sides. Perhaps the *aliptae,* as the slave masseur was called, worked on patrons while they were standing in the water, or sitting or lying on the ledges or steps. In the later baths, which were quite large and palatial, warm oil massage was given in the *aleipterion,* the heated room, after exercise in the gymnasium. Massage was also given within the steam rooms, hot bath rooms, or the lounge areas where skin scraping and anointing with oil and powder were offered.[21]

Some evidence from architectural remains point to a table made of marble, slate, or other stone being used for massage. Massage—called "frictions" by Johnson in his detailed description below—was applied to prepare the young men for exercise, refresh them afterward, and as an accompaniment to their bath.

> The usual routine was this: The youth was first rubbed by the paidotribes with oil; this process was called the preparatory rubbing—*tripsis paraskeuastike.* He then proceeded to some of the lighter exercises, as playing at ball; after which he sprinkled himself with Egyptian dust, and sought a companion (sungumnastes) to wrestle with. When sufficiently exercised, he passed into the room of the anointer (aleiptes), who by aid of the stlengis, or strigil, as the Romans called it, helped him to scrape off his dust, oil, and sweat, and then rubbed him again with oil, which process was called apotherapeia. This done, he entered the warm bath, and after a short stay proceeded to the cold bath, and from the cold bath he returned to the aleiptes, who anointed him a second time, and sent him about his business. It ought never to be forgotten that the aleiptes regulated the diet of every pupil, prescribing in the exact quantity and quality and time of every meal. It is not my intention to enter into details on the subject of the gymnasium; but I am compelled thus briefly to allude to it in order to render intelligible what remains to be said about gymnastic friction. Gymnastic or hygienic friction, then, consisted in the preparatory friction—tripsis paraskeuastike—and the friction which followed the exercises—apotherapeia.[22]

Massage, or rubbings, were also performed in Greek culture during the time of Hippocrates as part of the ritual preparation for incubation, or "temple sleep," whereby the ailing person would sleep in the temple and dream that the god Aesclepius and his daughters, Hygeia and Panacea, would appear to cure him. Aesclepius (or Asklepios) was a mythological figure whose father was Apollo and his mother the maiden Coronis. Homer called Aesclepius "the blameless physician." He is known more commonly as the god of medicine or god of health. Temples were erected throughout Greece in honor of Aesclepius.

Like their father, Hygeia and Panacea were worshiped at many temples in Greece, and later in Rome. Hygeia was the goddess of health whose characteristic quality was symbolized by the serpent, representing perpetual renovation. *Hygeia* means "the practice of cleanliness in the maintenance of health." Her domain was both physical and mental health. Panacea had a less prominent role than her famous sister, but her name, meaning "a remedy for all ills and difficulties," continues in the word *panacea,* a word still used universally. Many statues of Aesclepius and his daughters, especially Hygeia, also adorned the gymnasiums built in honor of the gods. Hygeia is depicted in a variety of healing manners. In some statues she assists her father; in others she has a basket of food, or the serpent is being fed from a bowl; and some show her tending to children.

Roman Medical Practice

In *The Concise Encyclopedia of World History* editor John Bowle states that the first physicians in Rome were slaves. Most were of Greek heritage, many of them freed slaves originally taken from Greece when Rome conquered it.[23] Because of their heritage, the social standing of Roman physicians was quite low. Also, as many early physicians were charlatans, offering ineffective cures, there was a deep mistrust of doctors. One citizen commented that the new doctor in town was previously an undertaker and that what he was doing as a doctor wasn't much different than his work as an undertaker. Another contended that the doctor charged too much, used worthless medicines and drugs, and attempted to treat diseases for which he had no training or understanding.[24]

Before the Greek physicians arrived, medicine was dispensed by a variety of Roman practitioners. Healing cures and surgery were administered by family slaves, often trained only by experience; by barber-surgeons, who used bleeding as a common practice; by priests, who exorcised or cajoled demons from the patient; and even by the slave masseurs, known as *aleiptes*. This latter category, like the family slave, was knowledgeable only through experience. These were times with no licensing (medical licensing would not arrive until 200 C.E.), and anyone who was willing to wield a scalpel did. The "masseur," working without limits and established within the gymnasium or the facilities of a rich householder, was able to dally in the medical "sciences" without much fear of reprisal, except a diminished reputation if he failed too often.

Into this environment came the astute and educated Greek physicians, who eventually took over the treatment of Roman citizens and their leaders. But their rise to acceptance was not an easy one. It wasn't until Julius Caesar "granted freedom to all freeborn Greek physicians practicing in Roman territory" in 46 B.C.E. that they were able to escape from the domination of their rich household owners and the general scorn of the Romans and rise to the heights of social and professional status.[25] Clear evidence of the role of massage in Roman medical treatment can be found in a letter to the emperor from physician Pliny the Elder (23–79 C.E.) about how his life was saved by the ministrations "of a medical practitioner who cured many of his patients by the process of rubbing and anointing." He derived so much benefit "from the remedy that he asked the emperor to grant the physician, who was either a Jew or a Greek, the freedom of the city and the privileges of Roman citizenship."[26]

The influence of Hippocratic medical practice, including massage, continued in the work of a number of prominent Greek and Roman physicians. Thus medical

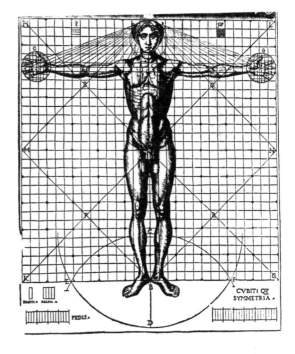

"The Proportions of Man," a first-century B.C.E. drawing by Lucio di Vitruvio. From *Anatomy Illustrated* by Emily Blair Chewning and Dana Levy (New York, 1979).

MASSAGE IN THE
ANCIENT WORLD:
GREECE AND ROME

practices of the time were built, as exemplified by the Hippocratic model, upon observation, trial and error, and especially on prescriptions for rest and proper diet. The theory of the four humors was still a working concept for most physicians, and the effects of massage fit well into their theories of circulation.

The Roman physician's knowledge of anatomy was very limited, because the study of anatomy through human dissection was prohibited in the Roman empire. Whatever human dissection was performed at the time was done primarily in Egypt, under the authority of the conquering ruler Alexander the Great. A man named Marinus, of Alexandria, is most often cited as the "expert dissector" of these times.

At the beginning of the third century B.C.E. the bodies of condemned criminals were made available to physicians, such as Herophilus and Erasistratus in Rome. The nervous system, and especially the human brain, received the greatest attention, and it was during this time that many advances were made in the knowledge of human anatomy. Despite these early studies of anatomy there is no evidence that anatomical knowledge played any part in the physicians' use of massage, and anatomy was certainly unknown and irrelevant to those working in the baths and gymnasiums, because they received no medical education, nor did they treat any diseases.

Asclepiades (124–40 B.C.E.) was a Greek physician who settled in Rome to practice and teach medicine just before the dawn of the Christian era. Asclepiades was a most favored son of Greece and Rome; he was not a follower of Hippocrates and did not subscribe to Hippocrates' natural medicine. The most famous story about Asclepiades is one in which he supposedly brought back to life a Roman citizen being carried to his grave in a coffin. His "cure" for the apparent dead man has been described as "several minutes of manipulation." Perhaps Asclepiades' success is related to his "corpuscular theory"; Asclepiades believed that life was the result of "atoms" constantly on the move within the body. Disease or death were caused by an obstruction of this movement. Thus his "manipulation" may well have been a simple jostling massage that woke up the "sleeping atoms" to bring his patient back to life.[27] In writing about Asclepiades, Sir William Osler states: "Diet, exercise, massage, and bathing were his greatest remedies."[28]

Kamenetz reports that massage was the third most important therapy used by Asclepiades, "after hydrotherapy and exercise. . . . For abdominal pains Asclepiades said that the suffering parts should be rubbed with oil long and energetically to tolerance. To dispel the frigid torpor he advised that the parts be massaged with warm hands and then wrapped in cloth. For convulsions he rubbed the vertebral column day and night in the hope of dissipating spasms. He did not advise massage in fever except during its remission, but he prescribed it in dropsy and leucophlegmasia."[29]

Kellogg claims that Asclepiades "held the practice of this art in such esteem that he abandoned the use of medicines of all sorts, relying exclusively upon massage, which he claimed effects a cure by restoring to the nutritive fluids their natural, free movement. It was this physician who made the discovery that sleep might be induced by gentle stroking."[30] Kleen acclaims Asclepiades as the Father of "Mechano-therapy" for the invention of several devices designed to produce fluid movement through swinging, vibration, or violent motion.[31] Kamenetz informs us that Asclepiades called this form of motion treatment *gestation;* it also included the use of a swinging bed, which was Asclepiades' own invention.

The Roman encyclopedist Celsus, writing about Asclepiades, said "Asclepiades speaks of friction as if he were the inventor of it. According to him there are only three therapeutic agents: first is friction, to which he devotes most space, then water and gestation [meaning "to bear or carry," not "pregnancy"]. No doubt we should not take away from the young the glory of their discoveries, but that is no reason for not leaving to the older what they have established in their writings. Assuredly, no one has presented more precisely and clearly than Asclepiades how and at which parts of the body friction's [*sic*] are to be applied. However, in this respect he has added nothing to what Hippocrates expressed."[32]

Aulus Cornelius Celsus (25 B.C.E.–57 C.E.) is credited with scribing the first organized medical history, tracing the development of healing practices from the simple remedies of "barbarous" nations to Hippocratic and Alexandrian medicine. He was a faithful follower of Hippocrates, known less for his medical practice than for the advice he recorded as a medical encyclopedist. He wrote about many subjects, especially agriculture and medicine, but only his *De medicina, libri octo* has survived. He "divided therapy into three forms: dietetic, pharmaceutics and surgical."[33] Massage was considered a part of the last form. Surgery comprises quite a bit of the text, osteology is covered, and detailed descriptions of amputation are given. Celsus also wrote about therapeutics; his advice in cases of phthisis (pulmonary tuberculosis or atropic diseases) includes "light massage, and warm baths." He also recommended a long trip to Egypt, which would have been by sea, advice often given and called "climatotherapy" well into the nineteenth century. His therapeutic remedy for headaches, to which he devoted quite a bit of attention, also includes massage in addition to an exacting diet, bleeding, and mustard plasters. His other recommendations incorporating massage included remedies for problems with the stomach and the overweight patient.[34]

Celsus provides the following remark, quoted by Kamenetz, which expresses the thoughts of Hippocrates regarding massage. "Vigorous friction's [*sic*] harden the fiber, light friction's [*sic*] loosen it. When pursued a long time, weight is lost; applied with moderation they increase weight."[35] Then Celsus adds the following exposé of his own, clearly based on Hippocratic anatripsis, and provides many of the details not found in the general aphorisms of Hippocrates.

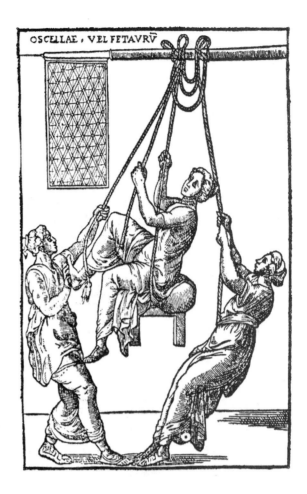

OSCILLAE . VEL FETAVRV

Asclepiades, considered by some to be the father of physical medicine, utilized motion by various means, such as swinging. This was one of a number of movements Asclepiades classified under the title of *gestation.* From *De Arte Gymnastics* (1573) in *The Muscles and Their Story* by E. J. Chapman and L. Hall (London, 1864).

MASSAGE IN THE

ANCIENT WORLD:

GREECE AND ROME

Consequently, friction's [*sic*] are indicated to strengthen relaxed organs, to relax those which are too tense, to dissipate detrimental plethora or to add weight to lean subjects without strength. If we try to determine how these different results are produced (which is beyond the physician's realm) we see that they all consist in the removal of the noxious principle. Indeed, tightening occurs with elimination of the cause of relaxation. Relaxation of the parts results after what made them hard is removed. Gain of weight does not result directly from friction's [*sic*] but with the help of friction of the skin, which becomes more supple, becomes more permeable to nutritious substances. The difference among these results depends upon the procedure used. Both inunction and light friction may be used in acute disease of recent onset provided they be applied during the remission and with an empty stomach. However, prolonged friction's [*sic*] are contraindicated in acute diseases, particularly during their *anabasis,* except as a soporific for a madman. By contrast they are useful in chronic diseases during remission. . . . Friction's [*sic*] are as favorable when the disease is beginning to decline as they are detrimental when fever is increasing. Thus, as far as is possible we should, before using them, wait for the fever to subside or at least for a moment of remission. Friction's [*sic*] are applied either to the whole body, as when we wish to invigorate a debilitated person, or only to a part, in order to remedy the weakness of a limb or some other local condition. Friction's [*sic*] may alleviate inveterate headaches, provided that the treatment is not applied at the acme. Friction's [*sic*] also give strength to the palsied limb. Most often, however, we should apply friction's [*sic*] at a distance from the painful regions; thus, when we wish to draw matter from the upper or middle parts of the body we rub the lower limbs.

It is difficult to determine the exact number of friction's [*sic*] to apply to a person since this will depend upon the strength of the individual. A weakened subject might not stand more than fifty, while a more vigorous one might take two hundred. . . . Thus, we must be more careful in applying them to women than to men and to children and older people more than to young adults.

Finally, if we rub certain limbs, we proceed vigorously for a long time, for, acting on one of its parts, we do not fear to weaken the body soon, and the noxious matter should be resolved as much as possible, be it to remove it from the limb we treat or to divert if from another area. However, if a weak constitution necessitates friction's [*sic*] of the entire body, we rub for a shorter time and less vigorously with the thought of softening the skin so that it can draw new material from the nutrients taken more easily. I have already noted as untoward signs the chilling of the surface while heat and thirst are experienced internally. The only thing to do in such a case is to rub the patient, and after having succeeded in producing warmth exteriorly, we can then apply other therapeutic agents.[36]

According to medical historians, the greatest physician of antiquity, second only to Hippocrates, was Galen (130–201 C.E.), also a Roman. He wrote many volumes of medical and philosophical texts and was an ardent disciple of Hippocrates. He had extensive experience dissecting animals, even the Barbary ape, and was one of the first to correlate anatomy and physiology, which is an ongoing theme in his writings. At age twenty-eight he was physician to the gladiators of Rome and gained a considerable reputation for his treatment of open wounds and tendon injuries. Later he was physician to a number of Roman emperors. His work on anatomy is his greatest contribution, especially his descriptions of bones and muscles and their attendant tissues, such as ligaments and tendons. One medical historian tells that Galen had the rare opportunity during his career to observe the beating heart in two live patients.

A brief remark in Galen's book *Hygiene* reveals his deep feelings toward massage and his disdain for those who would attribute a less than professional—in this case sexual—meaning to its use. This quote is taken from the opening paragraph of the chapter entitled "Morning and Evening Massage." "It still remains, therefore, to discuss morning and evening massage, but not, verily, in the manner in which they say Quintus replied to a gymnast who enquired what was the value of anointment, 'It makes you take off your tunic.'" Galen responds by writing, "These are all wanton witticisms, not at all befitting a man learned in so august an art."[37]

Galen elaborated upon Hippocrates' simple description of anatripsis, including the variety of possible hand directions: "And the rubbings should be of many sorts, with strokes and circuits of the hands, carrying them not only from above down and from below up, but also subvertically, obliquely, transversely and subtransversely. . . . But I direct that the strokes and circuits [*sic*] of the hands should be made of many sorts, in order that so far as possible all the muscle fibers should be rubbed in every direction."[38] Many other references to massage can be found in Green's translation of Galen's *Hygiene,* such as the following:

> If, therefore, he is completely rested, it is superfluous to massage or anoint him, unless it were necessary to overcome extreme cold; for then we shall prepare him with massage, just like those who are going to employ cold bathing. . . . But if there should be any sense of fatigue, it has been said before that then it is necessary to anoint and to massage gently. And so also if he were drier than desirable, he should be anointed with sweet oil; for this moistens the dry skin. And he should be massaged little, but with neither firm nor gentle massage. For we want the administration only to favor digestion, not to change the condition of the skin or of the flesh [muscle], nor to eliminate any of the excrements in them. But gentle massage does both, and firm massage the former, for it thickens and toughens the skin, whereas gentle massage purges and makes the body relaxed and soft.[39]

Galen wrote much more on this subject, describing the details of preparatory massage, the duration of massage at each stage of exercise, and finally "the rubbing of the body—which ought always to follow the exercises." He concludes with an application of massage techniques and their staged applications to the health and well-being of nonathletes, or those exercises not for competition but for their health. Galen was a student of Hippocratic medicine, and his writings, as they relate to massage, can be considered as representing five centuries of Greco-Roman anatripsis theory and practice.

Greco-Roman Midwifery

In cultures around the world, the midwife of ancient times was usually a woman with personal experience bearing children of her own who subsequently helped others within her own village or community. Lay midwives and birth attendants throughout history form a sorority of caregivers that offer very personal care, with special attention paid toward the mother, birth at home among friends and relatives (mostly females), and constant attendance during the pains of labor. Soothing massage was applied to the abdomen of the mother to be, or to her low back and legs, where birthing pain is commonly experienced. Men, usually shamans, priests, or physicians, became involved only when complications arose.

This pattern continued in Greco-Roman times. It was only when complications arose during the birth that a physician might be called in. According to historians of midwifery, these higher class men considered it below the dignity of their position to provide prenatal and delivery services unless an emergency required their educated services.

Midwifery in the Roman empire was almost entirely within the domain of birth attendants and family practices. Birth attendants were usually slaves or former slaves, daughters taught by their mothers, or women who apprenticed with a local midwife. They were rarely educated, because men did not allow women access to medical education. There appear to have been only rare cases of women midwife professionals who enjoyed a status similar to that of male physicians. Their services were cheap, but the poor could not afford even the midwives' low fees. They turned to either "wise women" (sagae) or to other women in the family willing to help.

Hippocrates was reportedly the first to offer women birthing training sometime in the fifth century B.C.E. They were taught almost exclusively by men physicians, and the training was aimed primarily toward Cesarean section and other surgical methods needed in critical situations of childbirth. Women physicians did write, but mostly about abortions, and their practice was largely patronized by prostitutes and ladies of the court.[40]

Soranus, who lived and wrote extensively about midwifery in the second century C.E., provides the most reliable and certainly the most prolific Greco-Roman accounts related to midwifery. His book, *Gynecology,* is a strictly medical approach to the subject. He writes at length about the qualities and qualifications of a good midwife, one of which is that she "keep her hands soft." Soranus describes the equipment needed for the delivery procedure: "olive oil, warm water, warm fomentations, soft sea sponges, pieces of wool, bandages, a pillow, things to smell, a midwife's stool or chair, two beds, and a proper room."[41] Soranus provides instructions to the midwife for easing labor pains by giving gentle massage, administered with a cloth soaked in heated olive oil, to the abdomen and genital region. Hot bags of water and oil were also recommended for application to the sides of the expectant mother's torso.

Unlike Soranus's writing, most writings on midwifery by physicians of the time contain no references to massage. Although some physicians may have used it in the manner described by Soranus, massage was typically not a part of their training or their practice. It was the female midwife who brought massage to the birthing room.

Massage was recommended for breast care after the baby was born by Pliny, who prescribed "rubbing the breasts with sow's blood, goose grease with rose oil and a spider's web, or the fat of bustards," to relieve swelling. Because most medically trained midwives were more expensive and less common than the midwife learned in folk ways, it is generally assumed that most mothers received their midwife care in the manners described by Pliny.

Roman Bath and Gymnasium

For nearly a thousand years before the Christian era a debate raged among Greeks and Romans. The lofty ideals of education and the benefits of physical fitness often clashed. Some thought that education should be strictly academic, while other great and influential thinkers, such as Aristotle and Socrates, believed the liberal arts and music should be accompanied by physical training, as long as it was fitness benefiting military purposes. The gymnasium as an institution of civic and academic activity was eventually transformed by the Romans' increasing emphasis on the hot bath. The other civic functions were reduced to secondary roles as bathing facilities and elaborate competitions became "an epidemic" in first-century B.C.E. Rome. Existing facilities were changed, and many new facilities were being built solely for bathing and exercise. Each incorporated new thermal technologies, such as different materials for making cauldrons in which the water was heated and various methods of heating the water—from wood and coal to dried manure—all while admitting more and more citizens. Hot baths and exercise were becoming a part of daily life.

Most wealthy Romans had baths built into their estates; according to numerous accounts these were often extravagant facilities, usually made of marble with decoratively painted ceilings and walls, and almost always with a lot of sunshine pouring in. Even within the suburban home, small makeshift steam rooms or hot water baths were used. But it was the public baths that provided the most pleasurable sensory experience for Roman citizens and its visiting guests: large, sun-filled, open spaces; exotic marble bathing tubs filled with clean, warm water; soothing gentle massage at the hands of adept slave girls; oils, essences, and powders, their scents augmenting the excitement in the air; and towels of linen and cotton, freshly laid out. The Baths of Caracalla, established circa 212 C.E. in Rome, featured facilities to handle three thousand bathers, a swimming pool, parks, a sporting area, and an extensive library. The Baths of Caracalla are often shown as the prime example of Roman bath architectural achievement.[42]

Roman baths were very similar to the Greek gymnasiums at their peak of popularity. The grandest of the baths, the "thermae," had libraries, lecture rooms, and promenades. They were facilities where athletes trained and competed. Masterpiece statuary of Greek gods adorned the hallways and promontory. Statues of local dignitaries or patricians were, unlike the others, shown fully clothed. A census in the year 33 B.C.E. shows 170 small baths in the city of Rome; barely four hundred years later that figure had increased to 856.[43] But the baths were not limited to the city of Rome. All large cities of the Roman empire, and Italy in general, had their baths; even the small villages in remote areas were proud of their bath facilities. Historians reveal that one of the greatest punishments that could be laid upon a village or city was to have its public baths closed.

The Roman baths were very popular for more than six hundred years, but it was during the last century B.C.E. that they took on an importance unparalleled in human history. The Roman bath was so popular that it was a social institution attended daily—you were nobody if you weren't at the Roman bathhouse. One author writes, "The baths embodied the ideal Roman way of urban life."[44] Roman vase paintings depict scenes from the open-air space known as the loutron, showing men and women (in separate facilities) showering, washing, rubbing, scraping their skin with strigils (metal blades used to scrape excess oil from the body), and anointing each other.

The Golden Ass, by Apuleius, provides a second-century glimpse into the hospitality of a householder toward his visiting guest. "And he called his maid . . . and said: 'Carry this gentleman's packet into the chamber and lay it up safely, and bring quickly from the cupboard oil to anoint him and towel to rub him, and other things necessary; and then bring my guest to the nearest baths, for I know he is very weary of so long and difficult travel.'"[45]

The changing face of the baths and gymnasium also demanded changes in the massage services offered. In the first Greek baths and gymnasium massage was not so much a primary service offered, and it was done, not by adept slave girls, but by captured slaves.[46] Slaves were the predominant providers of massage, and even they likely administered its prescription upon orders from the gymnasium physician.[47] Later, as the Greeks built more and larger facilities and the hot bath became more popular, a profession of bath attendants developed that brought the standards of the services offered, including massage, to a higher level.[48]

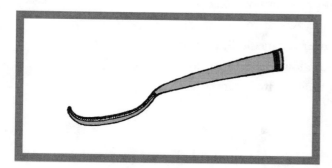

The athletes' strigil, a device used by Roman athletes or their aliptae ("rubbers") (circa 175 B.C.E.) to scrape the skin of dust, oil, and sweat after physical exercise. Modern rendering, from written accounts. Courtesy of World of Massage Museum

MASSAGE IN THE
ANCIENT WORLD:
GREECE AND ROME

It is clear from the literature that the slave girls of Roman times were highly regarded. However, it is very difficult to determine the quality of massage and the advancement of its technique in ancient Greece and Rome, precisely because it was the province of slaves, who kept no records, wrote no books, established no educational institutions, and passed no oral traditions along. Massage was a job to do, like stoking the fires at the hot baths or hauling dead animals and humans from the floor of the Coliseum. As the Roman armies conquered all of Italy, annexed Asia Minor, Syria, Britain, Greece, and the Hellenic states, and eventually overtook Egypt, they captured residents of those areas and forced them into slavery. Slaves were abundant in the Roman society. Some estimates are that a middle-class citizen might own about eight slaves. A wealthy man could own from five hundred to one thousand slaves, and an emperor would engage as many as twenty thousand slaves to serve his palatial household. Nearly four hundred thousand slaves are believed to have lived in Rome at one time.

We do not have a clear picture of massage as it was practiced in the bath, the gymnasium, people's homes, on the battlefield, or in the competition of sporting events because we can't hear from the slaves who provided these services. We must rely upon the limited material available from the Roman physician, who was preoccupied with studying anatomy, doing surgery, and treating the wealthy with newfound cures and remedies. Massage was one of the physician's tools, but it was a tool that received little attention compared to the rest of medicine. Still, massage was clearly an integral part of the success and popularity of the Roman baths. Graham writes:

> Among the old Greeks and Romans, massage in some primitive form or other was extensively patronized by people of widely different classes, from the patricians, the wealthy, and the learned downward to poor, decrepit old slaves, and for the most diverse purposes; with some as a means of hastening tedious convalescence, with others as a luxury in conjunction with the baths, and with others still to render their tissues supple and enduring preparatory to undergoing severe tests of strength, so that strains and ruptures would be less likely to occur. It was also used after the exercises and struggles, especially by the gladiators, in order to stroke away the ecchymoses and to relieve the pains of the bruises as well as to reinvigorate them. Those who applied the rubbing and anointing were as different in character and qualification as those who received it. Sometimes it was done by medical practitioners themselves, sometimes by priests, at others by slaves, but probably more often by those called *aliptae* (from alipes, swift of foot, nimble), whose business it was to anoint the wrestlers before and after they exercised, and who took care to keep them sound and in good complexion.[49]

It seems evident from Dr. Graham's comments here, and from many other references to Roman baths, that the aliptae was more than a rubber of bodies. Perhaps she was the precursor to modern-day *swaneirs*, who provide massage and almost valet-type services to elite European bicycle racers. Certainly the aliptae provided towels, oils, powders, essences, and maybe even drinks and food for bath patrons.

In Greek baths one would likely bathe and exercise in the nude, but in Rome they wore tunics or other garments suitable for exercise and bathing. Exercise was not like that of the Greeks, either, but was merely a prelude to the bathing experience. It was considered a form of preventive medicine to do a bit of exercise, like playing ball or running. The physicians' recommendations that diet, exercise, massage, and bathing were good for one's health were widely accepted. A light sweat was recommended by Celsus, among others; the "athlete" was not to be too strenuous in his or her exercise routine. Galen prescribed that all exercise should be followed by massage with oil, and sometimes by hot bathing. The actual bathing proceeded through a series of tubs or pools, always shallow, of increasingly hot water. The final plunge, called the *frigidarium*, was in cold water. Steam chambers were also available during the bathing process, and a stop in one of them produced profuse sweating.

Anointing with oil was an important function, done before or after a bath, or both. Some baths had designated rooms for anointing and massaging, called *aleipterion* or *unctorium*. But the final step in the whole routine was getting your massage with oils, perfumed unguents, or specially prepared cosmetic treatments. The order and time of your bath experience was often that prescribed by your physician and tailored for your particular health needs, depending on your condition, age, and ailment, if any.[50]

Even though a number of other writers have told the following humorous anecdote, it is well worth repeating here, both as a funny story and as an indication of massage's place within Roman culture.

> The wise and able Emperor Hadrian, A.D. 76–138, who will be so well remembered as having built the wall from the Solway Firth to the Tyne, and whose reign was distinguished by peace and beneficent energy, one day saw a veteran soldier rubbing himself against the marble at the public baths, and asked him why he did so. The veteran answered, "I have no slave to rub me," whereupon the emperor gave him two slaves and gold sufficient to maintain them. Another day several old men rubbed themselves against the wall in the emperor's presence, hoping for similar good fortune, when the shrewd Hadrian, perceiving their object, directed them to rub one another![51]

The Hadrianic Baths, located at Leptis Magna and opened in 126 C.E., was one of the largest Roman baths, comprised of an extensive complex of buildings. In the palestra of the facility you might find entertainment or lectures being offered as you lounged after exercise or a hot steam or a soothing oil massage. The thermae of Rome also had food and beverages available, gaiety and lively discourse. They were the venues to make known your presence and place in the Roman empire. But not everyone was pleased with the thermae's grand architecture, decadent slave girls, food and wine, and general excess. Roman emperor Marcus Aurelius, living in the latter part of the second century, is believed to have said, "What is bathing when you think of it—oil, sweat, filth, greasy water, everything revolting." Only a few centuries later Christians reflected upon the decadence of the Roman baths as evidence of the moral collapse of Roman society and upon the possibility that humanity, too, would have fallen if such ways would have continued.

The Christian era marks the beginning of the Middle Ages, a time when medicine, exercise, and all therapeutic measures connected with them fell into disuse, and their associated institutions into disarray.[52] The Olympic games were terminated in 393 C.E., ending an era of importance for massage as well as for exercise. Even hygiene, written about so eloquently by Galen, fell from its position as a centerpiece of Greco-Roman health care. Kamenetz states regarding this time that "medicine and its literature declined, as did medical gymnastics and massage which probably fell rapidly to its former level of folk medicine. There is virtually no mention of massage in the medical literature for centuries after the fall of Rome; it was considered too commonplace to qualify for therapeutic mention."[53] But in the Arab countries, India, China, and in some surprising places in Europe as the Middle Ages unfolded, the spirit of massage stayed very much alive.[54]

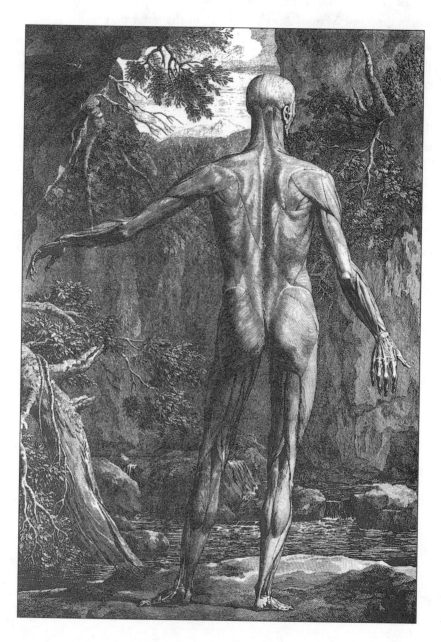

Sixteenth-century anatomical drawing by Andreas Vesalius (1514–1564). A professor at the University of Padua, Italy, Vesalius is known for providing the first significant anatomical studies of the human body in history. His study of human anatomy concerned the total "fabric" of the body; many of his drawings were set in natural surroundings. From *Anatomy Illustrated* by Emily Blair Chewning and Dana Levy (New York, 1979).

5 Keeping the Faith: Massage from the Fall of the Roman Empire to the Nineteenth Century

Massage in the Middle Ages

For several centuries after the fall of the Roman Empire, medical education in most of western Europe took place exclusively within the convents and monasteries of the Church. In many ways, healing practices returned to what they had been before the Greco-Roman period.[1] For nearly a thousand years medicine was dominated by religious dogma, superstition, and magic. The advent of the Christian era brought dramatic changes that undermined the previous popularity of the Greco-Roman ideals of philosophy, government, the good life, and health. Christianity focused on the salvation of the soul and frowned on anything that glorified the human body. Disciples were taught to renounce material things, the vanity of beauty, and even the preservation of bodily strength. All forms of public exhibition, such as the gymnastic spectacles of the Roman Empire, became increasingly un-Christian.[2] Eventually everything having to do with exercise or the baths was banned.

However strange it may seem in a climate of such negativity toward the body, it was the Church that helped to preserve massage within the Western world during the Middle Ages. It found a new home in the emerging Christian environment, both as a part of Christian ritual and in the care of the sick and dying.

ANOINTING AND THE LAYING ON OF HANDS

Zach Tomas, the founder of the National Association of Bodyworkers in Religious Service, wrote in his book, *Healing Touch, The Church's Forgotten Language*, that the

Many a poor woman was burned at the stake in northern Europe during the Middle Ages because she knew a little more than other persons and cured suffering men by massage, a magic which was looked upon as a power of Satan.

—Hartvig Nissen, *Practical Massage* (1932)

Church continued the ancient tradition of anointing, drawing inspiration from the many Biblical references to anointing with oil, such as Psalm 23.

> 5. Thou preparest a table before me in the presence of mine enemies: Thou anointed my head with oil; my cup runneth over.
> 6. Surely goodness and mercy shall follow me all the days of my life: And I will dwell in the house of the Lord forever.
> —Psalm 23:5–6 (King James version)

Christians developed many rituals associated with their beliefs about the ministerial methods of Jesus Christ, such as the laying on of hands, anointing, communion, baptism, and exorcism. Thomas adds, "Technically, laying on of hands was used to convey power and authority to those who would mediate the Spirit and shalom to the people of God. However, laying on of hands was also used along with rituals of anointing and in ministry to those sick."[3] The anointing of the body with oil and the laying on of hands was a central part of the baptism rituals of the mainstream church, for both men and women, as described by Zach Thomas.

> The word Christ comes from the Greek *chriein*, "to anoint." The act of anointing (chrismation) with oil (chrism) served two main purposes in biblical times. It was used to consecrate kings, priests, prophets, or temple objects . . . and to aid in caring for the sick and wounded . . . and after death. . . . Gestures of healing touch, such as laying on of hands, anointing with oil, and signing of the cross, are meant to strengthen members of the body of Christ so they might "reclaim all that baptism promises both in life and death."[4]

Douglas Graham, M.D., provides an example of healing by the laying on of hands in the following story.

> Clement the Eighth, one of the greatest popes that the Church has ever had, was a great sufferer from gout in his hands and feet. His friend, Saint Philip Neri, was very fond of him and visited him as often as he could, but was frequently prevented from doing so by sickness or other causes. It was about Easter, 1595, that the Pope had an unusually severe attack and was ordered by his physician to keep his bed. When Philip heard of this he had a great desire to relieve him. He first prayed for the Pope with great fervor and then went to visit him. When he came into the room Clement was in so much pain that he could not bear anyone to touch the bed he lay upon, and begged Philip not to come near to him. But Philip moved gently towards him and Clement again entreated that no one should touch him. With a smile of affectionate sympathy Philip replied: "I am not sorry for the gout, Holy Father, for that compels you to rest; but I am very sorry for the pain you suffer. Your Holiness need not fear; let me do as I please." And without another word he seized the

suffering hand and pressed it with great affection. The pain immediately disappeared, and Clement cried out: "Go on touching me, Father, it gives me the greatest relief." The Pope was thus healed, so it is said, and spoke of it as a miracle to the cardinals for examining bishops, and often adduced it as proof of Philip's sanctity.[5]

If a friend of the pope, Saint Philip Neri, knew how to administer healing massage in the sixteenth century, it is easy to imagine that within the Church the tradition had been kept alive since the fall of the Roman empire. And if the pope himself received massage, however reluctantly from his friend, it seems plausible that others were receiving massage as well. The unbroken stream of tradition is evident in this story and continues into other Church activities.

Touch was used not only for healing in the laying-on-of-hands practices, but extensively in the rituals of baptism and ceremonial rites of passage. New rituals were established for installation of bishops, kings, and popes, all conferring upon the recipient divine rights and the sanctity of spiritual leadership.

WOMEN OF THE CHURCH

In the palatial Roman baths female slave adepts administered massage during the last several centuries of the empire. In the medical and athletic arenas massage had predominantly been a male domain in the ancient world. In the Middle Ages it was the women of the Church who helped to keep the power of touch alive at the most basic level of human need. Many new healing establishments were established by women. Led by the sisters of various religious orders, the facilities were staffed by royal and wealthy volunteers, as well as by women who sought to become part of the order. Deserted ancient temples, no longer used for rituals, sacrifices, and social activities, were converted to hospices and hospitals. The Greek temples of healing had excluded the terminally ill and those with severe diseases or disorders. The women of the Church welcomed them—despite some opposition from their male counterparts—in their new healing centers. With the financial support of wealthy patricians, dedicated labor, and many prayers, the women managed to allay the suffering of many.[6]

The therapeutic methods used in these facilities ranged widely, but massage, baths, and other natural methods were the most predominant, because they were the cheapest and the easiest to provide.[7] This was a time of strict Church doctrine—the ways of the past were held in suspicion, and the women who managed these facilities had to operate within the knowing approval of Church authorities. But little attention was given to them because this was the work no one really wanted, except those dedicated women who acted selflessly in caring for those who needed it the most.[8]

SPAS AND THE CHURCH

The marriage of baths and religion predate the Christian era by hundreds of years. Deities of Greek and Roman antiquity presided over the public baths throughout the

Mediterranean region, as well as in England and Germany, but their placement within the bath did not serve as a religious reference in a Christian sense. History professor Fikret Yegul writes that "poetic and formulaic expressions connecting baths with the deities presiding over fire and water, the nymphs, the Graces, and Eros represent a fairly common theme among bath inscriptions and epigrams during late antiquity; although they reflect the public's appreciation of their baths, they should not be taken to imply a serious sense of religosity."[9]

In an unpublished manuscript by Jadi Campbell, a contemporary writer about massage around the world, she tells us that the fall of the Roman empire brought with it the deterioration of its great bathhouses. Many were destroyed by the invading barbarians from the north, but most fell into ruin through disuse and the natural elements of time, rain, and wind. Even so, for quite a long while they continued to be used by travelers and by the residents nearby.

Numerous attempts were made to restore the baths from simply being places to bathe and refresh for a few hours before getting back on the road to one's destination into their former places of learning, culture, and healing. King Charlemagne (742–814), crowned Emperor of the West in 800 C.E. by the pope, led the revival of many declining baths in his realm that is now France, Germany, and northern Italy.

Other baths were run and maintained by religious sects, such as the Benedictine monks who founded the spa at Bad Ragaz in northeastern Switzerland in 740 C.E. The French order of Capuchin built convents at nearly all the spas in France. At this time, nuns, priests, and physicians could receive special permission to visit one of these spas for healing treatments. In this way the old spas were used for both housing of the religious orders and healing facilities for the sick and dying.

ARAB HEALERS AND HORSES

While Europe in the Middle Ages turned away from classical learning and science, massage traditions in other parts of the world continued unhindered. The thread of the Greco-Roman medical and massage traditions was kept alive by the Arabs for several centuries. One of the most significant of the Arab scholars was Avicenna (980–1037), a devout follower of Aristotle who wrote a hundred volumes on topics ranging from medicine to philosophy. As the chief physician at the Baghdad hospital, Avicenna was second only to Galen in his influence within the medical field. Avicenna's *Canon Medicinae* was an encyclopedic attempt to collect all known medical knowledge. Interested in physical treatment, Avicenna wrote on massage, exercise, and hydrotherapy. The influence of the Greek medical tradition is evident in his writing, such as the following passage, which echoes Hippocrates:

> One kind of friction is hard, which enlarges or thickens: another is gentle, which loosens. One is prolonged, which causes thinness; another is moderate, which fattens. When these are combined, corresponding results will be produced. . . . There is also a friction which is rough, as with

rough clothes, which quickly draws the blood to the outward parts, and one which is smooth, as with the palm or with soft cloths, which collects the blood and keeps it in the part. Now, the objects of friction are:—the thickening of thin bodies, the softening of hard ones. Besides there is a friction of preparation, which comes before exercise, and is begun gently; this, when the desire to rise is felt, braces and hardens. Then there is a friction of restoration, which comes after exercise and is called rest-inducing friction. The object of this is the resolution of superfluities retained in the muscles, not evacuated by exercise, that they may be evaporated, and that fatigue may not occur. This friction must be done smoothly and gently.[10]

Avicenna also wrote: "As a sequel to athletic, restorative friction produces repose. Its object is to disperse effete matters formed in the muscles and not expelled by exercise. It causes them to disperse and so remove fatigue, the feeling of lassitude. Such friction is soft and gentle and is best done with oil. It must not be hard or heavy or rough, because that would roughen the members."[11]

The Arabs also continued the Greek equestrian practice of grooming their horses by applying friction with the hands. They were very much devoted to their horses. They fought wars on horseback, played games with their horses, and exercised with them. The care and affection given a horse by the Arab man was not second to that given to his wife, but usually came first. Like their Indian counterparts, Arab men affectionately rubbed their horses with bare hands. The earliest mention in an English text of this practice is from Walter Johnson. He writes, "In ancient, as in modern times, friction was considered very conducive to the health of animals. The horse, as everyone knows, is much improved in condition by regular friction. In England this is accomplished by the curry-comb, or a wisp of straw, but in India, as in ancient Greece, the groom rubs his horse with his own naked hand. My Indian friends assure me that their horses have, in consequence, a far finer coat than English horses."[12] Several historians and the ancient Greek geographer Strabo (23–79 C.E.) provide additional evidence for Johnson's claims. Strabo writes that the Indian and Arabian horses have much finer coats than their English counterparts due mainly to their being rubbed by hand.[13]

The Renaissance Period

With the Renaissance came exploration and innovation in all fields of endeavor, including medicine. The medical thinkers of the time looked back to the ancients and at the same time moved forward in a new understanding of the anatomical and physiological grounds of medical science.

By the sixteenth century there was a body of written work on "mechanical treatment" from a variety of European countries, including France, Germany, England, and Italy. In 1569 Italian physician Hieronymus Mercurialis (1530–1606) published a treatise entitled *De Arte Gymnastica.* The book deals extensively with exercise and movements, but also includes sections on manual therapies based on Galen's views. French physician Ambrose Pare (1510–1590), renowned as the Father of Surgery, was a strong advocate of mechanical treatments that included massage and exercise. He is credited with utilizing frequent friction treatments on patients who could not have physical therapy applied to them after surgery.[14] Many books published between the sixteenth and eighteenth centuries dealing with movement and exercise began their titles with the words *de motu,* which translates as "on the motion of." Dr. Douglas Graham tells us that "Fabricius ab Aquapendente . . . was the author of a treatise, 'De Motu Locali Secundum Totum,' in which he again brought massage to honor. He most warmly recommended this treatment by rubbing, kneading, and scientific movements as a rational measure in joint affections."[15]

In 1780 Swiss-born Simon Andre Tissot published a work on gymnastics that encouraged physicians to utilize manual therapies in conjunction with exercise and movements. Friction was the primary method Tissot prescribed; he defined it as "the action of rubbing some parts of the body with the hands, a sponge, flannel, new linen, a brush or horsehair." Tissot describes friction as "alternate pressures and relaxations of the external parts which should cause a movement of the solids and liquids of the body and thus increase circulation. . . . Of the many cures suggested for this condition [sprains] there is one to which there has been too little recourse. It is a kind of kneading (petrissage) of the involved parts. In what we may call pounding (en broyant), however, with a certain precaution; in grinding (en triturant) the viscous juices which are arrested in the ligaments of the joints, we give to the circulation an activity which it was about to lose. Thus we may say that we prevent all these ligaments from becoming an obstructed lump in which motion would become lost entirely. Do we not all know how rather large ganglions are removed by kneading them several times daily?"[16]

We'll look here at a few whose work was particularly influential during this time.

PARACELSUS

Born in Einsiedelin, Switzerland, Paracelsus (1493–1541) was a medical doctor, alchemist, and philosopher, sometimes called the Father of Chemistry but most often called eccentric. An outspoken and sometimes abusive orator, Paracelsus was not shy about speaking out against the dogma of his day. He denounced quacks and the medical establishment in general, saying, "Quacks found their way into medicine, seeking money rather than following the law of love."[17] Because of his outspokenness and his proclivity toward

An early fourteenth-century diagram of the human muscle system. From Ashmolean Codex, in *Anatomy Illustrated* by Emily Blair Chewning and Dana Levy (New York, 1979).

MASSAGE FROM THE FALL OF THE ROMAN EMPIRE TO THE NINETEENTH CENTURY sensational stunts to prove his beliefs, Paracelsus traveled quite a bit to avoid the criticism he received from his peers and the authorities. He defended his travels by saying, "It is impossible that it [all the learning to be gotten from the world] will come to us."[18] He was a staunch believer in the medicinal value of hot and cold natural springs (balneology) and the value of bathing. In 1535 he visited the spa at Bad Ragaz in Switzerland and wrote a study of its hydrology. He believed in the value of massage because of its effect on the circulation of the blood and its curative qualities in giving care to the sick and needy. Several centuries ahead of the discovery of germs, Paracelsus is credited with recognizing the value of keeping wounds clean so as to avoid infection. He believed in treating the mentally ill and wrote this about holding emotions in the body: "A man who is angry is not only angry in his head or in his fist, but all over . . . all the organs of the body, and the body itself, are only form-manifestations of previously and universally existing mental states."[19]

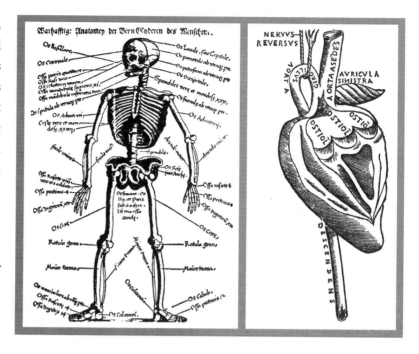

Medieval German diagrams of the human heart and skeleton made from woodcuts. From *Anatomy Illustrated* by Emily Blair Chewning and Dana Levy (New York, 1979).

VESALIUS AND EARLY ANATOMICAL STUDY

Although today the study of anatomy is considered essential to the practice of both medicine and massage, until the time of the Renaissance the study of anatomy had never advanced very far because of the taboos of religious and cult beliefs. Even the Egyptians, known for their embalming procedures, gained little anatomical knowledge because they were not studying the human body; they were merely preparing it for the afterlife. Their work was limited primarily to removing organs from the abdominal and brain cavities. The famous Greek physicians, not being allowed except on very rare occasions to dissect prisoners, learned most of their anatomy from animal dissection and the observation of human anatomy in bodies opened by war wounds.

By the end of the 1400s the study of anatomy began to rise out of the ashes of the preceding Dark Ages. Most universities in Europe once again recognized the study of anatomy as part of their curricula. Yet, despite increasing acceptance of human dissection in the universities as a method of studying anatomy, it would be three-quarters of a century before any real advances beyond previous knowledge of anatomy were made.

When we think of the Renaissance and the study of anatomy, the first figures that come to mind are the famous illustrations of the human body by Leonardo da Vinci (1452–1519). Human dissection was not yet openly allowed during Leonardo's time;

MASSAGE FROM THE FALL

OF THE ROMAN EMPIRE TO

THE NINETEENTH

CENTURY

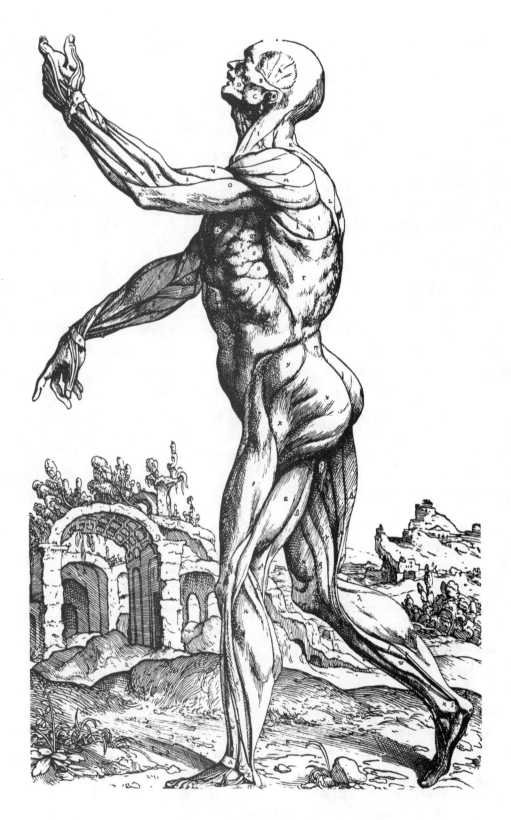

The human musculature by anatomist Andreas Vesalius, drawn
in 1543. From *Anatomy Illustrated* by Emily Blair Chewning and
Dana Levy (New York, 1979).

Leonardo did most of his work secretly and wrote his notes in mirror script. Leonardo's drawings and anatomical notes were lost after his death and not discovered for nearly two hundred years. They were the most detailed and complete to his time.

It was Andreas Vesalius (1514–1564) who provided the first significant study of human anatomy. Born in Brussels, Vesalius began his study at a young age by dissecting animals. A natural and gifted artist, his drawings are masterpieces of artistic achievement, precisely detailing human anatomy and form. Vesalius also wasn't completely free to do his work; he earned the scornful attention of religious leaders by cutting down the bodies of hanged criminals. After moving to Padua from his hometown of Brussels, he performed public dissections where large crowds observed his work and listened to his lectures.

It is worthwhile noting that Vesalius was among the first of his time to break with the tradition of "secondhand" operations and dissection. Since the early days of the Christian era, physicians had begun to disdain doing their own preparatory work in surgical procedures; they would instead have advanced students or physicians of lesser status prepare the patient. This led eventually to the study of anatomy, and some surgery, with the doctor in charge merely directing the procedure as the student or assistant did the actual work, the academy of physicians and other students sitting back watching from a distance. Vesalius disliked watching from the stands and so went down onto the operating floor and got his hands into the job.

One of Vesalius's books on anatomy described in detail the muscular system, including its actions and attachments. It would be about three hundred years before the study of anatomy would become a part of the training of massage practitioners, beginning with the training of nurses and doctors receiving instruction in massage.

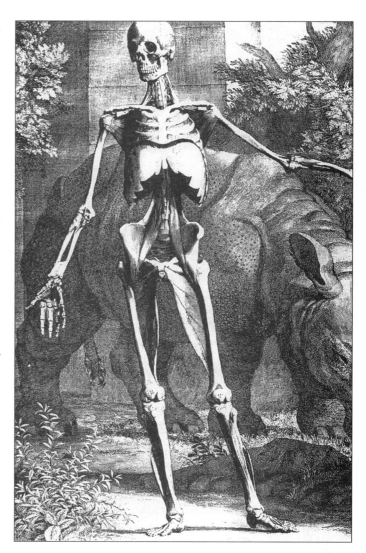

The human skeleton, a drawing by anatomist Bernhard Siegfried Albinus, 1747. From *Anatomy Illustrated* by Emily Blair Chewning and Dana Levy (New York, 1979).

Massage in the East

Unaffected by the advent of the Christian era in western Europe, massage continued to be practiced in China, India, and the rest of the East much as it had always been.

In Japan two ancient traditions were combined—Chinese anmo therapy and

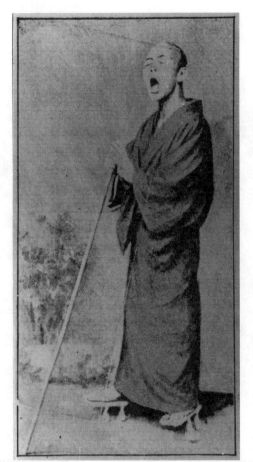

"The Blind Japanese Masseur Soliciting Patronage," from Dr. Kellogg's 1895 book, *The Art of Massage.* Typically the blind practitioner would walk through a local neighborhood at dusk calling out, "Amma, amma." The neighborhood masseur was for centuries in Japan the exclusive domain of the blind, their occupation sanctioned by the government as a way to provide the blind with a means of income.

Korean amma massage—resulting in Japanese amma massage, a tradition with ancient roots that persisted into the nineteenth century.

A friend of Dr. Kellogg's provided a description of a massage received in Japan "for the relief of a severe cold accompanied with fever." The description can be regarded as a valid description of massage in Japan for several hundred years before the good doctor's friend experienced this session in the late nineteenth century.

The shampooer sat in Japanese fashion at the side of the patient, as the latter lay on a futon (thick comforter or quilt) on the floor, and began operations on the arm; then took the back and the back of the neck, afterward the head (top and forehead), and ended with the legs. On the arms, back, back of the neck, and legs, he used sometimes the tips of his fingers, sometimes the palms or the backs of his hands, sometimes his knuckles, sometimes his fists. The movements consisted of pinching, slapping, stroking, rubbing, knuckling, kneading, thumping, drawing in the hand, and snapping the knuckles. The rubbing in the vicinity of the ribs was slightly ticklish, and the knuckling on the back of the neck, and at the side of the collar bone, a little painful. On the head he used gentle tapping, a little pounding with his knuckles, stroking with both hands, holding the head tight for a moment, grasping it with one hand and stroking with the other. The operator seemed to have a good practical knowledge of physiology and anatomy, and certainly succeeded in driving away the headache and languor, in producing a pleasant tingling throughout the body, and in restoring the normal circulation of the blood. He is to be criticised, however, for one serious fault in his operations—that of shampooing down, instead of up. A portion of the good done is thus neutralized, one object of scientific massage being to help back toward the center the blood which is lingering in the superficial veins.[20]

Dr. Kellogg relates his disagreement with the criticism because he says, "The limbs should be rubbed down, rather than up, for the relief of the condition of feverishness and irritation from which his patient was suffering."[21] Dr. Kellogg's disagreement is not an idle one; it demonstrates his knowledge of both the ancient and indigenous techniques of the shamans' way of rubbing down and out, as well as a method for releasing energy from the extremities by rubbing down and out. His use of the word *irritation* indicates his knowledge of moving pent-up energy from the body via this method. Today a brushing technique would be used to remove the "irritation" of energy buildup in the extremities.

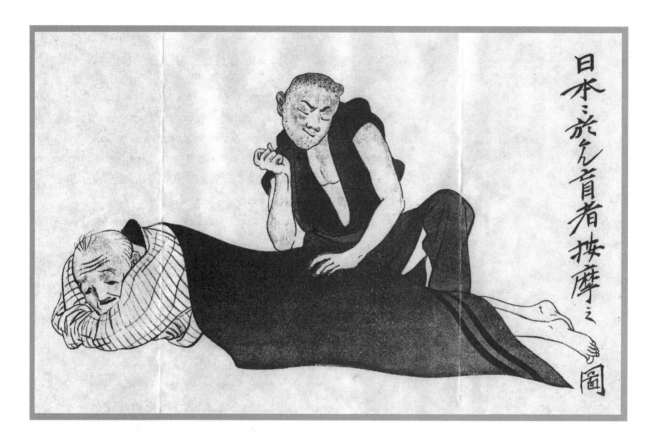

日本ニ於ケ
ル盲者按摩ノ
圖

The Continuing Legacy of Massage in Midwifery

The use of massage as part of the practice of midwifery—primarily to alleviate pain prior to the actual birth—persisted from ancient times through the eighteenth century and beyond. In the Middle Ages midwifery continued to be the province of the wise woman of the village or town, although women were occasionally afforded the opportunity to be educated and to practice their medical skills as midwives. Trotula of Salerno (1058–1097), an Italian noblewoman, learned her trade from the writings of Galen, Soranus, and Hippocrates. She wrote about the cravings of pregnant women and gave advice in matters of pregnancy, including the use of massage: "If she craves strange foods, like potter's earth, coal or chalk, let her be given beans cooked with sugar. As the time of birth nears, let her bathe often and her abdomen be massaged with oil of violets. Give her light, easily digestible food, like oranges and pomegranates. If her ankles swell, massage them with oil of roses and vinegar. If she suffers from wind, give her mint, mastic, cardamom and carrot root."[22]

Some physicians of the time also mentioned massage in their treatises on midwifery. Kamenetz reports that "Aetius of Amida [Turkey], who lived in the 6th century . . . [i]n his last book, devoted to gynecology and obstetrics, provides instructions for the pregnant woman with swelling of the feet, to 'massage or rub with rose water and vinegar and a modicum of salt.' In 'strangulation of the uterus' he advised the midwife to 'rub the part gently and for a long time, so that the thick and irritated

"Practice of Massage by the Blind in Japan." This drawing is located in the Dittrick Museum of Medical History in Cleveland; the Japanese inscription to the right of the drawing reads: "In Japan, a picture of a blind man giving a massage." Pictorial #79 from the *German Medical Weekly,* 1913, no. 1 (Leipzig).

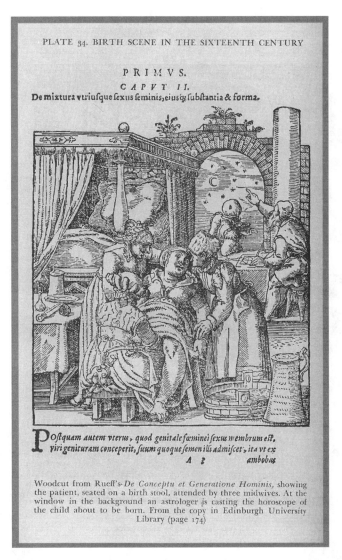

Woodcut from Rueff's *De Conceptu et Generatione Hominis*, showing the patient, seated on a birth stool, attended by three midwives. At the window in the background an astrologer is casting the horoscope of the child about to be born. From the copy in Edinburgh University Library (page 174)

Woodcut from Rueff's *De Conceptu et Generatione Hominis*. The two midwives at the birth mother's side were aides to the midwife; they would have provided massage to the mother-to-be if needed. At the window an astrologer is casting the horoscope of the child about to be born. From *A History of Medicine* by Douglas Guthrie (Philadelphia, 1946).

humor which clings to the uterus may come out.' He also ordered massage for 'those who do not conceive on account of humidity of the uterus.'"[23]

Although most births were attended not by physicians but by poor women who provided their midwifery services to neighbors and relatives, continuing a tradition as old as humankind, severe conflicts arose between midwives and physicians in the beginnings of the medical establishment. Midwives were also in conflict with the Church, which had declared midwives to be witches. Midwifery began to be a dangerous calling. Reportedly nearly sixty thousand people accused as "witches" were executed between the mid-1400s and the mid-1600s in Europe. Estimates are that approximately 80 percent of these were women, and more than half of those were midwives.[24] This period of immense fear drove midwives underground, inhibiting the development of the profession. The scant training that was available to raise a midwife from above suspicion of being a "witch" was mostly available in Paris, where during the 1500s licensing and regulation of midwives existed. However, most of these trained and licensed midwives worked primarily for the emerging middle class. The noble and wealthy received care from upper-class physicians, such as Louise Bourgeois (1563–1636), who was a midwife to the queen of France. She was, according to women's historian Elisabeth Brooke, "assistant to Amroise Pare, head surgeon at the Hotel de Dieu." In 1609 Bourgeois wrote a book entitled *Several Observations on Sterility, Miscarriage, Fertility, Childbirth, and the Illness of Women and Newborn Infants*. She was considered the foremost authority on midwifery in all of Europe during her time.[25]

The first book written on midwifery was a German text dated 1513 by the physician Rhodion. In 1554 Jacob Rueff published an improved edition of the book; it is from this text that the illustration on this page is taken. The two midwives at the side of the woman giving birth were aides to the midwife who actually delivered the child. They would have provided massage to the mother-to-be if needed.

In the 1700s women began to be allowed to attend training in midwifery in a number of countries in Europe. Russia established schools for midwifery as early as 1754, with lecture classes but no practical instruction. It is unknown whether or not massage was a part of this early midwifery training, but it certainly continued as part of the practice.

In the North American colonies midwifery played a central role in medical practice. For the first 250 years the colonists had very few trained physicians; as most colonists were themselves poor and uneducated, midwives held a respected position in their communities. Many of these midwives delivered thousands of babies during their careers, attesting to the small number available. In the early years they usually practiced without formal training and in isolation, often traveling hundreds of miles on horseback to deliver babies. Slavery brought the black midwife, serving black and white families alike.

The folk medicine passed along through the midwifery traditions included abdominal massage, massage of the legs and back, and of course the medical uses of massage for turning a breech baby in utero or vaginal massage for certain difficult deliveries.[26] Then in 1703 a law was passed in England requiring midwives to be literate, married or widowed, obtain training from a physician, and request a physician for problem births.[27] However, most physicians were not adequately trained, having learned what they knew about childbirth from theoretical lectures, barber-surgeons, or other secondhand sources. There were no medical schools in the early colonial days; like their midwife counterparts, most doctors were trained as apprentices or were self-trained. Doctors were not afforded much recognition or trust, and most medical practice was in competition with self-administered care or that given by midwives. The first medical schools weren't opened until end of the eighteenth century, and only males were allowed to attend.

The first midwifery chair established at an English university was occupied by a man, Joseph Gibson, in 1726. Gibson was, according to medical historian Douglas Guthrie, "the first professor of Midwifery to hold office in any university."[28] This marked the beginning of a new era—that of the male midwife.

Prior to the late eighteenth century most physicians were loathe to do births, attending only the difficult and complicated ones. The introduction of forceps in medical practice in the eighteenth century provided physicians with a new role in the delivery process. The use of the forceps to pull the newborn from the mother's womb extended the role doctors played in birthing and serves as a historical marker of the progressive dominance of medicine over childbirth. By the beginning of the 1800s obstetrics had emerged within the medical schools as a medical specialty. In 1816 Germany's midwifery law defined birth as an illness.

To put it mildly, massage as a part of the practice of midwifery suffered in this environment. A midwifery textbook was available as early as 1746, but if it is anything like the text of 1823 that I have, it contains nothing about massage. There is no mention of massage in the midwifery histories I've read to indicate how its role might have changed as midwifery began to be controlled more by government and the medical community. Although midwifery was one of the human activities that preserved the legacy of the healing power of massage through many centuries both before and after the fall of the Roman empire, it eventually fell away due primarily to the fact that

75

MASSAGE FROM THE FALL
OF THE ROMAN EMPIRE TO
THE NINETEENTH
CENTURY

physicians overtook the practice. However, another area of human activity in which massage was integrally involved persisted—that of exercise and movement therapy.

The Early Development of Exercise and Movement Therapy

Since the days when primitive man and woman gained their exercise from the chase of the hunt and the dance of its celebration, exercise has been both incidental and formal. Peoples of the earliest civilizations in Mesopotamia, Egypt, China, India, Greece, and Rome, as well as the Aztecs, Incas, and Polynesians, all gained the benefit of exercise by playing physical games.

Because the ancients were keen observers and noted well the successes and failures of trial and error related to health and disease, they came to value the curative powers of exercise. In fact, some of the first and most prevalent of remedies throughout history were based on the value of exercise, or movement. The early Greeks believed that riding a horse or swinging by a rope were treatments for a wide range of diseases. And hardly needing mention were the exercises performed for health at the Greek and Roman gymnasiums.

The ancient Chinese are thought to be the first known civilization to have developed a formal preventive, or medical, exercise program designed to prevent diseases caused by inactivity. Their system, known as kung fu, was primarily composed of stretching and breathing activities. The Chinese found that gymnastic dance alleviated the effects of diseases caused by humidity and stagnant water. Some movements or exercise systems were first ritualized as religious ceremony—martial arts were initially ritual practices that were later developed into self-defense systems.

In ancient India yoga developed as a spiritual practice that included meditation, breathing exercises, physical movement, and austerities. In the contemporary West yoga has lost much of its spiritual focus, becoming primarily a form of physical stretching and exercise. Breathing exercises—probably first developed in India but also used by the Greeks—continue to play a significant role in the many systems of yoga as a means of exercising the internal organs.

In ancient Greece great emphasis was placed on gymnastics. *Gymnos* translates as "nude." In the ancient gymnasiums exercise was performed in the nude; thus the word *gymnastics* literally means "exercises done in the nude." The Greeks took the basic concepts of kung fu to new heights by standardizing exercises and extending their range of activities to include boxing, running, wrestling, and jumping. Development of the body was thought to be significantly related to that of the mind and spirit.[29] A healthy, robust body reflected an inner spirit of youth and vigor. Additionally, the performing arts and academic study were important qualities for the Greek citizen. An *ascete* was someone who exercised both body and mind, while one who exercised merely to win prizes was called an *athlete*. Some exercise was strictly for the hearty, like wrestling or the gladiator's circus, games of the small ball (handball), and running both long distances and fast-running (sprinting). But playing ball (kick and throw), dancing, and pushing a wheel with a stick could be played by nearly anyone and were usually considered games for women or young girls. Unlike the Romans, who followed their example, the Greeks exercised with physical objects, such as slings, balls, bows and arrows, javelins, and spears, whereas the Romans utilized wooden horses, swings, and combative fighting in their training exercises.

All the ancients knew the value of exercise to vitalize their patients and themselves; as a preventive remedy against obesity, fatigue, blood and joint diseases, and complications arising from dislocations; and a wide range of other applications. Dr. Kleen calls Asclepiades the Father of Mechano-therapy because he invented several devices designed to produce fluid movement through swinging, vibration, or violent motion and recommended walking and running for dropsy (morbid accumulation of fluids, or edema).[30] These were the first expressions of a philosophy recommending the use of exercise as a remedy. The great ancient physicians and philosophers also proclaimed the benefits of exercise as a cure. Aristotle claimed: "The cause of disease is the excess of excretions which result from the excess of nourishment, or from the want of exercise." Galen wrote, "All the powers of the soul are increased and renewed by exercise. It is necessary to place health under the auspices of labor." Pliny writes, "The mind is stimulated by movements of the body." Hippocrates said, "He who eats without taking exercise can not be well. . . . Perfect health results from a just and constant equilibrium between alimentation and exercise."[31]

Exercise (from the Greek *ascesis*) was defined by the ancients as therapeutic motion of the body or parts of the body designed to alleviate symptoms or promote physical function. Massage could certainly be included within this definition. In fact, massage was a part of the systems developed for therapeutic exercise, a practice carried over well into the past century. George Taylor tells us that "friction may also be classed among exercises. . . . Pressures and pinchings also belong to the same class. Many other movements are included in the kneadings that the ancients employed so frequently."[32] Vibration therapy, used by the Greeks and Romans, can also be included in this list. The first vibration technique was jostling delivered from riding a horse or from riding in a cart with an uneven wheel over a rough stone road.

During the Dark Ages and the Middle Ages—beginning with the fall of Rome and the rise of the Christian era and ending about a thousand years later with the Renaissance—exercise in most of Europe was highly disdained.[33] During that time, however, the Arab physicians and encyclopedists kept the concept alive in their writings and in their translations of the Greek and Roman texts. Hygiene and moderate exercise, such as walking, were promoted by Avicenna, who wrote, "If men exercised their bodies by motion and work at appropriate times, they would need neither physicians nor remedies." Meanwhile, the Chinese continued developing their martial arts from ancient dance and ceremony, and the Indian culture advanced various forms of yoga as complete spiritual, mental, and physical endeavors. Most of these pursuits, though, were for the educated high-class citizens in these societies. They were not yet widely available to the general public.

Physical education declined in Europe during the Middle Ages but continued in such forms as rope climbing, ship mast climbing, walking beams and planks, and even using other people to climb upon. Vaulting was a popular form of prefatory exercise for fencing and knighthood.

In the Renaissance period the harmonious training of mind, soul, and body was once again valued. Educational gymnastic exercise began its revival in the fifteenth century largely due to the influence of the writings of Pietro Vergerio (1349–1428) on a number of physicians, some of whom started schools of instruction in educational gymnastics. The *Art of Gymnastics,* published by the Italian Hieronymus Mercurialis in the sixteenth century (translated into English in 1864), is considered by Kamanetz to be "the first important book in modern times on therapeutic exercise."[34] In 1708 Friedrich Hoffman published his *Dissertationes Physico-Medicae,* including a chapter entitled, "On Movement Considered as the Best Medicine for the Body." Hoffman wrote, "We can not perfect the art of healing till we learn to apply mechanics and hydraulics to medicine."[35] Hoffman's work was a purely scientific approach to exercise and established a model for the development of medical gymnastics.

The eighteenth century was marked in Europe by natural disasters, such as devastating earthquakes in Portugal in 1755, and by revolution—a Cossack uprising in Russia and the French Revolution in 1789. In Asia the seventh Dalai Lama was enthroned in Tibet. China extended its borders to its farthest reaches, annexing Tibet in 1750. India was invaded by Afghanistan in 1755, and Delhi was plundered; then in 1763 the British became the dominant power in India. Persia was united at the end of the century under Aga Mohammed of the Kajar dynasty. The eighteenth century was also the Age of Reason, an age of inquiry. An agrarian revolution in Europe and Great Britain, spanning three centuries and made possible by dramatic population increases, profit farming, new forms of land ownership and new crops imported from the Americas, altered the economic and political landscapes forever and eventually led to the Industrial Revolution of the nineteenth and twentieth centuries. Steam power had been developed, and there was a growing knowledge base in medicine and the sciences.

According to Sidney Licht, it was Swiss-born philosopher and writer Jean Jacques Rousseau (1712–1778) who "sparked the revolution in education."[36] Rousseau wrote, "It is a sad error to think that exercise of the body is bad for the operation of the mind, as if these two could not proceed simultaneously. . . . Exercise the body continually, render it robust and healthy to render it wise and reasonable."[37] Rousseau's writings were widely read and valued, inspiring the establishment of schools called *philantropinons.* One of the first was built in Dessau, Germany, in 1774. Licht tells us it was "a model training school, where for the first time in the Christian Era physical and mental education were fully integrated."[38] Johann Basedow (1723–1790), the school's creator, experimented with many devices, and received wide acclaim for his work in physical education.

The institutions and activities that had helped preserve massage in the West after the fall of the Roman empire—midwifery, healing and ritual in the Church, and physical education—gradually gave way to advances in medicine. Massage within midwifery declined as the practice of birthing moved into the domain of medicine. The healing rituals of the Church contained in the laying on of hands were replaced by more symbolic and relic rituals. Physical education minimized the use of massage, as the movement cure sought to address disease through exercise. Yet, even though in each of these areas massage gradually fell from disfavor, that trend only helped to bring it into its own in the twentieth century.

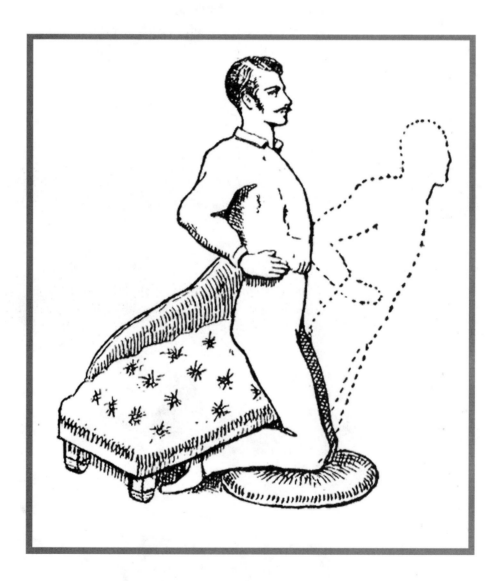

A medical gymnastic exercise for developing the muscles
of the trunk. From John Harvey Kellogg, M.D.,
The Home Hand-book of Domestic Hygiene and Rational
Medicine (London, 1899).

6 Nineteenth-century Massage in Gymnastics and Movement Therapy

Exercise and the Movement Cure

The revival of the ancient Greco-Roman philosophy of physical exercise for the prevention of disease and the maintenance of health, begun in earlier centuries, flowered in the 1800s. The movement cure boom of the nineteenth century was a trend to retrieve the ancient ideals, as evidenced by the following comment by George H. Taylor, M.D., a leading proponent of the movement cure for the treatment of disease. Taylor gives credit to those who came before him while at the same time chastising the public for its failure to keep active with exercise.

> The principle of cultivating the body along with the mind, so as by preserving the health to render mental culture available, is far from being new. It has been often recognized and put in practice; and laudable and successful examples have existed both in ancient and in modern times. But it has been culpably overlooked or slighted.[1]

Natural remedies, along with a conception of the body as a self-regulating system—some even likened it to a machine—were also gaining popularity among health practitioners, both medical and nonmedical. A number of practitioners believed in the movement cure as a means of preventing disease and maintaining health, not in conjunction with the drugs and surgery of medicine, but in spite of it. This perspective was clearly voiced by Taylor, writing in his book *Health by Exercise: Showing What Exercises to Take*. In the passages that follow we find Taylor lamenting that the movement cure had received little attention compared to drug therapy and chemistry. His

Movement is one of the primordial products of life and the regulator of all vital conditions. Artificial movements are the agents most specially adapted to excite natural, physiological, vital, organo-biological action, by which the human machine performs its functions, is developed, preserved, and repaired.

—French writer N. Dally, *Science of Movements* (1857)

Chart of terms

Exercise: "All voluntary motions of the body whatsoever, without any reference to the object or objects had in view. Thus labor and recreation, practiced by either body or mind, whether general or partial, are exercise."[2]

Movement: "Every exercise of which the direction and duration are determined, is a movement."[3]

Movement cure: A specific system of movements designed to treat disease and disorder.

Gymnastics: "The means of developing the corporeal frame, whereby it is fitted for the business of life, or for any special purpose, by means of certain exercises."[4]

Medical gymnastics: Gymnastics applied in the treatment of medical conditions.

Educational gymnastics: Gymnastics applied as a part of an educational program, to enhance mental and physical acuity in the pursuit of academic achievement.

Military gymnastics: Gymnastics as utilized in the training of military personnel, aimed at improving physical strength, performance, and mental discipline.

strong belief in the value of exercise as a therapeutic modality brings him to prophesy the exercise revolution that began almost one hundred years later.

In glancing at the history of movements, the reader will wonder why an art so easily practiced . . . should not in modern times have come more generally into popular favor. The answer to this inquiry will be found in the fact of the maze of obscurity that has prevailed in the general mind in regard to the true curative value of drugs. But while all possible things have been both asserted and denied in regard to drugs, the value of movements has never been denied or questioned, but only at times neglected, in the general interest with which the popular mind has invested the other questions. In the last few centuries, chemistry has . . . furnished medicine with the means of toying with the credulity, the hopes and fears of the suffering public; and it requires all of the present amount of knowledge, and more time than has elapsed, to enable the scientific, supported by the popular mind, to turn the influence of the full-fledged science into its proper channels, and consummate a revolution that may be delayed, but must eventually be realized.[5]

That all may have to a certain and sufficient extent the control of their own physical systems, will scarcely be denied; for it is on this fact that human actions and human responsibility are based. The acknowledgment of this evidently throws the responsibility for his health, efficiency, and happiness upon his own shoulders, where every man should feel that it belongs. . . . Physical culture, then, should be promoted both as a science and as an art, in all the numerous applications of which it is susceptible, till it assumes a position in the public esteem commensurate with its importance.[6]

NINETEENTH-CENTURY

MASSAGE IN GYMNASTICS

AND MOVEMENT THERAPY

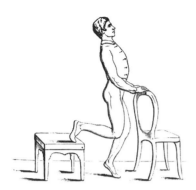

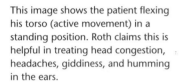

This image shows the patient flexing his torso (active movement) in a standing position. Roth claims this is helpful in treating head congestion, headaches, giddiness, and humming in the ears.

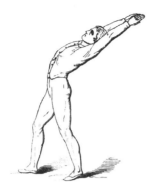

This graphic shows a "commencing position" described by Roth as useful in treating many diseases. He does not mention any specific diseases, but only describes how these voluntary movements prevent, allay, and cure or suppress diseases by "neutralizing the bad effects of external injuries, partly by effecting a more favourable position of diseased parts, partly by removing fluids from the body, especially by inducing the excretion of injurious matters, and by increasing and diminishing absorption and reproduction."

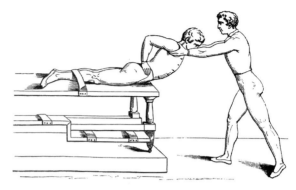

This image shows an active-passive movement performed by the operator with some assistance from the patient and the strap on the table. This movement was a part of a series of trunk, leg, and arm movements said to be helpful in treating congestion of the head and headaches.

Many physicians in the mid 1800s used drug therapy almost to the exclusion of other available remedies. Other physicians, in opposition to this movement, began writing about the inherent value and curative powers of exercise and mechano-therapy during this time. In his book *The Prevention and Cure of Many Chronic Diseases by Movement* (1851), Dr. Matthias Roth instructs readers in curative exercises.

In a later book, *Health by Exercise: The Movement-Cure,* Taylor expands upon this idea. "I have not endeavored to shake my reader's faith in the wise, prudent, conscientious, and learned physician. No one honors him more than the writer. Blessed, say I, is the man or woman who has a good doctor, but more blessed he who can do without him! To enable my reader to do so has been my main aim in the preparation of this manual."[7] Taylor's remarks are representative of a number of physicians of his time who spoke out about natural therapies.

Dr. Taylor, along with several other writers in the movement cure and gymnastic movements, shared the populist sentiment voiced by Dr. Neumann in 1851.

Every medical man who finds pleasure in study, will certainly be well pleased in being able to assist any patients whom he previously was obliged to leave uncured. The wish of professional as well as non-professional men to use less medicine is in part fulfilled by this method [Treatment by Movements], which for this reason deserves to be recommended. It may be made a great blessing to the poor especially, as being curative in many chronic diseases, whilst it would save them the material sacrifices [expenses] they have to incur when they are treated by means of medicines.

The assistance of one or two persons for the purpose of these movements is procured by the poor more easily than money, and almost every one has either a friend or relation who would bestow half an hour daily, in order to relieve him from his sufferings. Even the greatest stranger assists the poor if it costs nothing, and he can contribute to the alleviation or cure of suffering.[8]

Note especially Dr. Neumann's call for help with those less fortunate, a call for charity via the movement cure, because nearly anyone could perform the movements with little instruction. In the same vein, Taylor wrote:

This system regards man as a spiritual being—recognizes all the various influences that operate upon his intellectual and moral life flowing from physical causes, and the power of the mind over the exercise of functional acts of the body, of every kind. . . . The practice of duplicated movements, wherein the mental powers of both the invalid and friend co-operate to the production of certain effects, affords many new facts and interesting illustrations of the control of the mental and nervous states over those functional acts of the body that constitute the health; and such as may lead to higher results than have yet been conceived—in building up, indeed, what may be called a system of *moral* medicine.[9]

With this statement Taylor takes the issue of morality within medical paradigms directly to the physician and the general public.

The Ascent of Ling's Medical Gymnastics

Although some writers have given credit for the renaissance of exercise and movement—presented as medical gymnastics—to Peter Henry Ling (1776–1837), Ling didn't create medical gymnastics. Rather, he coalesced earlier knowledge into a systematized method. A contemporary of Ling's, Johann Muth (1759–1839), is credited with establishing an outdoor gymnasium featuring power lifting and apparatus to develop balance, grace, and sensory acuteness. His classes included dancing, fencing, climbing, walking, and running. Muth published a book in 1804 on the subject and has since been given the title Great Grandfather of Gymnastics.[10]

According to historians in this field, the title Father of Gymnastics belongs to another German, Friedrick Ludwig Jahn (1778–1852), a priest. Father Jahn took very seriously the manifesto of building a better Germany through education.[11] Along with his countrymen, he helped usher in a new era in German academic and physical education. Jahn's system, called Turnen ("movement"), quickly became utilized by citizens and educational leaders.

The Turnen system can be considered the precursor to every other modern gymnastic exercise system, including that of Peter Ling. Jahn's slogan was "Strong in body,

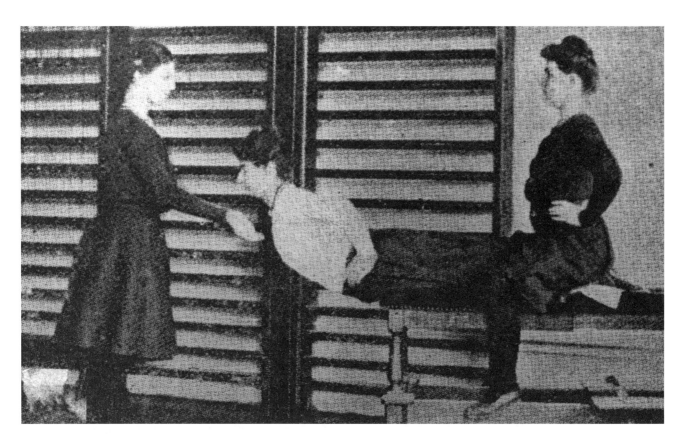

Swedish medical gymnastics'
"arch-leg forward-lying
position," an exercise for
treating scoliosis. From
*Massage and Medical
Gymnastics* by Emil Kleen,
M.D. (London, 1921).

free in spirit, cheerful, intelligent, good." But not all was good for Jahn; he was arrested and accused of plotting against the Prussian government in 1819 and jailed a few years later. Fearing the strength of any organizing initiative, the reactionary government outlawed the Turnen movement in 1819.

Turnen was criminalized until 1842. The system was revitalized later but in different form, eventually becoming the domain of strict formalization, a rigid military regime of exercise.

Ling, a Swede, distinguished the field of medical gymnastics from the educational and military gymnastics prevalent at his time. Even though gymnastics and exercise were popular long before Ling came along, his contribution was in creating an overall system, based on the principles of anatomy and physiology, that applied gymnastics and exercise to the treatment of specific diseases and disorders.

Unlike Jahn, who built his system of exercise from playground experiences, Peter Ling developed his system of gymnastics from a theoretical framework of speculation based on a scientific foundation. Ling did not include an exercise in his system until he knew its exact effects, whereas Jahn developed a therapeutic exercise or apparatus from experimental movements of children, without regard to its scientific effects.[12] Ling, although he held no degrees in science, was an avid student of the sciences. He described his system of the movement cure thus: "The movements are based upon an understanding of the human organism as a self regulating system in which Dynamical,

Chemical and Mechanical agents harmonize to maintain a healthy condition. All aspects of the individual including the moral, intellectual, nutritional, muscular, etc., must therefore be developed in balance in order to avoid weakness and disease."[13] In 1851 Matthias Roth, an English physician, wrote about Ling's system.

> The subject [gymnastics] may be divided into two parts, hygienic and medical, having the closest relationship with each other.
>
> 1. The hygienic, which should form, as in Sweden, an essential feature in our general education, comprehends the healthy development of the body, and, by strengthening the system where constitutionally weak, the prevention of many diseases.
>
> 2. The medical, or that treatment of diseases in which movements are the sole curative agent, or form a very important accessory.[14]

The first part, hygienic, came to be known as educational gymnastics, while the second developed as medical gymnastics. Ling's intention, according to Dr. Roth, "was to make gymnastics not only a branch of education for healthy persons, but to demonstrate it to be a remedy for disease. . . . Ling's gymnastics were introduced many years ago, not only into all the military academies of Sweden, but into all town schools, colleges, and universities, even into the orphan institutions and into all country schools. In the rooms of the Central Establishment at Stockholm, persons of every age, the healthy as well as the sick, executed, or were subjected to, the prescribed movements."[15]

Despite the fact that Ling was not a medical doctor, his Royal Central Gymnastic Institute, established in Sweden in 1813, was an attempt to give exercise and the movement cure system a solid place in medical practice in Europe. Ling laid the foundation and his successors achieved that goal. Perhaps the crowning achievement of Ling's more than two decades of work was attained years after his death, when his work was hailed as a new medical system, and the Swedish Royal Medical Association made public acknowledgment of the high importance of the "treatment by movements." The following is an extract from the medical association's report dated May 22, 1849.

> Many members of the Association, from the knowledge that the medical treatment by movements, according to Ling's system, has proved very effective as a curative means, and has produced extraordinary and most satisfactory results in many chronic diseases, are convinced that this method, developed with the scientific and practical clearness which is required for the adoption of any new medical system, and practised in harmony with other medical sciences, under the special direction of, or in conjunction with, the physician, will take a high standing in medicine.[16]

Ling was praised for his personal qualities as well: "Ling was a man of high moral tone, pious, sincere, honest in all his dealings with his fellow-man. His intellectual

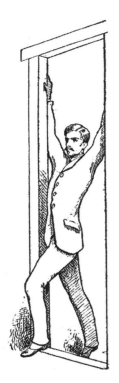

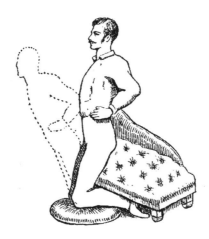

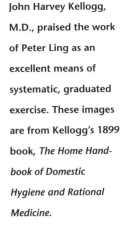

John Harvey Kellogg, M.D., praised the work of Peter Ling as an excellent means of systematic, graduated exercise. These images are from Kellogg's 1899 book, *The Home Hand-book of Domestic Hygiene and Rational Medicine.*

Another "Swedish movement" or medical gymnastic exercise, this one to develop the muscles of the trunk.

One of many "medical gymnastic" movements developed by the Swede Peter Ling. In this movement the chest is thrust forward and suddenly "arrested" to produce "a strong strain upon the muscles of the front of the body . . . a most excellent means for strengthening the chest."

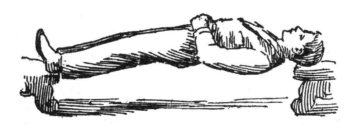

About this movement Dr. Kellogg writes, "This movement calls into vigorous action all the muscles of the neck, trunk, and legs. The position should be maintained for a few seconds, and then the body may be let down to the floor to rest. Care should be used not to strain the muscles too violently."

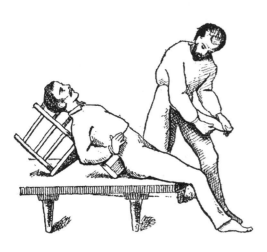

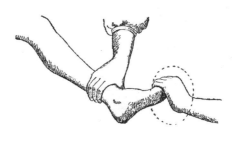

An active-passive movement demonstrated on the foot.

This illustration shows an active-passive Swedish movement exercise, where the subject is lying passive while the operator actively manipulates a body part. The movement is usually a range of motion around a joint.

powers were of a very high order; he loved with the same energy with which he worked, the objects of his home-affections, his friends, the poor, his country, and mankind. His life is another proof to be added to many illustrious examples, that learning, science, and genius shine most when associated with moral worth, generous affections, and piety. The best praise of Ling is that he was a genuine humanist."[17]

The same combination of qualities can be seen in Ling's own comments about anatomy.

> Anatomy, that sacred genesis, which shows us the masterpiece of the Creator, and which teaches us how little and how great man is, ought to form the constant study of the gymnast. But we ought not to consider the organs of the body as the lifeless forms of a mechanical mass, but as the living, active instruments of the soul.[18]

Ling earned the respect of many physicians for his work, although the praise of some was not undiluted. Dr. Taylor wrote in 1879, "The system of Ling, though probably invented by him, is really but the collecting together, on a philosophical plan, of the fragments that had long existed. It comprehended, as it were, by an instinctive grasp, all the truth that had been previously realized at various times and places. What in China, Hindustan, and Greece had been but empiricism, he put upon the ground on which his successors and followers may hope to build a system of philosophical accuracy."[19]

Dr. Kellogg, in 1895, wrote, "As a means of systematic, graduated exercise the author especially commends the excellent system of medical gymnastics developed by Ling, of Sweden. . . . It ought to be in the hands of every masseur."[20]

Douglas Graham, M.D., wrote extensively about Ling in his 1902 history of massage.

> Some regard him as the inventor of this system of treating certain maladies, while others considered that he only made rational that which had been in use for many centuries amongst the Chinese and other Eastern nations. The latter is doubtless the more correct view, for one of his disciples states that Ling thought not, like his predecessors, of merely imitating the gymnastic treatment of the ancients, but he aimed at its reformation and improvement. But the former view served a useful purpose in stirring up the critics and opponents of Ling's method, who adduced testimony to show that the method of Ling is that of the Brahmins of India; is that of the Egyptian priests; is that of Asclepiades, of Pythagoras, and of Herodicus [sic]; is that of which Hippocrates, Celsus, Galen, Rufus of Ephesus, and other physicians, Greek and Roman, have preserved fragments for us; and that all the movements which Ling has indicated are described in an ancient book of the Chinese called the "Cong-Fou of the Tao-Tse.". . . However . . . there seems to be no doubt as to the merits of the system which he rescued from oblivion and by all accounts put upon a scientific basis.[21]

NINETEENTH-CENTURY

MASSAGE IN GYMNASTICS

AND MOVEMENT THERAPY

Dr. Kleen is less favorable in giving credit to Ling. He wrote in 1892, "Ling's activity suffered from certain unfortunate defects. He lacked scientific training, and was ignorant of medicine. He was able, indeed, by reason of his conscientiousness, his enthusiasm, and his strong will, to do good work himself. But he was not able, properly speaking, to advance his science. In the name of truth, I am forced to say that nothing—absolutely nothing—of what Ling left was new. All that he employed and taught, existed long before his time; and, though it is possible, or, indeed, probable that Ling did not know of the documents in Chinese, his own writings testify that he was familiar with the ancient, European works on mechano-therapy. Neither his gymnastics nor his massage can be considered as more than a modification of the same."[22]

Kleen received considerable criticism for his comments about Ling, for Ling (posthumously) enjoyed a devoted following and widespread acclaim even late into the nineteenth century. Dr. Kellogg, for example, doesn't mention Kleen by name, but does admonish those who have attempted "to discredit" Ling even while qualifying his own praise for him.[23] In the 1921 edition of his book, two years before his death, Kleen, while continuing his sharp criticisms of Ling and his followers, seems to have softened his earlier remarks by adding passages that praise Ling for his contributions to gymnastics, and especially to massage. "I have written as I have about him, not to disparage a justly famous name, but because I believe a more sober estimation of his service will, in certain relations, be for the good of his art."[24]

Ling's system has been variously referred to by medical and massage historians. Kleen uses the term "mechano-therapy" in his reference to Ling's work, while others refer to it as "Swedish manual treatment,"[25] "gymnastics or medical gymnastics,"[26] "series of movements,"[27] "passive or communicated movements,"[28] and "therapeutic movements."[29] Dr. Graham uses the term "Swedish movement cure" in his reference to Ling's work.[30]

Ling's system spread from Sweden throughout Europe. The French reaction was very positive, but because of the fallout from the French Revolution in 1830, which stymied medical gymnastics in favor of military gymnastics, his system gained little acceptance. In England several publications based on Ling's system met with success. It was introduced in Russia in 1837, and in 1847 the positive results of an inquiry into its effectiveness were given to the Supreme Medical Board. "Ling's writings were first mentioned in [Germany] in 1830. In 1847 . . . Lieutenant Rothstein . . . induced the Prussian ministry to send [himself] and another gentleman to Sweden to examine personally Ling's system."[31] Rothstein published his very positive findings in 1849, and introduced the Swedish system of gymnastics into the Royal Prussian Institute of Gymnastics. Most histories of massage refer to this— and the introduction of Ling's system into similar institutions in Europe—as landmark events. But another side of this story reveals a tumultuous reaction at the Prussian Institute. A fierce controversy arose between the followers of Ling and those of Jahn. A commission was formed to investigate the controversy, aimed

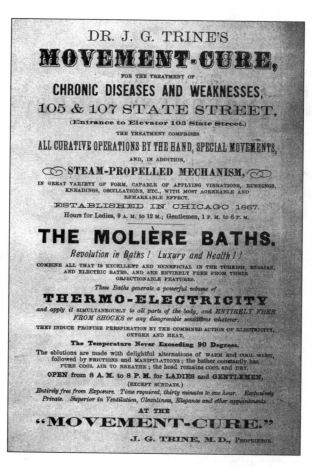

particularly at the use of parallel bars, an apparatus included in the Ling system. Those at the institute loyal to Jahn believed that they were detrimental to physical development, but the commission upheld their usefulness and they were allowed.

The system of Swedish movements and the movement cure also spread to the United States. The former was primarily medical gymnastics, while the latter included some elements of the Swedish movement system along with a strong emphasis on diet, rest, and hydrotherapy. Great interest was shown in these therapies by some members of the established medical community, as well as by the general public. According to Patricia Benjamin, writing in the summer 1986 issue of *Massage Therapy Journal,* Swedish immigrant Baron Nils Posse came to Boston, Massachusetts, in 1885 to establish a practice in medical gymnastics. Posse's was not a novel idea; he had likely read the German text of Johann Muth, published in Sweden in 1813, which had become the text for physical exercise in the schools of his homeland, and the numerous other texts advocating this approach in the school systems. Through his work and the efforts of others, Swedish educational gymnastics was soon adopted in the local public school system in Boston. This prompted Posse to open a training institute, the Posse Gymnasium (later called the Posse Normal School of Gymnastics), to train physical education teachers in the method. Benjamin claims that this school "also offered courses in Swedish massage . . . and so it was that massage and corrective exercise came to be taught in physical education in schools, a practice that continued up through the 1940s, when special schools of physical therapy were opened."[32] By 1928 Posse's course was three years in length, with one year devoted to massage and corrective gymnastics.

Massage in Movement Cure

Ling's system addressed the mechanical aspect of movement, provided a curative means in the form of medical gymnastics, and included passive movements later known as massage. The movements were carefully classified by studying their effect on specific diseases and deformities, thus forming a system of specific actions performed in various combinations to produce a desired remedy. It was not until well after Ling's death in 1837 that any substantial writing about his life's work was published. But it is clear from what little he did write that the manipulations of friction, kneading, stroking, cupping, clapping, and others were included within his exercise system known as Swedish, medical, or rational gymnastics. These manipulations were not, however, called *massage* or *rubbing*.

Ling's system of exercise gymnastics consisted of a series of movements labeled active, active-passive, and passive. Active exercise was done solely by the efforts of the patient. Passive exercise was applied by an attendant, and active-passive was a combination of the two, the patient and attendant working together in the exercise movement.

The active portion of Ling's exercise regime was comprised of isometric exercises or specific bending and lunging movements done by the patient under the direction of a physician or attendant. These regimes were performed in near military style, with participants standing in rank-file order and moving only when given specific commands.

The active-passive exercises—now known as range-of-motion movements—were done by the attendant upon the patient. The active-passive exercises were later extracted from Ling's medical gymnastic system to become the Swedish gymnastics that were taught at nearly every massage and physical therapy school in America from about 1921 to 1975. These movements comprise the attendant moving a foot, leg, or arm in a circle, or range of motions, around the joint.

The passive movements were the manipulations that we now know as massage, such as clapping, stroking, friction, kneading, shaking, and vibrating. One of the first to write about Ling's system after his death in 1837, Matthias Roth, M.D., lists the passive movements as spanning, stemming, holding, balancing, rocking, Russian swinging, peripherical, pendulum, swinging, pressing, squeezing, ligature, shaking, knocking, tapping, clapping, chopping, sawing, kneading, stroking, frictions, standing, and walking.[33] These movements were called passive because the patient would passively allow the attendant to perform each movement. Roth provides this footnote in his attempt to clarify the term: "As the term passive may occasion some confusion, I consider it necessary to be somewhat more explicit. In using the term passive, reference is invariably made to an external agent, though this is in itself really active."[34] An example of the description of a technique and its effect is given by Roth:

> Kneading is a repeated movement, by which the skin of a certain part is acted upon by softer and stronger, but not painfully pinching and griping movements; the skin is then alternately held and let loose, as we are accustomed to do when kneading a mass of dough.

Effect. Kneading increases the nutrition, retroformation, and the circulation of the blood in the muscular substance and other tender parts; the hyperaesthesis of the nerves of the muscles is diminished, which is probably the reason of its popular use in rheumatic pains; also the morbid products, as for instance, the rheumatic swellings under the skin, between the fasciae and fibres of the muscles, are more quickly and easily absorbed. Kneading of the abdomen is executed in the same manner, and is only a kneading of the skin; but if we wish to communicate the effect to the bowels, then we do not pinch more strongly, but we take a larger grasp, whereby we include the bowels. In this case the movement is called *peristaltic kneading.*[35]

In Ling's medical gymnastic system these movements were applied only on specific body parts and most often in conjunction with the active and active-passive movements. George H. Taylor provides a clear description of the movement cure system and why the manipulations of massage are included in it.

Movements, in short, are simply motions of specific kinds, having specific effects, practiced for specific purposes, and intended to secure definite results. Movements are mechanical agencies, directed either upon the whole

Was Peter Ling the Father of Swedish Massage?

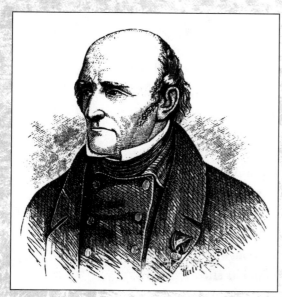

Peter Henry Ling (1776–1837)

According to Dr. Emil Kleen, the "Swedish tradition . . . began with Per Henrik Ling."[36] From the 1930s through the 1960s, Peter Ling's reputation spread throughout America along with the growth of several dominant massage institutions. Those institutions, along with their prolific correspondence courses, supported Ling's role as the creator of Swedish massage, the form of massage that is in large part defined by the use of four movements—effleurage (stroking), petrissage (kneading), frictions (rubbing), and tapotement (striking). One example of such support comes from an unpublished textbook by Dr. Esther C. Swanson, proprietor of the Chicago-based School of Swedish Massage. In the 1957 edition of her textbook she writes, "P. H. Ling, the Swedish fencing master, was the first person to succeed in putting these forms of treatment on a scientific basis. He opened a School of Swedish Massage, in Sweden, hence the name."[37] A well-known and influential contemporary author, Gertrude Beard, writes, "In the early part of the nineteenth century we see a definite change in terminology, evidently due to the influence of Peter Ling of Sweden, in the beginning of the use of French terms. Ling, to whom credit has been given as the originator of the Swedish system of massage, traveled widely over all Europe and incorporated the use of the French terms effleurage, petrissage, massage a' friction, and tapotement into his system."[38]

It is unclear why Beard came to believe this about Ling, because no French terms related to massage were used by Ling or the Royal Central Gymnastic Institute or any of Ling's followers. Patricia Benajmin discovered the truth from translations of Peter Ling's *Notations to the General Principles of Gymnastics*. In an article published in 1986, Benjamin, too, had stated that Ling's medical gymnastic system was the seed of Swedish massage brought to this country in the early nineteenth century. Then, in an article published in 1987 in the *Journal of the American Massage Therapy Association*, Benjamin cleared up several "misconceptions we have had about his work." She wrote, "Considering this traditional belief, it was amazing to find that there were no French terms used in the Notations written by Ling either to denote soft tissue manipulation in general, or to describe any techniques. Ling refers to this system of treatment as a whole as 'medical gymnastics' and to the techniques within medical gymnastics as active, active-passive, and passive movements (passiva rorelserna). He used all Swedish words to describe a total of about nineteen separate techniques."[39] She went on to explain that the misconception came about because the first books written about Ling's system of medical gymnastics utilized the French terms and were subsequently attributed to Ling. Given this discovery by Patricia Benjamin, and the fact Ling did not create an institute in Sweden (or anywhere else for that matter) called the School of Swedish Massage, it is clear that Swedish massage as we know it today did not originate with Peter Ling, and therefore we must question his title as the father of it.

Dutch practitioner Johan Georg Mezger (1838–1909) might be a more likely candidate for the title. Many authors give Mezger credit for simplifying the passive movements of the Swedish gymnastic system into the four categories so well known as Swedish massage. Mezger wrote a doctoral dissertation in 1868 entitled "The Treatment of Foot Sprain by Friction," as well as a small book on massage. His fame as a successful practitioner was widespread in Europe, especially after he successfully treated the Danish crown-prince for chronic joint trouble. Kamenetz tells us that Mezger's influence also spawned "the oldest association of masseurs [Dutch Association for Medical Gymnastics and Massage] . . . founded in Holland in 1889 and the oldest periodical of the profession 2 years later."[40]

Kleen credits Mezger with even more. "We find no essential advance on Ling's mechano-therapy in the first half of this [nineteenth] century. In France this form of treatment, after a short period of florescence in the eighteenth century, declined. . . . In Germany and Scandinavia, the medical gymnastics were active in a more or less rational way, but massage, on the whole, received little attention. Finally, in England, where sports fill the place of gymnastics . . . mechano-therapy made no especial progress. . . . The new era of mechano-therapy begins with the middle of this century. . . . Prior to this time—beyond receiving slight attention from a few scattered physicians—mechano-therapy was in the hands of laymen who were unable either to comprehend its real significance, or to introduce it to the scientific world. . . . It is to Teutonic peoples, especially the Germans, that we owe the greatest achievements in this as in so many other fields. A strong impulse was first given by the famous Dr. Mezger, of Amsterdam, who was already an active masseur in the early sixties . . . [and who] through his German and Scandinavian pupils has exercised a powerful influence upon the standing of massage in the medical world."[41]

Ling can be credited with bringing together some of the manipulations we now classify under the name of massage and incorporating them into his medical gymnastics as a coherent and teachable set of passive movements. It must be kept in mind, however, that the passive movements were a small part of the larger set of active and active-passive exercises that comprised his gymnastic system. Those that followed him, such as Mezger, always gave Ling credit for his work. But it was Mezger and his followers who organized the manipulations into simpler divisions and labeled them with the French terms *effleurage, petrissage, frictions,* and *tapotement,* and it was Mezger who created the first system of massage therapy as a stand-alone healing art. Thus he may be more deserving of the title Father of Swedish Massage.

system or a part of it, for the purpose of inducing determinate effects upon its vital actions, and generally having reference to its pathological state. . . . The division of movements into active and passive relates to the sources whence the moving power is derived. The motion of riding, for instance, is passive, if the body be supported. So also are the clappings, knockings, strokings, kneadings, pullings, shakings, vibratings, etc., . . . because both the motion and the will that gives it energy are derived from another person.[42]

Distinguishing Between Massage and Exercise

Massage historians have reported that prior to the eighteenth century little distinction was made between massage and exercise. This situation continued well into the nineteenth century. It wasn't until the middle of the nineteenth century that massage techniques began to be separated by description—but not practice—from the movements of therapeutic exercise. Techniques we now attribute to a system of massage—such as kneading, stroking, slapping, and cupping—were not considered distinct therapeutic measures, but were included as part of an overall exercise or movement regime. Many of the writings about exercise do not contain references to massage; in fact, most of them do not. But many of the individual techniques that make up massage were included within exercise systems. For example, the ancient Greek physicians prescribed horseback riding as a form of vibration therapy, or recommended violent shaking or riding in a wagon on a rough road to induce the effects of percussion. Typically, the use of friction following an exercise routine was considered a part of the exercise, although this does not mean that massage was exercise.

Kleen explains that massage and exercise (gymnastics) have been like Siamese twins, joined at the hip throughout history. "It is impossible to separate the history of massage from that of gymnastics. . . . On the whole, gymnastics have emerged within the domain of science earlier than massage, since the scientific requirements of the first are much more easily fulfilled than those of the latter. Men have been quicker to learn the worth of muscular exercise, to set forth its indications and to prescribe it, than in attaining a comprehension of the physiological effects of massage and of the meaning of its various manipulations, which presupposes a far wider knowledge of anatomical, histological and physiological facts."[43]

Kamenetz, writing in 1980, confirms Dr. Kleen's statement. "We found particularly in ancient literature that exercise and massage were mentioned without sufficient differentiation between the two. In fact we know of no history of massage of any importance, which excludes the subject of exercise."[44] It seems odd that Kamenetz would make this last statement in light of the work of Walter Johnson in 1866 called *The Anatriptic Art: A History of the Art,* a book devoted to the history of massage. Nowhere does Johnson mention exercise; his book is exclusively about "medical rubbings." Evidently, Kamenetz did not consider Johnson's history "of any importance," which is even stranger because it was used by Graham, Taylor, and others.

An example that demonstrates the trend of confusing massage and gymnastics comes from Kurre W. Ostrom, a Swedish practitioner of the Swedish movement system. The word *massage* does not appear in his 1912 book until the third chapter, where he defines it as "a scientific treatment, by certain passive systematic manipulations, upon the nude skin of the human body." Ostrom uses the words *manipulation, movement,* and *gymnastics* in his brief historical review of the subject of massage. It appears that Ostrom and others classified massage as a passive movement or manipulation within the Swedish gymnastics or movement cure because, in his words, "all manipulations are passive—i.e., applied to the patient without his assistance or resistance."[45]

Writing in 1892, Kleen—a strong proponent for massage as a stand-alone therapy—argued for its separation from gymnastics in order to keep it viable, instead of being suffocated under the medical gymnastics movement. His writing offers some clear guidelines for distinguishing between exercise and massage. He differentiated the types of movements based on whether they are done by the patient or done by others to the patient, regardless of the similarity of effects.

> For the proper limitation of the conception of massage, it is of paramount necessity to discriminate between it and gymnastics, which involve the exercise of the organs of motion. At first sight it seems unlikely that the definitions of these terms should be confused or misleading. Both forms of treatment, however, have many points in common; both, of necessity, are often employed simultaneously in medical practice; they have, likewise, very frequently been practiced by the same professional persons—and herein . . . lies the reason for the failure of almost all writers, earlier and later alike, to distinguish between gymnastics and massage. In concrete cases, however, the distinction is often so striking that it is scarcely possible to escape grasping it. For instance, one may massage an exudation or a haematoma, since they are soft tissues, at least in a sense, but one cannot give them gymnastics, for they are not organs, least of all are they organs of motion and capable of being exercised as such. On the other hand, a muscle can be given both gymnastics and massage: in the latter case it plays either no part or an utterly inconspicuous part as an organ, being treated as a tissue simple, e.g., in the removal of an infiltration by friction's [*sic*]; while in the first case it is always treated as an organ and must function as such. The fact that massage, through the removal of the infiltration, heightens the functional power of the muscle, and so far forth, in this same case, has the same end and the same influence that gymnastics have—and the further fact that gymnastics, when employed simultaneously with massage, in their turn assist in removing the infiltration, in no wise detracts from the propriety of drawing a sharp distinction between the two methods of treatment.
>
> I have emphasized the distinction between massage and gymnastics,

95

for the reason that the attempt to blend the two, or rather the inability to separate them, still continues. Messieurs the gymnasts, in their zeal to secure all possible recognition for medical gymnastics—and in their not unusual confusion of ideas as to their office, will have it, perforce, that massage is "only a part of gymnastics," and declare that the "passive movements" of the latter include the former. . . . My criticism on this is that when for the sake of clearness one undertakes to divide a subject into parts, he should be careful not to transgress the limits of his subject-matter; and when such a division of gymnastic movements is attempted, one must, to be consistent, take into account only the movements (be they passive or active, be they made with or without assistance or resistance) of him who exercises his own organs of motion, of him who takes gymnastics, of the gymnasticizing patient—in the case of medical gymnastics—for these are the movements which constitute gymnastics, and without the same there are no gymnastics. It does not answer to have reference to the movement of the patient one moment, and in the next instant to have reference to those made upon the patient by another person, e.g., by a gymnast or masseur; nor, by the way, can these latter movements be called passive—neither do they belong to gymnastics more than any other movements. However, in order to leave no room for the common misapprehension, and for the sake of consistency, I think it best to speak of the *manipulations* of massage, and of the *movements* of gymnastics.[46]

Kleen considers gymnastics and massage separate divisions of a larger field called "mechano-therapy," in which he includes orthopedics. Kleen stood nearly alone in his attempts to separate gymnastics and massage. His remarks above were written in 1892, well after the development of medical gymnastics, and it's the time when its considerable following in Europe and America had established it as a viable movement cure system. However, his perspective slowly spread.

Taylor, writing in 1860 on the movement cure, did not mention massage, but in the next edition of his book (1883) he included an entire chapter on massage apart from the active and passive movements of the gymnastic routine developed by Ling. I have also discovered another book written by Dr. Kellogg that does exactly the same thing—separates massage from the gymnastic movement system we now call Swedish gymnastics. In 1895 Kellogg wrote: "When the first edition of this work was published [1880], many of the measures therein recommended were looked upon with more or less distrust by a large proportion of the medical profession, as they were at that time little known in this country."[47] Although Kellogg's section on massage—separate from the section on passive movement—is small, it is distinct from the gymnastic movement exercises. Unlike Kleen, who argued for the separation of massage from gymnastics or exercise systems, Kellogg merely presents it as such: "This mode of treatment [massage] . . . is really nothing more nor less than a combination of a number of the above-described forms of treatment [kneading, stroking, pulling, clapping, chopping, and knocking]."[48] This statement by Kellogg places massage as a part of the gymnastic movement in a different context. He explains that massage is the application of a combination of manipulations upon the whole body. The significance of this is that the individual manipulations were not considered massage when used individually within Ling's Swedish gymnastics system; they only became massage when used together upon the entire body during one treatment. No other author has described massage in relation to the gymnastic movements in this manner.

To say that the history of massage has always been a part of the history of exercise is a limited perspective. The distinctions between massage and exercise made by Kleen, Taylor, and Kellogg counter the claims made by Kamenetz that they were always commingled. But even their comments are pertinent only from the limited perspective of the medical point of view. Most writers on gymnastics and massage believed that the value of massage rested in its reflex and mechanical effects alone; the merits of passive movements beyond the measure of science were rarely discussed. They failed to see the value rooted in the inherent human need for touch, or its moral value as a part of medicine, as expounded by Taylor.

As we have already seen, massage has long been a part of activities other than gymnastics or exercise—such as midwifery, the practice of healing arts by Christian nuns, and the healing rituals of shamanic cultures—where massage is employed with a broader sense of its value. It is more accurate to say that massage and exercise have a shared history, just as massage has a shared history with midwifery and medicine.

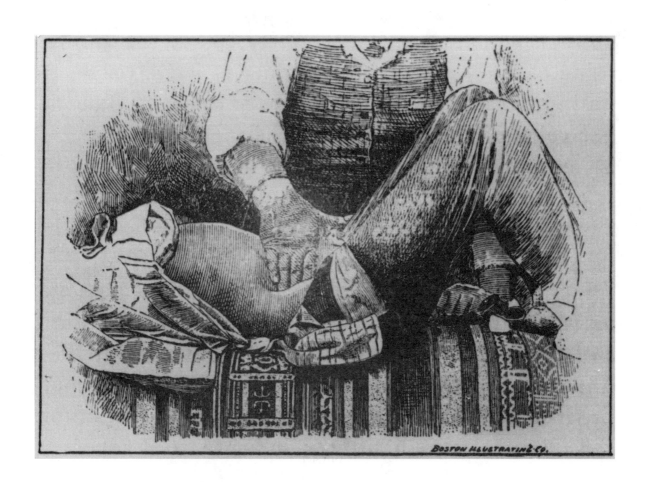

The belly-kneading movement, "chiefly employed in cases of
habitual constipation, or of dilation of the stomach." From
Handbook of Massage by Emil Kleen, M.D. (Philadelphia, 1892).

7 First Steps to Credibility: Massage in Nineteenth-century Medicine

Medical historian Felix Marti-Ibanez, M.D., described the tenor of the nineteenth century in this way. "The leaders of this age were supremely optimistic, sturdily confident in human progress, and imbibed with a broad humanitarianism in place of the cruel passions of the preceding century. The universe was looked upon as a gigantic machine; all that was required was to discover the immutable laws that governed its operation. This was the era that deified science, seeking to reduce all intellectual and moral processes to precise Newtonian principles of matter, motion, space, time, force."[1] The development of medical gymnastics, the movement cure, and scientific massage were in tune with the times—their proponents believed that by applying scientific principles to the age-old methods of exercise therapeutics, medicine would rise to new levels of achievement while also adhering to the ways of nature.

There was considerable diversity among those preferring the natural way of healing in the mid– and late nineteenth century. Some physicians felt assured that gymnastics or exercise, which included certain massage manipulations, was not only enjoying a resurgence of its ancient and historical place in medicine, but that it held more promise than drugs and surgery. One institute went so far as to claim medical gymnastics as "new medicine." Some physicians with a populist bent believed that medical gymnastics and movement cure systems were the medicine of the future that would serve all, rich or poor. One of the advocates for massage, George Taylor, M.D., wrote that "the fundamental principles underlying massage are natural, having their type and exemplar in those involuntary motions of the organism which afford the primary impulse to nutritive acts. Nothing can therefore be more natural and timely than the contributions of the abundant power of the strong and well to supply the defects of the weak and infirm." The "nutritive acts" he mentions refer to the circulatory system as it corresponds to the ebb and flow of the assimilation of food and the elimination of waste products. He felt that massage provided the same beneficial

Why is the masseur not more generally and confidently employed? . . . When massage first came to our attention, experts who offered themselves were mostly Swedes and Germans. . . . They were used where trained only under the direction of physicians themselves skilled in the principles of hand treatment and able to direct efficiently. In America, not only is the physician not so instructed, but scarcely one in hundreds has any clear or competent conception of the scope and applicability of these measures.

—J. Madison Taylor, M.D., *New York Medical Journal*, 1912

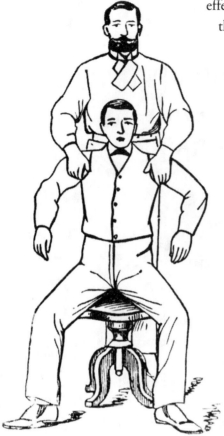

A passive-movement exercise of the late nineteenth century, called "shoulder rotation and chest lifting—sitting." The teaching text states: "This is a mild but effective movement in weakness of the lungs and heart, as it deepens the inspiration followed by a stronger expiration, thereby stimulating the flow of venous blood to the heart." From *A Manual of Instruction for Giving Swedish Movement and Massage Treatment* by Hartvig Nissen, Ph.D. (Philadelphia and London, 1889).

effects on the action of the cells as did the treatment by movements, the difference being that massage was given by those better off to those needing its application.

Many proponents of natural healing methods believed that massage should no longer be considered only as an adjunctive therapy; they thought it could stand on its own merit as an important option in treating illness and injury. Dr. Taylor appears to be the first physician of his time to write about massage as a stand-alone therapy. In 1887 he noted that massage had not received the acknowledgment it deserved as an independent therapeutic tool, even while most other professions were dividing into specialties.

It is, therefore, in furtherance of progress in the healing art that it spontaneously divides itself into well-known specialties. Such division affords opportunity for extended research, and the consequent development of facts and principles that otherwise must remain unknown. The profession and the public unite in fostering these specialties, which are therefore multiplying. The remedial specialty which has received the appellation of MASSAGE has unfortunately failed to enjoy the advantages to be derived from separate, careful, special investigation, whereby its facts and principles might be assigned their true place; and whereby these might be properly applied and controlled by themselves, and unconnected with any other system or theory.[2]

The proliferation of books written about massage during the 1800s were in part a result of this broader period of specialization. Most of the massage literature written by physicians expounds the virtues of massage, but many of them are defensive, eager to separate physician-approved massage from that found outside medical practice. Their attempts were largely unsuccessful because the majority of the medical community pretty much ignored them. Despite this, the zeal of writers such as Roth (1851), Johnson (1866), Mitchell (1875), Taylor (1879), Billroth (1880), Murrell (1886), Nissen (1889), Graham (1890), Kleen (1892), Kellogg (1897), Haehl (1898), and others for their subject was not diminished, nor was their success at using massage for the benefit of their patients.

In 1892 Kleen wrote, "The new era of mechano-therapy begins with the middle of this century [nineteenth]. Its history conveys the same impression as the history of medicine in general, namely, that the greater part of what has been gained, has been gained within this period. Prior to this time—beyond receiving slight attention from a few scattered physicians—mechano-therapy was in the hands of laymen who were unable either to comprehend its real significance, or to introduce it to the scientific world; from this time dates its more frequent appearance in the service of science."[3]

Massage in Nineteenth-century European Medicine

During the nineteenth century massage in Europe was described in the medical literature, practiced in select doctors' offices, and taught at some institutes in addition to being offered by lay practitioners. It was initially a part of the medical gymnastic and movement cure systems but gradually began to be studied and written about as a separate subject within medicine. In Russia, M. Y. Mudrov, M.D., a doctor of internal medicine, began using massage and movement exercises in his adult medical practice in the middle of the nineteenth century. Later it was applied toward children's development and health in Russia.[4] Vibrational massage was also developed and studied, and by "the end of the 19th century centers for massage studies were developed all over Russia and the Ukraine."[5]

One British author notes that "from the end of the eighteenth century a great revival in massage [in England] really began. Many authorities wrote and expounded their theories on the subject. One extremist advocated that massage should be given with great violence, and all had different ideas about the terminology, pressure, rate, rhythm, and medium, such as oil or powder to be used, position of the patient, and the duration of treatment. Some advocated dry hands; one used a metal object covered with leather. Some suggested that four minutes' massage to any one area was sufficient; another stated that up to forty minutes could be given. . . . In 1894 a group of women joined together to form the Society of Trained Masseuses, in order to try to raise the standard and reputation of massage in this country."[6] This was the world's first professional association of massage practitioners, founded by five female nurses.

Great Britain had a system of "health visitors" who worked in the homes of the poor, offering midwifery and other health services. Massage was a part of their training, because it included some instruction in medical gymnastics. Kellogg confirms this in his chapter on obstetrics in *The Home Hand-book on Domestic Hygiene and Rational Medicine*. "When the patient is for any reason too feeble to walk, ride, or take much vigorous exercise of any kind, daily passive exercise should be given in the form of massage and Swedish movements."[7] But the majority of massage practitioners were either barber-surgeons who dabbled in many areas of medical practice, or immigrant Indians who practiced their form of massage, called shampooing. (The barber-surgeon tradition began during the fifteenth century when plagues killed off a great many physicians and surgeons. The surgeons guild, in a controversial act, joined in partnership with the barbers to become the barber-surgeons guild. Ambrose Pare was such a person who belonged to the barber-surgeons guild. Barber-surgeons worked throughout Europe even into the early twentieth century. Their craft included bloodletting, surgery, amputation, tooth pulling, and other medical and nonmedical procedures. Most had little or no training, and as massage came more into prominence they dabbled in that as well.) This form of massage was not well regarded by the medical community, who considered it "mere rubbing."

Perhaps the first English physician who, according to Walter Johnson, "made any considerable use of friction" was William Balfour, M.D.[8] His first book, which covered percussion, compression, and friction techniques, was written in 1819. English physician John Grosvenor, a hospital surgeon at Oxford who also visited patients at their homes by horseback, found the benefits of massage late in his career. He suffered from "a morbid affection of the knee" which he cured by self-treatments of "friction." He then began using friction upon his patients and soon developed a considerable reputation for curing joint problems.[9] It is worth repeating a report written in 1825 by his biographer, Mr. Cleobury, describing how these treatments were performed. Although Cleobury's description of medical rubbing is referred to as friction, it appears to be a kind of effleurage.

> Females were engaged, who supported themselves by this occupation. The female rubber, seated on a low stool, and taking the patient's limb in her lap (which position gave her command over it), so as to enable her to rub with both hands, proceeded to rub with extended hands, so that the friction should be performed principally with the palm of the hand; taking long strokes, one hand ascending as the other descended; keeping both hands in motion the whole time; and occasionally applying a small quantity of fine hair powder to the palms of her hands, to prevent the moisture from producing an erosion of the skin. After the friction had been continued in this manner for half an hour, the limb, if contracted, was taken by the female rubber at the ankle, and in the slightest possible degree an attempt was made to extend it. The friction was at first continued for one hour daily (more or less as the case would admit), and gradually increased till the patient could bear it to be rubbed an hour at a time three hours in the day, observing always to rub by the watch.[10]

Balfour and Grosvenor had little influence on their profession, however, as Walter Johnson made clear in 1860. "The practice and writings . . . of these gentlemen failed to attract the attention of the profession, and from that time to this, rubbing has been left almost wholly in the hands of unprofessional persons; some of whom, as Mr. Beveridge, of Edinburgh, used simple rubbing, while others employed various kinds of liniments and ointments, as the once fashionable St. John Long, Mahomet of Brighton, Harrup, and others."[11] The Mr. Beveridge Johnson refers to published a pamphlet in 1859, entitled "The Cure of Disease by Manipulation, commonly called Medical Rubbing."

Johnson reflects the attitude of most of the physicians who wrote on the subject of massage during this time. They were enthusiastic about its benefits but had a limited notion of who should be doing it. Many of the pro-massage physicians were highly critical of the common rubber, masseur, masseuse, gymnast, or Turkish rubber who did massage for a living, many of whom were immigrants simply doing what they knew best. They often went so far as to say that only someone working under the direct supervision of a physician was qualified to do massage and that receiving a massage from those whom they regarded as untrained or inadequately trained was a waste of time and might even cause serious injuries.

Physicians who were proponents of massage firmly believed in its value; however, they often found themselves in the minority of medical opinion, as medicine raced toward a new future with microbiology and advanced pharmaceuticals and surgical techniques. Most of their concern about massage not being a larger part of medicine no doubt stemmed from their zeal to distinguish massage as an important medical tool; at the same time, their criticism of those who had not received "proper" instruction from a physician also reflected class prejudice. The mid– and late nineteenth century was a time of enormous civil unrest and social upheaval in both North America and parts of Europe. Class consciousness and labor strife reflected the growing divisions in society. Massage was performed in the bath houses and in private and health homes, primarily by immigrants with little or no formal training who cared little for what the physicians thought.

English physician William Murrell can be seen as a representative voice of the massage-friendly physicians who viewed their struggle from a class perspective. In his 1886 book, *Massage as a Mode of Treatment,* Murrell writes,

> I'm afraid that a good deal of misconception exists in this country on the subject of Massage. Many people think that it is only a kind of "rubbing" or "shampooing," whilst others associate it in their minds with the idea of a Turkish bath. . . . Another common mistake is to suppose that anyone can "do massage," and that the whole art can be acquired in one or two easy lessons. . . . I constantly see nurses and others who think they are thoroughly competent to undertake Massage, but who have not the dimmest idea even of the meaning of the word. . . . The ignorant rubber of course thinks that it will cure everything, but as a matter of fact its sphere of action is very limited. If carried out under the direction of a scientific physician, who has had experience in this mode of treatment, it yields excellent results, but if allowed to drift into the hands of an ignorant empiric it soon degenerates into the most arrant quackery. . . . I do not think that a man-rubber should ever be employed for ladies or children. For them it is absolutely necessary to obtain the services of an educated and accomplished masseuse. It is a safe rule to have nothing to do with the people who advertise.[12]

Murrell can be credited with distinguishing true massage, as he referred to Massage with a capital M, from massage with a little m, the improper and "simple act of rubbing."[13] In his quest to interest the medical field in the significance and utility of massage, his criticism ranged from other practitioners to authors of dictionaries. He was so critical of English massage he went so far as to write, "There is as much difference between Mezger's Massage and the so-called English Massage, as there is between champagne and gooseberry. It is oysters and macrobrunner versus ginger-beer and whelks."[14]

Another English physician, Mathias M. Roth, directed his 1851 book, *The Prevention and Cure of Many Chronic Diseases by Movements,* primarily at physicians in an attempt to advance the movement cure system. He included excruciating detail about the many movements of Ling's system. But the medical community's reaction to his book was dubious, as shown by a review in the English medical journal *Lancet* in 1852. "The work before us proposes to cure . . . diseases through the beneficial influence of movements and mechanical appliances. . . . In certain chronic and functional maladies, physic alone will not achieve the results desired. . . . The most rational section in the work is that on dress . . . Dr. Roth insists, and very properly, on the ill consequences of stays; and when the matter is seriously considered, we believe that an immense amount of human suffering, and even great saving of human life, would be consequent upon the total discarding of stays."[15]

This review reveals much about the attitude of the conservative population of physicians toward the movement cure system. Although movement cure advocates stressed the scientific nature of their work, it seems evident that the medical establishment considered their work less than rational. The mention of stays refers to a small chapter in Roth's book that tells about the most common faults of clothing; in focusing on it the *Lancet* reviewer completely disregarded the majority of Roth's work. It must be noted, however, that the *British Journal of Homeopathy* and several newspapers gave Roth's book laudable reviews.

In 1892 Emil Kleen, M.D., writing in his *Handbook of Massage*, presented the perspective of the European physicians who believed in proper training and supervision for massage, apart from gymnastics.

> In one respect massage holds an extremely peculiar position; it is very frequently practiced—in some countries almost exclusively—by persons who have had little or no medical education. I pass by the troops of "wise men," barber-surgeons, and the like, who occasionally try their hands at massage, and propose to devote a few words to a particular class of professionals who are now quite numerous in all Germanic countries, and who devote themselves as well to gymnastics as massage, but usually call themselves "gymnasts."
>
> Obviously, the gymnast occupies a favorable position which cannot be compared with that of the quack-doctor who meddles with internal medicine. The former has no need of using medicines, which, though highly prized by the public are a source of danger to the quack, and, on account of the innocent nature of his manipulations, and the peculiarity which they posses [*sic*] of seldom leaving any visible traces, he is not nearly so often, or in so high a degree obliged, as is the quack-doctor, to exercise caution in displaying his ignorance. Moreover, the gymnast can always make capital out of a lucky cure, which the discriminating public pronounces an extraordinary achievement, though a physician under similar circumstances would "only be doing his duty." Let us admit that the gymnast often has had a special, though meager training for his work, and also that he belongs, in contrast with the quack doctor, to the better educated classes.[16]

In 1891 a Swedish ordinance was passed into law prohibiting nonphysicians from doing mechano-therapy unless they had taken appropriate training at the Royal Central Gymnastic Institute in Stockholm. But Dr. Kleen made it clear that the training given at the institute was not well regarded by physicians. "As soon as the large number of completely uneducated gymnasts shall have died off, mechano-therapy will stand much better in Sweden than formerly, so far as the degree of education possessed by its practitioners is concerned."[17]

According to Kleen the Royal Central Gymnastic Institute was a nonmedical institution that did not appreciate the distinction he made between gymnastics and massage. Kleen wrote: "Leaving out the noisy advertising and 'puffing' of Swedish gymnastics by Ling's followers, it was chiefly massage which gained for this form of therapy the prestige it has won. Moreover, among the workers trained by the Royal Central and other institutes, massage forms a more important and essential part of their work, both for themselves and their patients, than gymnastics. It is worth noting that Ling himself included massage manipulations among passive gymnastic movements, and that the Swedish gymnasts, partly in reverence for their idol, partly from a practical motive, have done their utmost to eradicate the term 'massage' and to represent the use of movable pressure on the soft parts as a special part of gymnastics."[18]

Kleen's statement about the role massage played in Ling's gymnastic movement system is quite different from Ling's successors, who did not attribute the success of their methods to the massage manipulations. Kleen can be considered a representative voice for those who believed it was time to separate massage from the movement system. He points out that Ling's Royal Central Gymnastic Institute was originally considered a fringe organization that did things on its own without regard to accepted medical practice. He supports this point of view by noting that Ling had to make several attempts to gain government funding of the institute before it was finally approved in 1813, and that one presentation to the Minister of Public Instruction in 1812 received the following response. "There are enough of jugglers and rope-dancers, without exacting any further charge from the public treasury."[19]

Gustav Schutz, M.D., who translated Dr. Kleen's writing from Swedish to German, wrote in 1890, "Kleen's clear, scientific manner of statement, and his independent, critical sifting of the material, are especially praiseworthy. Kleen's book therefore seems to me to be of value to the practicing physician, in that it is free from all specialistic narrowness and enthusiasm for massage; does not run into extravagance in setting up indications for it; or into parsimony in showing its contraindications; and always assigns massage its place among the other adjuvant measures of therapy."[20]

A few further examples demonstrate the range of criticism leveled by physicians at those who did massage. Axel V. Grafstrom, M.D., a Swedish physician who also practiced in the United States, wrote that his colleague, Kurre W. Ostrom, M.D., very correctly remarked: "Let me now say a few words about educated operators. Some of them, and especially females, have been accused of thinking too much of themselves— of being too independent. Masseurs and masseuses should remember that they are only using one special remedy that nature has taught man to employ to arrest disease. Persons who are properly trained will not attempt to enter into competition with medical men, but confine themselves to the scientific treatment that we have endeavored to analyze. . . . Were it not for abuses that have prevailed, the manual treatment of disease would, no doubt, be more universally adopted and recommended by the medical profession and the general public."[21]

In 1898 Richard Haehl, M.D., of Hahnemann Medical College in Philadelphia wrote a book for medical students about massage. In the preface he states that "among the adjuncts to therapeutic effort, none are of more value than the subject to this present treatise. The importance of it has become so universally recognized by practitioners in every branch of medical art, and the technique of the masseur has put on such a highly scientific finish, that massage has come to be regarded as one of the 'Long Toms' of our therapeutic armamentarium."[22] But in the first sentence of the very next paragraph he seems to alter his view of massage within medicine.

> Massage is rather neglected in this country; it is often mentioned in our lecture rooms as a valuable means to combat certain diseases and conditions, but no instruction, as far as I know, is given on this subject. What student of our College, after finishing his junior course, does not know that massage forms an important part of the treatment of fractures, especially fractures of the patella? . . . Still, most of the students, after leaving the College, do not know any more in a practical way about massage than the general meaning of the word itself. For this reason its employment is sometimes not as successful as we are led to anticipate. Massage is not a drug which will act, after the patient had his prescription filled and had taken it "as directed." Massage treatment should either be done by the scientific and educated physician himself, or at least the administering Masseur should be under his immediate observation and supervision. It is then, and only then, that the beneficial results can be obtained.[23]

The underlined emphasis is original. Haehl added, "Massage, however, must not be used all by itself, regulation of diet, exercise, indicated remedy, and at the beginning of the treatment even enemas and in severe cases purging drugs may be necessary."[24]

There were well-educated voices speaking for the other side of the argument, such as Professor Hartwig Nissen, writing in his 1889 book, *A Manual of Instruction for Giving Swedish Movement and Massage Treatment.*

> It has happened more than once to the author of this book that he has been called in by physicians to apply "massage" to patients who were already suffering with a high fever, and he invariably declined to do so. In one of these cases the patient died the following day. Had the physician's request been acceded to, the massage treatment would have been accredited with hastening or causing the sick man's death. . . . At

MASSAGE IN

NINETEENTH-CENTURY

MEDICINE

other times the writer has asked the physician in charge what the illness was, and has been told that it was unnecessary for him to know.

Some physicians seem to have the idea that we specialists are their rivals and their opponents. Still, we have frequently repeated that we are not physicians and do not practice medicine.

We are specialists, and, as such, necessarily physiologists, and have the practical experience gained by the practice of many years in this one branch. . . . But it is co-operation between the medical profession and the specialists which is desirable and necessary in order to produce the best results.[25]

Nissen's plea for cooperation is based on his desire to help the patient. The placement of his work as a specialty is perfect for the times. With these two arguments he hoped to draw respect to the practice of massage as an adjunctive but distinct healing art. He delineates his specialty within medicine by knowing when to treat and when not to treat.

Massage in Nineteenth-century American Medicine

The early period of massage practice in nineteenth-century America was marked by great enthusiasm, as well as a general lack of unification of definition, technique, and application. Many physicians devised and proffered massage systems; these were typically local or regional and often known by the name of the physician.

In 1902 Douglas Graham, M.D., of Boston, Massachusetts, published what he claimed was "the first book on Massage in point of time in the English language." His book, *Manual Therapeutics, A Treatise on Massage,* focuses on the treatment of specific diseases and disorders by the method of massage. Graham also addresses the lack of trained operators giving massage: "Benefit or harm may follow from the roughest kind of scraping and pounding, and in a matter of such great importance as recovery from chronic and often hitherto regarded as hopeless invalidism, the means employed cannot be too carefully selected, especially when it is a question of such a potent agent as massage, which affects, either directly or indirectly, every function of the human body."[26] He proceeds to provide a discourse on the influences of massage on the skin and the physiological effects of massage on the many systems of the body.

Professor Silas Weir Mitchell (1829–1914), a Philadelphia neurologist, is credited by some authors with being the first to bring massage to the attention of the United States' medical community. Medical historians applaud him for his contributions as a man of letters and as a distinguished neurologist who first described causalgia (burning pain), erythromelalgia (skin neurosis), and postparalytic chorea (nerve pain). In 1877 Mitchell published an article entitled "Fat and Blood, and How to Make Them." His therapy is generally known as the rest cure, or the fattening, rest, and isolation cure. Mitchell's work was highly criticized as well as acclaimed. Many physicians deplored the use of massage in any circumstances, which they considered quackery. At the same time, his article was widely circulated and was written about in medical journals.

Dr. Kleen, writing in 1892, states that Mitchell was using massage "of the general sort," while Kamenetz claims Mitchell's book "gave much respectability to the field of physical therapy—especially massage and electricity."[27] According to Dr. Graham, Mitchell treated "thin, nervous, anaemic, and bedridden patients, usually women. The methods comprise an original combination of previous well-known agencies: namely, seclusion, rest, and excessive feeding made available by rapid nutritive changes caused by the systematic use of massage and electricity."[28] He goes on, "It has always seemed to me that 'Nerve and Muscle and How to Strengthen Them' would have been a much better and less sensational title for Dr. Mitchell's book . . . for the reason that there are cases that lose adipose tissue to their advantage under massage."[29] Graham believed that all the attention given Mitchell's article and the cure associated with it was misplaced. But he also made it clear that he thought it was absurd of critics to throw out a valuable therapeutic means just because those administering it were unqualified from a medical standpoint. He pointed out that Mitchell's early work using massage during the Civil War did not have the trappings of the rest cure given to the upper class women of the day. "Even Dr. Mitchell's own valuable testimony in treating some of the consequences of nerve injuries by massage during the war in the United States from 1861 to 1865 has been entirely lost sight of in the burst of blind enthusiasm over his more recent experience."[30] Dr. Graham admonished those physicians who disdained massage because of Mitchell's rest cure, ignoring its more important benefits proven in the treatment of war patients.

Patricia Benjamin writes that Wier's "work was so influential that he was described by another physician as having 'introduced this science (massage) on [sic] America, of grasping it, as it were, from the hands of quackery and bringing it under the control of the medical profession.'"[31] But long before 1877, the date of Mitchell's article, massage was being used in Turkish baths, rest homes, sanitariums, and a few medical establishments—places where it was not usually done under the supervision of a physician and hence was labeled quackery. It may be that it received wider attention in the medical community as a result of Mitchell's article, but its investigation as a treatment modality had begun long before this time in Europe and within some institutions, such as the Battle Creek Sanitarium run by John Harvey Kellogg, M.D.

In 1895 Dr. Kellogg published what was to become a classic textbook on massage, *The Art of Massage, Its Physiological Effects and Therapeutic Applications.* In 1897 he had a second edition published, followed by editions in 1909, 1919, 1923, and 1929. A total of 27,000 copies were printed. For later editions the subtitle became *A Practical Manual for the Nurse, the Student and the Practitioner,* but the text changed very little. The book is still used today in some massage schools. In the preface to the first edition Kellogg gives us a bit of a view of massage in the period in which he was developing the Battle Creek Sanitarium.

Massage is a subject which to the rational physician is one of greatest interest and importance. Twenty years ago its employment, as well as the use of electricity and hydrotherapy, was generally regarded by the profession as closely allied to quackery. Up to that time, scientific massage was almost unknown in this country, although various rude manipulations were practiced by bonesetters, so-called "magnetic healers," and a few superannuated nurses who claimed to be specially gifted in "rubbing." Twenty-two years ago, when the writer first made a study of massage and passive movements as a therapeutic means, even the term "massage" was as unfamiliar to the medical profession of this country as it still is to the majority of the laity. . . . I visited Sweden, Germany, France, and other European countries, with the purpose of becoming acquainted with the methods employed by the most expert manipulators abroad. . . . Added to my personal experience in the constant employment of ten to twenty masseurs and masseuses, in the treatment of patients suffering from a great variety of chronic ailments, I have endeavored to summarize and condense in this little work the facts which are essential to a scientific knowledge of the art and science of massage and its rational employment.[32]

Physicians such as Kleen, Graham, Taylor, and others—each strong proponents of massage—are not mentioned by medical historians. Even though some of these massage advocates write about the state of medicine during their time as if they are in the middle of it all, it seems evident that they were working outside the mainstream of medicine. But Ling's legacy of medical gymnastic exercises did gain wide appeal among mainstream physicians.

In 1897 Frank Foster, M.D., an editor of the prestigious *New York Medical Journal* and *Foster's Encyclopedic Medical Dictionary*, wrote an interesting section on exercise. First he writes, "Exercise is not a remedy which in some mysterious way may prove beneficial in disordered conditions of the system, still less a specific in any given disease, but it may be made the means of producing gentle or powerful effects of a definite kind, which vary with its form, intensity, duration, time of application, method of administration, and the condition of the patient. The problem presented to the physician in a given case is not merely the prescription of exercise, but rather such proportioning and contrasting of the muscular activity to periods of rest that the total result shall be beneficial; here, as always, the patient is to be treated rather than the disease. . . . Though most of the useful effects of exercise can be obtained under skilled supervision with little or no apparatus, its practical importance is ignored in hospitals, but little recognised in asylums, and imperfectly appreciated in private practice."[33] Then Foster says, "With the Swedish system of exercises, devised by Ling and elaborated by his pupils, totally different ground is reached . . . in exercise as a stimulus to development and as a remedy from observing its beneficial effects on his own health . . . which remains to-day [*sic*]as the basis of the most valuable procedures in therapeutic kinesiology. . . . He also devised systems of educational, military, and aesthetic exercises

MASSAGE IN

NINETEENTH-CENTURY

MEDICINE

. . . consist[ing] in free voluntary movements executed by the patient in different positions and in a determined order. The remedial movements include, in addition, passive movements executed by a manipulator, and assistive and resistive movement, in which the operator opposes resistance to the movements of the patient, or vice versa. To these are added the various manipulations of massage."[34] The term *therapeutic kinesiology* was derived from the writings of one of Ling's most famous pupils, A. Georgii, who in 1847 published a book on Ling's system under the title *Kinesitherapie.*

Dr. Foster seems to show some ignorance of massage in his last statement, "to these are added the various manipulations of massage," because massage *was* a passive movement. He falters in the same manner when he writes, "The extraordinary prominence in recent years of massage as a remedial agent, in so far as it is justified by results, rests largely on the employment with it of passive movements."[35] The passive movements he refers to were a part of the medical gymnastic system devised by Peter Ling, the division of movements devised by Ling called active, passive, and combined. As described in chapter 6, active movements are those rendered by the patient. An example of an active movement is doing a jumping jack or swinging along the metal rungs of an apparatus. Passive movements are those conducted by another person or an apparatus upon the patient, or the patient applying a movement with one hand to another part of the body, and combined movements are those that are either combined-active or combined-passive. Foster's remark is a redundant statement because massage is a passive movement and cannot therefore be employed with itself.

Massage for the Treatment of . . .

The doctors who chose to use massage as a therapeutic tool advocated its use in many areas of medical practice. It was used in the treatment of chronic conditions, such as diseases of the circulatory system; anaemia; dropsical and hemorrhagic exudates; certain diseases of the nerves and muscles; a number of organic diseases; hyperaemia of liver and spleen; emphysema pulmonum; and some diseases of the heart. For diseases of the nose and throat, neck massage was used to increase the venous and lymphatic flows and vibration to stimulate the mucous membranes. Chronic constipation was a common ailment, and very often massage was the treatment of choice because it stimulated the peristalsis of the intestines and stomach.

Dr. Karnitsky, quoted in the International Medical Annual of 1892, advises abdominal massage for children with constipation. Among several suggestions, he notes, "Habitual constipation may be easily cured by massage without the aid of purgatives. . . . The younger a child is the milder should the manipulations be and the shorter the seances."[36] (*Seance* was a word used to mean "session.")

Richard Haehl, M.D., recommended massage for treatment of indigestion, ascites, and edema, but found it contraindicated for "almost all the acute inflammations of the abdominal cavity, as acute peritonitis, typhilitis, round ulcer of the stomach, and appendicitis."[37]

Dr. Haehl provides a prescription for obese patients. "Obesity is a condition in which massage is often used as a sort of routine remedy. Some masseurs go even so far as to promise their patients an entire cure by massage treatment, without encroaching upon any of the patient's conveniences. This is, however, wrong. Restriction in diet, especially carbohydrates, fat and liquids is just as important as the mechanical treatment. The latter should consist in [sic] daily energetic massage of the abdomen, followed by Swedish movements of all conceivable kinds, particularly resisting motions. To this may be added a general massage every alternate day, plenty of exercise in the open air and mountain-climbing. The patient's weight should be taken once a week, in which time he should not lose more than about 2 pounds."[38] You can imagine how long an obese person would have to remain under the care of the doctor losing weight at that rate.

Also included in Dr. Haehl's list of treatment by massage are migraines, those caused by "dilatation of the branches of the carotid artery and congestion," with neck massage. If caused by "anaemia or nervousness," massage of the frontal, temporal, scalp, and cervical areas is recommended. But "a great deal of caution" is suggested "in hysterical cases" to prevent the onset of a "hypnotic condition." Massage was used to alleviate writer's cramp, telegrapher's cramp, piano player's cramp, spasms in the calf—to all massage gives "quick and prompt relief when effleurage, petrissage and tapotement are used." Sciatica was well treated with massage by German physicians, as was lumbago. But acute rheumatism "at first sight seems to be a disease in which massage could do wonders. This is not the case. . . . Chronic muscular rheumatism, however, can be greatly benefited by a systematic massage treatment."[39]

And in surgery, Dr. Haehl says, "The diseases and conditions in the domain of surgery, in which the most beneficial results can be obtained are: Inflammations, contusions, joint diseases, especially chronic synovitis, tendon diseases, distortions, tendencies to contractions, sprains, dislocations, and fractures."[40] Haehl is very progressive in his claims for massage in these areas, because they were usually considered contraindications. Although he doesn't describe the techniques used in these cases, it would appear that his knowledge must have included massage of the surrounding areas in the cases of inflammation, joint diseases, and fractures.

W. R. Latson, a New York physician and editor of *Health-Culture Magazine*, wrote a book entitled *Common Disorders with Rational Methods of Treatment including Diet, Exercise, Massotherapy, Baths, Etc.* Latson told his audience that massage was a substitute for exercise.

> Is there no other means by which the same results as regards the nourishment of the body may be attained without such muscular exertion as would be a dangerous tax upon a patient of lowered vitality?
>
> The question can be answered in the affirmative. In massage we have an agency which does for the tissues all, and in some respects more than mere muscular contraction can do. Proper massage, in addition to

normal diet and full breathing, will give results in improved nutrition which are obtainable by no other means.[41]

A popular book of this time was *The Care and Feeding of Children,* a small book by New York physician Emmett Holt. Another such book, *Advice to a Mother on the Management of Her Children and on the Treatment of the Moment of Some of Their More Pressing Illnesses and Accidents,* was written by English physician Pye Henry Chavasse. Originally published in 1868, this book was very popular in Britain and the United States. It answers mothers' concerns in a question-and-answer format. Question twelve asks: "Perhaps you will kindly recapitulate, and give me further advice on the subject of the ablution [washing] of my babe?" The answer advises details about the water temperature and states, "When he is thoroughly dried with warm dry towels, let him be well rubbed with the warm hand of the mother or of the nurse. As I previously recommended, while drying him and while rubbing him, let him repose and kick and stretch either on the warm flannel apron, or else on a small blanket placed on the lap."[42] For abdominal aches and pains the doctor recommends rubbing with "castor oil, or Dr. Merriman's Purgative Liniment, well rubbed every morning, for ten minutes at a time, over the region of the bowels," and "warm olive oil, well rubbed, for a quarter of an hour at a time, by means of the warm hand, over the bowels, will frequently give relief" for flatulence or excessive gas.[43]

Many magazine columns giving advice not only to mothers, but to all women on a wide range of social issues, were very popular during this period, and a few contain references to massage such as that above.

The People's Medical Advisor, published by the World's Dispensary Printing Office and Bindery in Buffalo, New York, was one of many ventures of a group of physicians and surgeons working in association with U.S. Congressman R. V. Pierce, M.D. *The Medical Advisor,* one of the first attempts to provide the general public with medical information on a substantive scale, covered physiology, anatomy, hygiene, temperaments, diseases, and domestic remedies. The section on human temperaments included an extensive section on marriage, procreation, and raising healthy and happy children. The book also covered hydrotherapeutic methods, such as cold, cool, temperate, tepid, warm, hot, Russian, and Turkish baths, as well as spirit vapor baths, sea bathing, shower bath, douche and sponge baths, foot, sitz, head, medicated, alkaline, acid, iodine, sulfur, and sulfur vapor baths. Massage is mentioned briefly, but it is used synonymously with the terms *shampooing* and *rubbing* when it is mentioned. A section on "The Turkish Bath and How it is Used" in *The People's Medical Advisor* reads in part:

> The Turkish Bath is a dry, hot-air bath. The bather passes from one apartment to another, each one being of a higher temperature than the preceding. He undergoes a thorough shampooing, and, although the person may be scrupulously clean, he will be astonished at the amount of effete matter removed by this process. . . . Lying upon a warm marble slab, *massage* is applied most thoroughly to every portion of the body.

Women as a new audience for exercise and massage

For one hundred years women strived to gain acceptance as equal citizens in the United States. From 1880 when the battle reached its zenith to 1920 when Congress passed a suffrage amendment to the constitution, many commercial companies adopted the pro-suffrage stance by marketing their products to the growing female audiences in America and Europe. Not only products but lifestyles were promoted; the following short article that ran in the March 1891 issue of *Ladies's Home Journal* is indicative of how women were being told they could exercise, get massage, and be self-sufficient without succumbing to preconceptions about being weak and feebleminded. This type of article also served to help women join the ranks of the nursing profession and learn about how they could help those in need. The article, entitled "Gymnastic Exercises for Women," reads as follows:

"Light gymnastics embrace the use of dumb-bells, barbells, Indian-clubs, wands, hoops and exercises without anything whatever in the hands. Marching, deep-breathing movements, poising, stretching and equilibrium exercises, all of which have, in a great measure, grown out of the Delsarte system, also come under the general term, light gymnastics. The beneficial results of all these are many and varied. Hardly any one is too weak for gymnastics. Gentle massage will start the muscles and send the blood into healthy circulation. Then the patient should help herself. One of the advantages of light gymnastics is that the sick and convalescent can make what appear to be trifling efforts, and by them, in time, be restored to active health. If too feeble to be practically able to make but little exertion, try what are known as deep-breathing movements. Lie flat upon the back, take as long and as deep breaths as possible, and while the mouth is closed, slowly throw the arms up in front and then at the sides. Rest for ten minutes. Try again the same inhalation and exhalation of air, the latter being pure and fresh. After awhile, attempt the same, sitting up. These exercises can safely be taken by the sick one every day, several times, and the whole muscular system will be improved, just as if some revivifying tonic had been given, a far better one than any charged with alcohol or some like stimulant."

The Delsarte system refers to a German method of calisthenic exercises used throughout Europe in schools and in military training. The "gymnastics" exercises were imported into the United States, primarily to the great sanitariums, where the wealthy would go for diet, exercise, and healthy lifestyle treatments. It is interesting to note the recommendation in the article about massage not as a means of giving relief from sore and tired muscles after exercise but as a way of warming the muscles by increasing circulation before exercise.

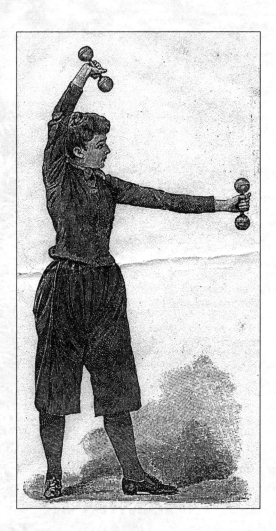

Graphic accompanying an article on exercise and massage for women from *Ladies's Home Journal,* March 1891.

By the *massage,* shampooing, or rubbing, the superficial veins are thoroughly emptied of their contents, the muscles are given elasticity and tone, and glandular activity is promoted. Innumerable dead epithelial cells, together with other impurities, are rolled off in flakes under the skillful manipulation of the attendant.

After a thorough shampooing, the shower bath is applied, to secure a contraction of the capillaries and a diminution of the perspiration.[44]

In the section entitled "Motion as a Remedial Agent" massage is once again mentioned, this time as "rubbing." It reads in part:

Rubbing is a process universally employed by physicians of every school for the relief of a great diversity of distressing symptoms, is instinctively resorted to by sympathizers and attendants upon the sick, and constitutes one of the chief duties of the nurse. Uncivilized people resort to this process as their principal remedy in all forms of disease.[45]

It must be noted that the authors of this book were alternative physicians, administering the rest cure and many other natural remedies before they would resort to drugs or surgical procedures. As such they must be considered out of the mainstream of medical practice. The section goes on to recommend both manual and mechanical rubbing; their preference, though, seems to be mechanical, as expressed in this statement: "The hands have not the power, by kneading, manipulating, or rubbing to impress the system except in a very mild degree, and deep-seated organs and parts are scarcely influenced by the comparatively slow movements thus administered."[46]

Early Massage Research

Part of the support for a scientific basis for massage came from research on its effects. The first rational approach to discovering the effects of massage were conducted by Hippocrates, who said that by ardent rubbing the body is hardened; if done gently, it is softened; if it is attenuated, the body is wasted, and if done moderately, the body is filled or enlarged.[47]

Asclepiades, a Greek physician who settled in Rome to practice and teach medicine just before the dawn of the Christian era, was also an advocate of massage and conducted years of anecdotal research into its effects on disease processes. Like Hippocrates, he used massage in mostly chronic cases, but also in the case of some acute conditions such as fevers, coughing, vomiting, and headaches. Asclepiades discovered that when one part is in pain it was helpful to rub another part of the body in order to "draw matter from the upper or middle parts of the body" by rubbing the extremities. Both of these great physicians conducted their research in the field of real disease processes; they used no laboratory except that afforded them by their suffering patients.

Keen observation was the first research method, followed by trial and error. Eventually clinical trials were conducted. The distance of time between these methods is great, clinical trials having been utilized only within the past hundred years. Despite some claims to the contrary, the efficacy of most medical practices of today has not been proved by clinical trials. Most medical procedures are based on the tried-and-true methods of observation and trial and error.

Many a writer discussing the beneficial effects of massage on specific disease processes bases his or her recommendations on these traditional methods. Only in the past decade or so have scientific clinical trials been conducted to demonstrate the efficacy of massage as a treatment modality. The proof of its value, though, rests solidly upon centuries of observation and trial-and-error experience that have discovered how and why it works. The contribution of modern research is primarily that of convincing the medical community of its efficacy as a treatment modality, while confirming what the rest of us already know about massage.

From Hippocrates to Walter Johnson in 1866, clinical results were presented via the case history method. The details of the case history provide an inside look at the symptoms presented, the diagnosis, the treatment applied, and the ensuing results. Galen wrote extensive case histories that read like the strictest clinical notebook. Johnson provides several chapters of case history spanning several decades of experience.

Among the first to conduct clinical experiments to test the effectiveness of massage in the treatment of disease were two women physicians, Drs. Jacobi and White. Their findings, published first in the *Archives of Medicine Journal* in 1880, were later presented as a medical monograph.

Dr. Kellogg also conducted research into massage as early as the 1870s at the Battle Creek Sanitarium facility. His results were published in several medical journals and eventually ended up as practical advice in his 1895 book, *The Art of Massage*. Kellogg says his experiments "repeated and verified," the "numerous investigations by able physiologists for the purpose of determining with exactness the physiological effects of various procedures included under the general term *massage*."[48] Kellogg goes on to explain each of the findings in his experiments. Although the effects of massage that he lists are not altogether new, they are, he asserts, based on sound scientific experiments in his physiological laboratory. "The various effects produced may be included under the following heads: Mechanical, Reflex, Metabolic. . . ." He then lists the effects on the nervous system as, "Direct Stimulating Effects . . . Reflex Effects . . . Sedative Effects . . . Restorative or Reconstructive Effects" and goes on to describe the effects of massage on the muscles, bones, ligaments, circulation, respiration, heat functions of the body, nutrition, and so forth.[49] Kellogg doesn't provide us with the details of his experiments in the book, but the massage textbooks written for the next sixty years continued in large measure to describe the effects of massage just as Kellogg had done. More is known today about the systems of the body, but little has changed about our understanding of the effects of massage on them. Since Kellogg's time this kind of information has become less relevant because today's practitioner is more interested in learning how do to a technique than the science behind how and why it works.

William Murrell, in *Massage as a Mode of Treatment* (1886), cites the work of several physicians as examples of "painstaking observations." He gives examples of several "experiments" to demonstrate, as he puts it, "exactly how these results are obtained. It is easy to theorise, but we want carefully observed facts and accurately recorded experiments."[50] He recounts an experiment conducted by a Dr. Gopadze on four medical students. We are not told whether the students were ill or healthy, or why the experiment was done.

Murrell writes, the "students . . . were kept in the hospital, and subjected to systematic massage for twenty minutes or more daily. The operation commenced with effleurage beginning at the extremities and working upwards. This was followed by petrissage, friction and tapotement, ending up with a second effleurage. In each case the appetite was decidedly improved, the patient—or victim—taking more food than usual, not only during the week that the operations were performed, but during the subsequent week as well. In the massage week two of the subjects gained slightly in weight, whilst the other two lost, but in the week following, that in which massage was resorted to, all four gained notably. It was found that the temperature in the axilla fell for above half an hour after each rubbing, but never more than half a degree. It then rose steadily, and an hour later was generally a degree higher than at the commencement of the se'ance [*sic*]. The respirations were always increased in frequency, and were deeper and fuller. The effect on the pulse varied with the kind of massage employed. With surface effleurage carried on lightly, the pulse became more frequent, but under the influence of petrissage it was rendered slower."[51]

The example that is perhaps the closest of those given by Murrell to an actual clinical experiment is the work of a German physician, J. Zabludowski, and Professor Von Mosengeil. About the latter Murrell writes, "He took a number of rabbits and injected into the knee-joints a syringeful of Indian ink. Massage was performed at intervals on the right knee, but the left was left untouched. At the expiration of twenty-four hours or more the animals were killed, and the tissues on both sides were carefully examined. The left knee-joints were distended with fluid, whilst on the right side which had been manipulated it had entirely disappeared. The lymphatic glands on the right were full of particles of Indian ink, whilst the corresponding glands on the untreated side remained unaltered. The differences were so marked as to be visible to the naked eye. The conclusion arrived at as the result of these, and a number of similar observations, was that massage promoted absorption by the lymphatics. It is probably in this way that effusions and other morbid products are removed."[52]

Although experiments on humans and animals had been conducted in the early part of the century—primarily on the effects of electrical current on the muscles and nerves—the experiments described by Murrell were probably the first real attempts to verify with more modern physiological testing the vast body of knowledge that had been obtained by observation and trial and error. Most texts of massage at the time simply asserted the effects of massage and proceeded to demonstrate how to obtain them through the application of techniques without providing the scientific data to back up the claims.

Murrell's work was perhaps the first serious effort to communicate the experimental basis for massage to the medical community. It was widely accepted, and the initial small book of about 80 pages grew to more than 250 pages by 1890, with editions printed in both London and Philadelphia. Taylor, writing in 1887, compared the effects of massage with those of exercise and distinguished between remedial and hygienic intentions. The only limit he placed on massage seemed to be in those effects which are "outside the range of the natural powers of the human hand."[53]

One result of massage research was a more systematic understanding of when massage was contraindicated. Graham cites "Indications and Contra-Indications" in the subtitle to his book *Manual Therapeutics*. In his extensive coverage of massage used in the treatment of a variety of diseases and disorders, he intersperses a wealth of information about how to, how not to, and when and when not to do massage. Graham also for the first time presents information related to the practitioner's body mechanics. But his description of body mechanics seems in direct opposition to what we know today.

> Many do not know how to do the kneading or malaxation with ease and comfort to themselves and to their patients, for in place of working from their wrists and concentrating their energy in the muscles of their hands and forearms, they vigorously fix the muscles of their upper arms and shoulders, thus not only moving their own frame with every manipulation, but also that of their patients, giving to the latter a motion and sensation as if they were at sea in stormy weather. By this display of awkward and unnecessary energy not only do they soon tire themselves out and fancy that they have lost magnetism by imparting it to their patients, but by the too firm compression of the patient's tissues they are not allowed to glide over each other, and hence such a way of proceeding entirely fails of the object for which it is intended. Surely, cultivation is the economy of effort, and the most perfect art consists in acting so naturally that it does not appear to be any attempt at art at all.[54]

Like Murrell, Dr. Kleen cites the research of professors Von Mosengeil and Zabludowsky. But Kleen also provides research from two others not mentioned in earlier works. Ludwig, Kleen tells us, conducted experiments in his laboratory which have been duplicated by another scientist named Lassar. Their work demonstrates that "all manipulations which bring pressure to bear upon the tissues are effective, though to a less degree than centripetal strokings; since the lymph-vessels are, like the veins, provided with valves which permit a flow in a centripetal direction only."[55] Zabludowsky explains the initial increase in lymphatic flow and its subsequent decline this way: "The augmentation is due to the livelier circulation; the diminution results from the mechanical irritation of the nerves of the skin, and these two factors strive with each other for the upper hand."[56] Kleen reports that Von Mosengeil's experiment with the rabbits was duplicated by Sturm and Sallis, two other research physicians in Europe. Other experiments were conducted on rabbits to test the concepts of fluid flows in their circulatory and lymphatic systems. All seemed to confirm the effects of the basic massage strokes of effleurage, petrissage, vibration, and friction in this regard to varying degrees.

Kleen also offered a short chapter devoted to contraindications to massage in his book. A few examples exemplify those found elsewhere in the literature of the time.

> In the first place, for massage the skin must be fairly normal, and therefore it cannot be given in several skin conditions. Unhealed recent injuries or burns, erysipelas [swelling associated with fever], . . . certain forms of eczema, herpes, acne, boils and carbuncles, lymphangitis, and gangrene preclude the possibility of massage within their area.
>
> [Dr. Kleen adds this footnote.] After acne, boil, carbuncle, erysipelas, and other processes have run their course, leaving behind inflammatory products and thickenings in the skin, massage may be used to get rid of these.[57]

He continues:

> Some diseases and changes in the blood-vessels contra-indicate massage in their area; others call for great caution in its use. . . . Aneurysms might easily be broken by manipulation, and embolism follow. Advanced atheroma [a sebaceous cyst] forbids local manipulations, which might cause detachment of particles from the inner wall of an artery and otherwise cause injury. Marked varicosity of veins, with or without phleboliths, for similar and obvious reasons does not allow any of the stronger manipulations in the immediate neighborhood. (On the other hand, cautious effleurage may be of use in many cases of chronic phlebitis and periphlebitis, with their accompanying evils; of which more anon.) . . . Pregnancy I consider a definite contra-indication to abdominal massage. It is certainly stated that cautious massage, even of the uterus itself, may be performed without shortening or otherwise unfavourably affecting pregnancy. For practical reasons, however, it seems best even during the early months to regard this as a contra-indication; during the later months it seems a great mistake not to do so. . . . In recent fracture there is risk of moving the fragments in performing massage. Effleurage, which is recommended by some to produce absorption of exudation, must be performed centrally from the seat of fracture; in some cases it may be performed with great caution also over the seat of fracture. Recent unreduced dislocations contra-indicate massage over them, and I consider the proposal to massage in these cases (to make reduction easier) quite unwarranted. Such treatment

could only cause unnecessary pain for the patient and make reduction more difficult, since it is always easier the earlier it is performed.[58]

Anatomy and Physiology and Massage Instruction

Massage practitioners of the nineteenth century—even those working under a physician—rarely studied anatomy or physiology. Those areas of expertise were generally left to the supervising physician. A quick survey of the major books on exercise and massage of the time reveals the lack of emphasis on anatomy training for gymnasts, masseuses, and masseurs. Wanting better-trained practitioners, it was the physicians who emphasized the need for some training in anatomy to at least familiarize manual practitioners with some general anatomical terms and landmarks. Among the most important books written on massage and the Swedish gymnastic system, only those of Taylor, Kellogg, and Kleen provided instruction in anatomy and physiology. Massage techniques were seldom related to anatomy. The inclusion of anatomy and physiology training in massage programs did not begin in earnest until the mid-1920s.

The Greek term *anatomy* originally meant "to cut" or "to dissect." The study of anatomy was later divided into that of vegetal bodies (plants), comparative (animals), human (healthy bodies), and pathological (diseased human bodies). Human anatomy is further subdivided into three categories: general, descriptive, and surgical. General anatomy covers epithelial tissues, such as mucous membranes, epidermis, and glands, as well as muscular tissues, nervous tissues, and connective tissues, including elastic, adipose, cartilage, white fibrous, and bone. Descriptive anatomy covers the territory of organs as they are arranged into systems, such as osteology, syndesmology, myology, angiology, neurology, and splanchnology. Finally, surgical anatomy is the study of the organs' positions relative to one another and their surrounding parts.

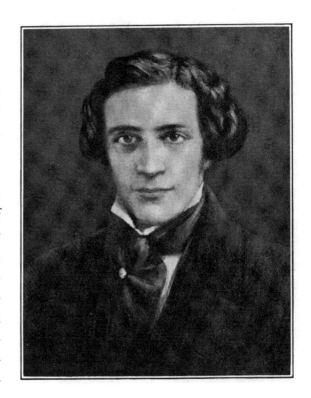

Dr. Henry Gray (1827–1861), an English physician and author of *Gray's Anatomy*.

While anatomy is the study of structures, physiology is the study of function in living organisms. Physiology studies the internal systems of the body, such the as circulatory, respiratory, digestive, reproductive, and endocrine systems.

One of the most enduring books of anatomy—*Handbook of Anatomy*—was originally published in Great Britain in 1889 and reprinted numerous times until its last edition in 1936. It covered visceral, surgical, and even dental anatomy. The authors, Drs. James Young and George Miller, were professors at the University of Pennsylvania and Jefferson Medical College, respectively.

The most widely known text of anatomy—*Anatomy of the Human Body* by Henry Gray—is known simply as *Gray's Anatomy*. In 1845 Gray began medical studies at St. George's Hospital in London and learned anatomy primarily through human

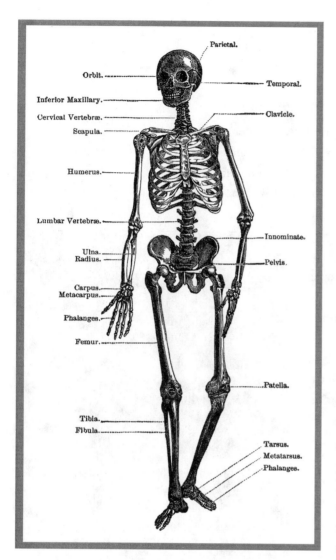

The skeleton, from an 1884 elementary textbook of physiology and hygiene. The book lists 28 skull bones, 52 bones of the trunk, 64 bones of the upper limbs, and 62 bones of the lower limbs for a total of 206. From *The Human Body and Its Health* by William T. Smith, M.D. (New York, 1884).

dissection. He was successful in publishing several papers of his anatomical studies in 1848 and 1852. Gray was both the curator of the museum at St. George's and a lecturer in anatomy; his career was cut short by smallpox, which killed him at the age of thirty-four. The first edition of *Gray's Anatomy* was published in 1858, a second in 1860. Much of its success was due to the quality of its illustrations, rendered by Gray's friend and colleague, H. Vandyke Carter, M.D. The first *Gray's Anatomy* featured 750 pages with 363 illustrations. In the ensuing years, various editors have continued to update the original body of anatomical knowledge with the latest findings of science, while maintaining Gray's presentation style. Later editions contain more than 1,600 pages and more than 1,300 illustrations.

The English physician Mathias M. Roth, writing in his 1851 book, *The Prevention and Cure of Disease by Movements,* makes no mention of anatomy but he does begin the book with a quote from another physician, Dr. Londe, which reads, "It is not enough for the physician to know that bodily movement is useful in a disease, but he must also be enlightened by physiology, in order to be able to prescribe what kind of movement must be used. . . . If he has not this indispensable knowledge, his remedy may become very dangerous, and will always be imperfect in its results."[59] This comment reveals something about the state of medical training of the times. There were no standards of education in anatomy and physiology, even in medical schools. Standardized education in American medical training institutions did not come about until after 1918.

Roth provides numerous other statements in his introduction which support the need for training in anatomy and physiology for movement cure practitioners. Most of these remarks are directed at institutions that teach gymnastic movements but provide no training in anatomy and physiology.

In Dr. George Taylor's *Health by Exercise*, anatomy and physiology are mentioned as the underlying principles upon which health by exercise is founded. He provided scientific principles from anatomy and physiology in his discussion of exercises as well as adding chapters on the history of exercise, hygiene, and hydrotherapy. His is the most complete picture of the system of movement cure yet written. Dr. Taylor took his work in *Health by Exercise* to another dimension when he wrote another book in 1887 simply titled *Massage*. In it, he clearly places massage in a category never before found in medical or movement cure literature, and he does so based on anatomy and physiology and the evolving sciences of neurology and motor-energy.

By localizing massage and concentrating the physical impressions at some special region of the body, the nutritive response becomes correspondingly localized. . . . Manual massage is much used remedially in affections of the nervous system, functional and organic . . . massage is easily . . . applied as to produce gradual division of separation, to the extent of destroying marked adhesions . . . No remedial effects should be expected of manual massage, either in degree or kind, that are outside the range of the natural powers of the human hand. The source of the operator's capacity for expenditure lies in the capacity of his vital system to evolve energy.[60]

Throughout the book Taylor provides no anatomy and physiology instruction, but does continually refer to the principles espoused above.

Emil Kleen's *Handbook of Massage* was translated from Swedish into English and German. Dr. Kleen's book is addressed primarily to physicians, evidenced by the many remarks against the "common" or "mere" masseur. The book is founded upon anatomical and physiological principles but does not provide any anatomical instruction. The physiological orientation is decidedly prevalent in discussions of the many diseases and disorders treated by massage. Dr. Kleen also provides an entire chapter on the contraindications to massage, something only mentioned briefly, if at all, by previous authors.[61]

The first text to address the anatomy and physiology of the human body as it relates to the application of therapeutic massage was Dr. John Harvey Kellogg's *The Art of Massage*. The book was aimed primarily at nurses, particularly those in training at his sanitarium. It covers the therapeutic applications of massage, including its procedures and joint movements; mechanical massage; the rules of massage; structures especially pertinent to massage (skin, connective tissue, muscles, nerve trunks, and so forth); and muscle physiology, including an extensive chart of the nerve supply and actions of muscles. It also provides an extensive section on the physiological effects of massage and many case histories. It is certainly the prime example of the first real textbook on massage anywhere.

One section covers the subject of touch, a treatment not found in any other book. Accompanied by photographs, this section of the book describes the kinds of touch to be applied under varying circumstances. There are illustrations of massage techniques, along with schematics of the skeleton, ligaments, muscles, arteries and veins, and nerves, and even the lymphatic system. Kellogg's text was so comprehensive that it was used by a large number of massage schools in America until the late twentieth century.

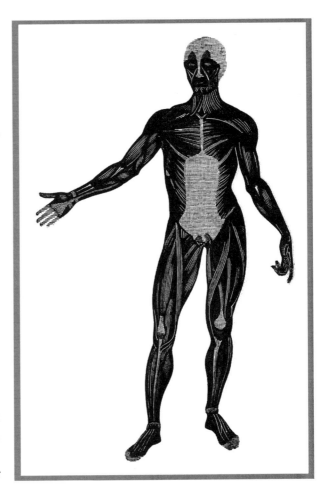

The muscle system. The caption to the graphic from this 1884 text reads: "The figure . . . gives a general representation of the muscular system." The author recommends that "a piece of fresh beef" provides a good example of the gross structures of voluntary muscles. From *The Human Body and Its Health* by William T. Smith, M.D. (New York, 1884).

Graphics from typical anatomical charts from the turn of the century; these became even more elaborate during the first two decades of the twentieth century. Notice that the skin of the hand has been folded back to reveal the inner structures of bone and muscle. Some of the later versions of this style of presentation were multiple page fold-outs providing intricate details; most were used for high school and college courses. Circa 1896, from the author's collection.

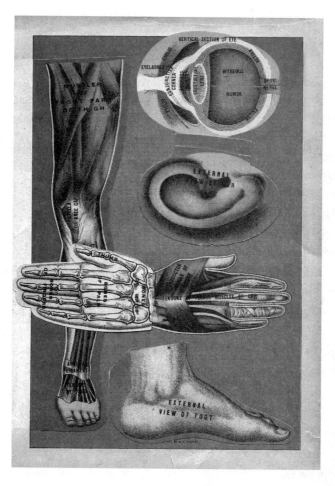

During the two decades following publication of Kellogg's book, numerous texts specifically designed to train massage operators in technique and the sciences were released, some of them no doubt the result of various articles in the medical literature calling for improved training in the manual therapies within medical colleges. This is interesting because, according to physicians such as Haehl, lectures were given in medical colleges regarding manual therapies but no classroom time was devoted to teaching it.

In 1884 William T. Smith, M.D., of Dartmouth Medical College in Hanover, New Hampshire, published an elementary text of physiology and hygiene entitled *The Human Body and Its Health*. The book was aimed directly at general college and nursing students. In the preface the author states the "little book" is an outline of the structures and functions of the human body. In one remark he states, "I have not mentioned the names of many of the muscles, because it is difficult and unnecessary to remember them."[62] The book covers the bones and joints; the muscles, blood, and lymphatics; respiration; and the nervous and sensory systems. There are nearly seventy illustrations; a few examples are provided here.

In *Manual Therapeutics* author Douglas Graham, M.D., offered an inspiring perspective on the value of the study of anatomy by massage practitioners. "A careful study of the structure of the human body, its contours and conformations, together with the most agreeable and efficacious manner of applying massage to it, results in proving that the Creator made the body to be manipulated and that He put it into the heart of man to devise massage as a means of arousing under-action of nerve, muscle, and circulation."[63] The natural theology expressed by Graham in this passage could be the rallying anthem of modern and ancient practitioners of the art of massage. Certainly the more a massage practitioner knows about the structure of the human body the better he or she can do the work. As knowledge of anatomy increased, massage tech-

MASSAGE IN

NINETEENTH-CENTURY

MEDICINE

niques became more clearly defined and described, directing the application of the art of massage to specific parts of the body to relieve the conditions from which it suffered.

Massage in Nursing

American nurse Minnie Goodnow, writing in 1916, reflects on the obscure history of nursing in ancient times in a way that bears directly on the history of massage. Caring for the helpless, hurt, and downtrodden was a common duty of those with compassionate hearts and the means to do it. These were not events that were written down as history; they were everyday occurrences, stemming from an instinctual source. "All men doubtless possess these instincts," she concludes, "until they lose them by indulgence in the abnormal habits that are the result of so-called 'civilization.'"[64] Goodnow taught her students an appreciation for the place of massage by emphasizing that the instinctual practices of people who care for the wounded and sick included nursing care, surgical procedure, medicinal preparations, and healing contact in the form of simple massage.[65] And that "nearly all primitive tribes practice massage in some form, with good results."[66] In shamanic/priestly traditions, the medicine man or shaman would determine a remedy and often have his assistant apply herbs, dressing, and relief from pain by massage. It is from these ancient traditions that nursing arose. Thereby, massage and nursing have—like massage and exercise—been joined throughout human history, but their joint stories were mostly unrecorded until each stood out on its own as a valuable and renowned therapeutic service.

Medical historians such as Sir William Osler (1921) and Walter Libby (1922) rarely mention the role of nursing in the history of medicine. Douglas Guthrie (1946), quoting Sir William Gull, does make one flattering statement on the subject, "Nursing, sometimes a trade, sometimes a profession, ought to be a religion."[67]

The first healing institutions were the temples of ancient civilizations. In China, "halls of healing" were established adjacent to the religious temples, and massage was a part of the treatment administered in these charitable establishments. In Egypt and Greece, people went to temples with their sickness or lameness more to pray to the temple gods than to seek healing care from other humans. But healing care was given, often by well-trained slaves under the direction of physicians. In Rome, philanthropic hospitals were established circa 225 B.C.E. where Greek physicians practiced their trade using mostly male attendants, but tendered their skills only to those thought to be curable.

Early in the Christian era the temples were utilized by the men and women of the Church to minister to the sick and wounded who could not get care from physicians, the latter wanting nothing to do with the penniless poor. With compassion and the spirit of their religion, the men and women of the Church nursed people with any kind of disease. Classical historian Peter Brown calls the early Christians' constant attention to healing an "obsessive compassion."[68] Zach Thomas, in his book, *Healing Touch, the Church's*

Forgotten Language, writes that "recipients of compassion were often those whom the Greek healing temples excluded, especially the dying. By the fourth century, Christians had established the first hospices and hospitals *(xenodochia),* sometimes in the remains of ancient temples. Christians also attended to the poor."[69] According to Thomas, healing touch in the Church can be "understood as an expression of a potential built into every one of us . . . This God-given capacity . . . develops naturally. We exercise heart/hand coordination whenever we communicate through touch the compassion we feel toward those receiving our care."[70]

As the disciples of Christ began organizing churches, deaconesses appeared. They were usually mature and widowed women who assisted the clergy. Included among their duties was nursing for the poor sick; over time their nursing duties became their primary job. In the example of their religious savior, their work was done in people's homes—thus emerged the first visiting nurses. It is believed that as the Christians established homes for the poor, sick, and orphaned, the deaconesses were in charge. Goodnow gives us an example of the women who were the first nurses circa 300 C.E.

> Paula [a friend of several well-known Roman Christian women who gave their time and resources to helping the poor and sick] . . . established hospitals in Rome and in Jerusalem. She was probably the first to train nurses systematically. An old English account, in quaintly vivid language, says of her: "She was marvellous, debonair, and piteous to them that were sick, and comforted them and served them right humbly; and gave them largely of such food as they asked. She laid their pillows aright and in point; and she rubbed their feet and boiled water to wash them."[71]

Unfortunately, little more than a century later the Church would abandon its idea of healing in terms of caring for the body, and the word *healing* would come to mean "save" instead, shifting the emphasis entirely to spiritual matters while ignoring the body and mind.[72]

No mention is made of massage in the history of nursing during the medieval period. This was a time of many wars, plagues, and religious fervor. It was women, especially women of the Church, who rushed without regard for their own safety to the aid of those who succumbed to the devastating effects of major epidemics in Europe. Medical care for wounded soldiers was practically nonexistent except that provided by so-called royal nurses. Several European queens used their station to provide at least some care to those suffering from the wounds of war and the plagues that besieged the growing population. From these royal efforts grew a brotherhood of male nurses, because it was considered improper for women to care for men unrelated to them. However, a number of religious orders that tended the sick included both men and women.

From the sixteenth to the middle of the nineteenth century the care and feeding of the poor sick received little attention. The Reformation—during which labor revolted against the feudal elite—forever altered the power position of the Church and those in it that had cared for the sick and poor. No longer was it a noble act to care for those less fortunate, especially when the Church had lost much of its wealth to the reformers' policies. Nursing care slipped back to its ancient ways, and only servants provided for the needs of the indigenous sick person. Certainly massage suffered as the profession of nursing fell into its darkest period. This is not to say there were no charity hospitals and other organizations operating during this time. St. Vincent de Paul and the Sisters of Charity began their work during the seventeenth century. But theirs was a harsh struggle and they were ill equipped to deal with the enormous numbers of needy. Even so, their examples spawned a tradition of charitable acts that continues today.

The Beginning of Modern Nursing

Modern instruction in nursing began during the middle of the nineteenth century, but it didn't come from hospitals, mainstream physicians, or even teaching institutions. Nurse training in modern times began in the tent wards found on the battlefield in the Crimean War from 1854 to 1857. No organized military institution existed to care for the wounded in 1854. Florence Nightingale (1820–1910) of England took it upon herself to provide nursing care to the wounded soldiers of the Crimean War, with little financial support and even less moral support from the powers that were. Her example sparked a new era in nursing still unfolding today. Although Nightingale is credited with establishing modern nursing practice, German pastor Theodor Fliedner (1800–1864) may have been the first to suggest that women should be trained in nursing. In 1833 he and his wife established a school specifically for that purpose in Germany. Florence Nightingale visited the school and modeled her English schools after Fliedner's.

In her *Notes on Nursing* published in 1859, Nightingale reveals her holistic approach to health care. She writes, "Shall we begin by taking it as a general principle—that all disease, at some period or other of its course, is more or less a reparative process, not necessarily accompanied with suffering: an effort of nature to remedy a process of poisoning or of decay, which has taken place weeks, months, sometimes years beforehand, unnoticed, the termination of the disease being then, while the antecedent process was going on, determined?"[73] In her writing about the benefits of fresh air, light, warmth, quiet, cleanliness, and diet, Florence Nightingale does not mention massage, but massage was included in her training school for nurses as early as 1860. L. A. Maule, writing in Cassell's *The Art and Science of Nursing* in 1907, informs us that student nurses were required to be proficient in thirteen skill areas. The fifth skill area is reported by Maule as friction of the body and extremities.[74]

Instruction written specifically for nurses on the subject of massage begins with Dr. John Harvey Kellogg's *The Art of Massage,* first published in 1895. His is the

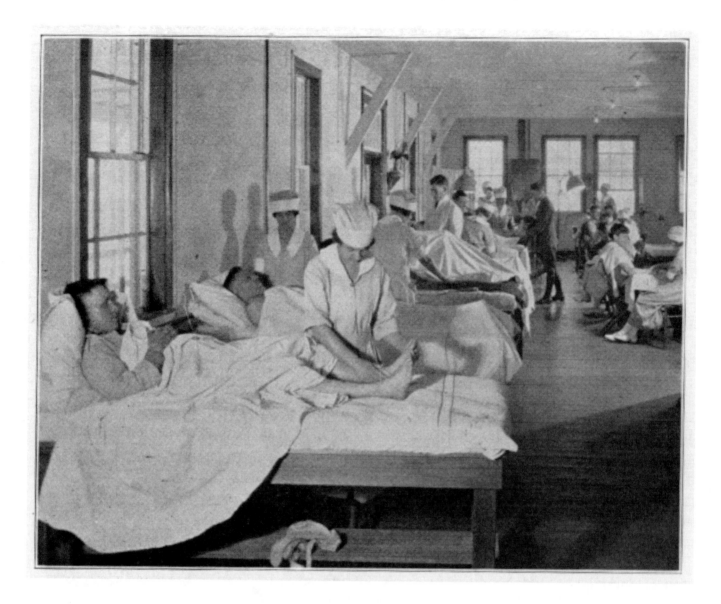

first true text on the subject because of its instruction in the techniques, effects, and applications of massage. He also included hygiene and contraindications and the sciences of anatomy and physiology.

In 1911 Irish practitioner Louisa Despard wrote an even more extensive textbook on massage. Her *Text-Book of Massage and Remedial Gymnastics* was very popular in English massage and gymnastic schools for thirty years, the third edition being published in 1932. Hers is also the largest volume of this period, with more than 450 pages of text and 222 illustrations. Her book was used in many English hospitals, where nurses were trained in massage technique. Despard's text compares very well with a modern-day book on the subject because it includes not only anatomy and physiology of each body system, but massage theory and practice as it was applied to a wide range of medical conditions proved effective during the time in which she wrote the book.[75]

German physician Robert Ziegenspeck's 1909 book was intended for those (obviously, nurses) who worked in the gynecology department of medical establishments. The book included considerable instruction in hygienic gymnastics, covering "percussion, chopping, compression, stroking, and even the simple laying on of hands."[76]

Nurse Nellie Macafee published a small book in 1920 called *Massage—An Elementary Text-book for Nurses*. The text was intended as a study guide for the Pennsylvania State Board of Registration for Nurses. Even though physicians were given no training in the practical aspects of massage, Macafee, like many others writing about massage for use in medical settings, claims at the outset of the text: "A general treatment of massage is never given without an order from the physician in charge of the case."[77] She provides a considerable amount of information related to the physiological effects of massage and its application to a range of diseases, such as lumbago, stiff neck, and sciatica, and for use after a leg or arm cast was removed. She also provides a section on the effects of working too long and too short a time on the patient, and other contraindications.

Nurse Mary McMillan, a woman I've dubbed the Mother of Massage in America, wrote *Massage and Therapeutic Exercise* in 1921. During World War I there was a high demand for women to work in army hospitals throughout America, as they had been doing in Europe. Mary McMillan's book was intended to teach practitioners in hospitals, in the military, and in private practice.[78] The first American physical therapist with a strong orientation toward massage, she served as the chief aide at Walter Reed Army Hospital after the war, and there helped to develop the Reconstruction Department of the United States Army, a program that included extensive use of massage treatments. Later, McMillan was director of physiotherapy at Harvard Medical School and a founder of the American Physical Therapy Association in 1921. Her influence spread across America, through Europe, and to China within the hospital establishments of her time.

Nurse McMillan's text integrated relevant anatomical and physiological information with procedures of massage and therapeutic exercise. Much of her instruction in massage technique is given in conjunction with the benefit of a physician's diagnosis, X-rays, and drugs that aid in the determination of a condition, such as joint stiffness. Hydrotherapy and other modalities are also integrated into the massage text.

Other texts available to teach nurses about massage came from other nurses,

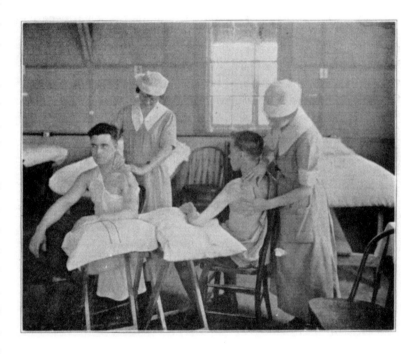

Massage for arm and shoulder injuries at an army barracks in America in 1923. From C. M. Sampson's *Physiotherapy Technic* (St. Louis, 1923).

physicians, physiotherapists, and nonmedical authors. From the on-the-job training provided in the sanitariums and health homes in the latter part of the nineteenth century to the complete texts of the early twentieth century, massage received more than ample coverage as a part of nursing training.

Nursing students were instructed in the art and science of massage between World Wars I and II as a standard part of nursing coursework. Nurses gave hospital patients back massages each night before they went to sleep, and massage was used as a remedy against bedsores. It was recognized in many hospitals that massage aided in the recovery from illness or surgery.

However, because of medical attitudes such as those expressed by C. M. Sampson, M.D., a contemporary of Nurse McMillan, massage gradually came to lose its place in nursing, and its status has been regained only recently. Sampson wrote, "Massage fills an important niche in any physical clinic and I would not attempt to do physiotherapy without it, but just as the ox cart was once the very best means of travel and still is a very sure means, although not so much used as formerly, it is no longer the very best way of accomplishing many of the things formerly given over to it almost exclusively. When it was the best known remedy for a given condition it was good therapy to make it the remedy of choice, but when advancement in knowledge of physics, biophysical or chemical reactions, appliances and technics [sic] for their proper use in producing them showed a better means of producing the desired reactions, then it ceased to be good therapy to use massage in place of the better procedure."[79]

Nurses in Massage

Through this section of the book the focus has been on massage in nursing, but the other side of this story is nurses involved in massage. This tradition began with Mary McMillan because she wasn't just a nurse who happened to do massage as a part of her nursing duties. McMillan was an advocate, teacher, and political activist on behalf of her belief in the value of manual therapies, massage being among her favorites.

Another massage advocate who happened to be a nurse was Maude Rawlins. Writing in 1933, she tells us that "about 1895, hospitals here and there in the United States conceived the idea that a few lessons in massage might be of value to nurses; so massage was adopted and six hours were devoted to the subject. As time went on, more and more hospitals added this short course to their curriculum. The hours were gradually increased to eight, then ten, where they remained until the close of the war when the New York State Nursing Department made it a compulsory, instead of a selective, course and demanded sixteen hours of elemental training in practical massage."[80] Rawlins book, *A Textbook of Massage for Nurses and Beginners,* was intended to provide this modicum of instruction.

Registered nurse Kathryn Jensen, having studied massage in Europe, wrote a text in 1932 for a course that provided more than "the seven classes in theory and seven laboratory periods" recommended by the National League of Nursing Education in that year. *Fundamentals in Massage for Students of Nursing* is addressed to both student and instructor, but the author's emphasis is clearly on the student learning the massage techniques. Jensen took her lesson from the institutions that taught massage in Europe during the late 1920s by including anatomy and physiology, emphasizing that the soft tissues should be noted on the body charts as the movements are practiced.[81]

Jensen especially wanted nurses to be trained in massage in the face of the trends of the time. She writes: "There is an effort by a small group in European countries to keep this branch of medicine, in practice as well as theory, in the hands of physicians."[82] She goes on to say there are two other groups with differing beliefs about who should practice massage—one that believes massage belongs in the hands of nurses, and the other, by far the larger group, that thinks it should be in the hands of specialists, neither nurse or physician.[83] In Jensen's remarks we see the first concrete hints of the emerging separation of massage from the medical field in America.

The legacy of Mary McMillan, Maude Rawlins, Kathryn Jensen, and others like them can be found today in the National Nurse Massage Therapists Association, established in the early 1990s, and the designation in that same decade of massage as an official nursing specialty within the nursing profession in America.

The emergence of massage from its historic connections to exercise, nursing, and medicine to a stand-alone therapeutic tool coincides with the advances of Western civilizations from predominantly agrarian cultures to a strong industrial base. Such advances in Western cultures have been accompanied by greater access to education, job opportunity, and the establishment of laws and equality.

Massage grew out of its integral relationship with other human activities to become an industry of its own, with advances in education, job opportunity, and practice development. And in both the advances of Western civilization and massage, the commercial aspects of a market-driven economy and representative government emerged as powerful influences.

Where before there was no organization of the massage field in terms of membership organizations and educational institutions, we find giant strides being made beginning at the turn of the twentieth century; perhaps most important, aside from the historic stance of massage standing on its own two feet, we find it being associated with a revolution in health and fitness in the new century. That association has further advanced its cause and its standing in the lives of many other cultures around the globe.

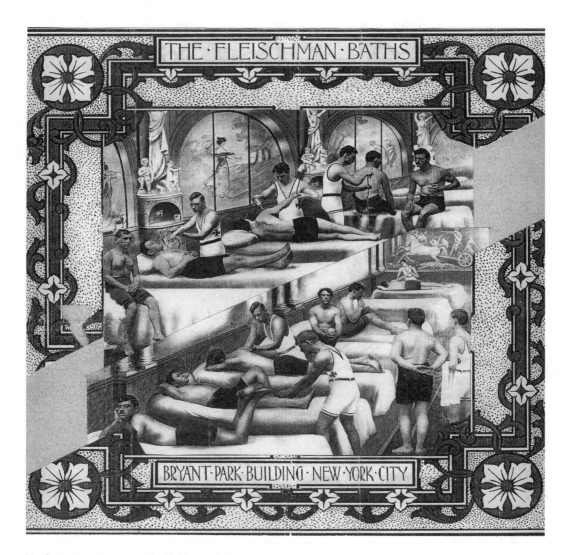

THE · FLEISCHMAN · BATHS

BRYANT · PARK · BUILDING · NEW · YORK · CITY

Men's treatment rooms at the Fleishman Baths, a private
New York club. Note the use of early 1900 electric vibrators
by the massage practitioners. The palatial surroundings re-
create the ancient Roman bath environment and the plush
decorative style of the late Victorian era. Collage created
from the National Museum of History, Smithsonian
Institute photographs. Courtesy of World of Massage
Museum.

8 Massage in Nineteenth-century Alternative Therapeutic and Restorative Cultures

In Europe and the United States, people living in the nineteenth century experienced a movement toward health and physical culture not seen since the days of the Greco-Roman period. For several decades, massage had a place in the gymnastic and movement cure systems and within some fringe circles of medicine. Exercise, including massage, became a way of fighting disease, getting and staying healthy, building the body to optimal health, and achieving beauty. Like with the gymnasiums in ancient Rome and Greece, indulging in the pleasures of spas, sanitariums, and similar institutions became a way of life espoused by the leading physicians. This gave rise to a plethora of health experts and treatment facilities, such as resorts, clubs, public baths, physical culture institutes, and health hotels, in addition to sanitariums and spas. While some physicians attempted with little success to assert the value of massage as a medical specialty, the practice and profession of massage was slowly growing within these alternative therapeutic and restorative cultures.

Health Publications at the Turn of the Century

Several publications that were founded in the late nineteenth century—notably *Physical Culture* magazine and *Hygeia: The Health Magazine*—were very popular. *Physical Culture* later produced *Physical Culture and Muscle Builder* magazine, and *Hygeia* eventually evolved into the *Journal of the American Medical Association,* or *JAMA,* as it is known today.

Articles and advertisements in these and other publications give clear evidence of the significant role of massage in the various types of treatment facilities. The October 1882 issue of *Popular Science Monthly* features an article by Douglas Graham, M.D., entitled "Massage: Its Mode of Application and Effects." The article is sixteen pages in length and contains much of the same material found in Graham's 1890 book. The very informative article covers a wide range of topics related to

The finger of a good rubber will descend upon an excited and painful nerve . . . as gently as dew upon the grass, but upon a torpid callosity as heavily as the hoof of an elephant. . . . The fingers of a good workman dart from spot to spot like flies upon the surface of a pool. They never stay long on the same place, but are here, there, and everywhere, now rubbing lightly, now pressing heavily, now coaxing an angry nerve, now digging into a refractory callosity.

—Walter Johnson, *The Anatriptic Art* (1866)

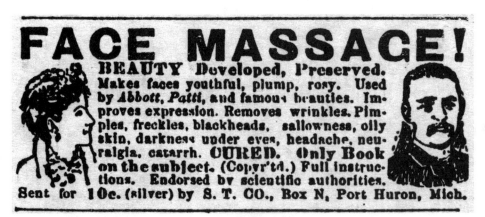

Advertisement for an instructional book on massage from the April 1891 issue of *Ladies Home Journal.*

massage, such as some of its history, its usefulness, its esteem in Europe and the United States among physicians, and its methods and effects. In the closing paragraph the author writes, "Discuss any therapeutical agent as we may, there is something still peculiar to each that evades expression by tongue or pen. Of what use is it to describe odors, tastes, sensations, sights, and sounds? They can only be comprehended by smelling, tasting, feeling, seeing, and hearing. Just so with the peculiar calm, soothing, restful, light feeling that so often results from massage, which can not be understood until experienced."[1]

A December 1891 issue of *The Medical Advance,* a monthly homeopathic magazine, displays a number of advertisements for sanitarium treatments. One, from Dr. Strong's Sanitarium in Saratoga Springs, New York, lists massage as one of its major treatment modalities.[2] An 1899 souvenir catalogue from the Mayfield Sanitarium in St. Louis, Missouri, lists the various treatments they offer. One section, entitled "Baths, Massage and Electricity," reads, "We have bath rooms on each floor for the accommodation of both ladies and gentlemen. Shower, needle and salt baths are given in the basement, two rooms specially constructed for that purpose, all of which are at the disposal of the patients and guests of the house. Massage treatment is given daily. We employ the best masseurs in the city and procure their services for half price for our patients."[3]

The newsmagazine of medicine, *Modern Medicine,* in October 1932 published a short newsbrief entitled "I Got Rhythm: Vascular Massage for Effusions, Circulatory Disturbances in Extremities." It reads in part: "Vascular massage, plus (1) gymnastic antics like bicycling or rolling over in bed without use of arms; (2) cold showers running up the legs to the spine, hot and cold foot-baths, alternately, and underwater massage (thermally stimulating hydrotherapies) & (3) medicines that dilate capillaries and arteries, are all cited and pinned with medals by F. Schede & E. Bettman, German M.D.'s, for gallant assistance in restoring order to circulatory disturbances of the extremities and chronic effusions of the knee joint, refractory customers when their etiology is unknown."[4]

From the June 1945 issue of *Physical Culture* magazine, with famed swimmer and actress Esther Williams on the cover, we can find an article entitled "Sciatica—Allopathy Fails—Drugless Methods Succeed."

Our family physician . . . explained that it was an inflammation of the large sciatic nerve . . . that no one had yet discovered the cause of these painful attacks and there was nothing he could do except to have me lie quietly in any position that was most nearly comfortable and to give me some easing tablets and some tablets to quiet my nerves. . . . Twelve miserable days and nights passed. . . . Both my legs had drawn so badly at the knees due to keeping them in a bent position so long, that I was unable to extend them out straight and the toes had drawn down and I hadn't enough muscular action to move them at all. . . . Finally we got an osteopath to come from a distant town and give me a treatment. . . . He pulled my legs in every direction and massaged the muscles. These exercises were followed by electrical massage which relieved the tension and helped to restore the tissue. . . . After the first treatment . . . I sat up on the bed and the next morning I stood up straight on my feet. It was little short of miraculous . . . Two days later I underwent a second treatment and . . . two weeks after the second treatment I made a 100 mile trip to the city, driving most of the way myself. . . . I can thankfully say I can still walk and work.[5]

Many of the advertisements in these health publications offered readers sales jobs, business opportunities, or schools and colleges related to the health field. Some ads mentioned educational opportunities in nursing and chiropractic or offered training at sanitariums in hydrotherapy, gymnastics, or massage. Such ads often served as a means of gaining new employees. An example of a classified ad in *Physical Culture* reads: "Crane Sanitariums, Elmhurst, Ill. We offer four weeks' residence course in massage, hydrotherapy and gymnastics for men. Diplomas granted. Write for particulars." Another, placed by the Kneippe Sanatorium in Minneapolis, Minnesota, advertised "free books on health and vigorous manhood." Free publications from the Cleanliness Institute were available to readers of *Hygeia,* such as a small booklet entitled "The Book About Baths" that promoted baths as a way to gain energy, foster sleep, avoid sore muscles, and head off a cold. The institute also offered booklets on "A Cleaner House by 12 O'Clock" and "The Thirty Day Loveliness Test." Outrageous claims were also made during this period for a great number of remedies, including massage, such as in the advertisement pictured on page 142 entitled "Massage Your Way To Health!"

These publications also advertised health resorts, such as Crane Sanitariums, the Rose Valley Sanitarium in Media, Pennsylvania, the Dr. C. O. Sahler Sanitarium, Kingston-on-the-Hudson in New York, Wilderness Heights in Olalla, Washington, near Seattle, The Caldwell Health Home in Pasadena, California, Heald's Hygeian Home in Wilmington, Delaware, Dr. Galatian's Sanitarium in Baltimore, Maryland, the Binghamton Water-Cure in New York, and the International Health Resort established by Bernarr Macfadden, self-proclaimed father of physical culture and publisher of *Physical Culture* magazine. Most of the advertisements for health resorts promised quick and permanent relief from constipation, stomach troubles, nervousness, kidney diseases, general debility, high blood pressure, emaciation, and other chronic diseases.

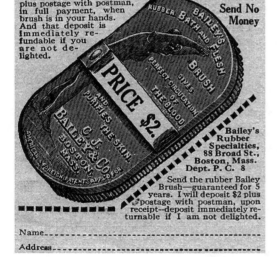

Massage *Your Way To* **Health!**

Dr. Edmund C. Gray, noted physical culture authority, writes: "*Massage* is one of the greatest natural curative agents. It benefits in cases glandular sluggishness, rheumatism, anaemia, tuberculosis, constipation: *banishes fat, builds tissue*: in fact, has an almost magical effect wherever *stronger circulation* is desired."

The Bailey Rubber Bath Brush

enables health seekers to give themselves professional massage with ease and privacy—*in the bath*. For over 40 years, physical culturists have used the Bailey Brush instead of the harsh bristle brush. The Bailey Brush is molded out of a solid block of pure red *rubber*. The 2000 tiny rubber studs stimulate with a *velvety* touch. Pores are purged of impurities. Fresh red blood races through your body. You glow with fiery youth from head to toes. Writes a user: "After using Bailey's Brush 3 months, I feel 100 times better and would not part with it." Raymond Nava, Austin, Tex. SEND NO MONEY. Simply mail the coupon. Bailey's Brush is *guaranteed for years*—but you need only deposit $2 plus postage with postman, in full payment, when brush is in your hands. And that deposit is immediately refundable if you are not delighted.

Send No Money

PRICE $2.

Bailey's Rubber Specialties, 88 Broad St., Boston, Mass. Dept. P. C. 8

Send the rubber Bailey Brush—guaranteed for 5 years. I will deposit $2 plus postage with postman, upon receipt—deposit immediately returnable if I am not delighted.

Name_____

Address_____

The Bailey Rubber Bath Brush espouses the virtues of massage as a curative agent. The ad goes so far as to claim that massage "in fact, has an almost magical effect wherever *stronger circulation* is desired" and that you can give yourself a "professional massage" with the Bailey Rubber Brush. Courtesy of World of Massage Museum.

A prominent example can be found in the full-page ads that promoted the "milk diet" created by Macfadden. While the rhetoric of the ads reads like the back of a magic elixir syrup bottle, it also mirrors the teachings of Hippocrates and Galen as well as the philosophy of many physicians and gymnasts writing about natural therapies during the first half of the nineteenth century. One ad reads, in part: "To-day [*sic*] any honest doctor of whatever school will tell you that nine-tenths of all effective medical or curative practice consists purely and simply in helping nature and that very, very few drugs have any real value as curative agents. The most that can be hoped for from drugs is to temporarily stay the progress of the disease. If nature does not seize upon the respite to begin active operations in casting out the ailment, the treatment is a failure, with valuable time and good money wasted. . . . In the final analysis it is you who must supply nature with the necessary assistance and that assistance must come in the form of increased physical vitality."

Sanitarium proponents and mainstream medical practitioners often demonstrated a mutual mistrust of one another's methods. Sanitarium publications were often dubious about the growing emphasis in the medical profession on drugs and surgery. The following is a typical comment from a sanitarium brochure of this period: "We do not use any one method of treatment alone, but a unique combination of all that is good in all systems, rejecting only crude drugs and surgery which we can positively prove only bring temporary results and are, in the end, really harmful."[6] On the other hand, mainstream physicians often were skeptical, if not derisory, about the care offered at sanitariums. In *Hygeia: The Health Magazine,* published by the American Medical Association (founded in 1846), we find an interesting exchange between a reader and the publication's editors. Both the question and the answer reveal something about the attitudes on both sides.

Sanatoriums, Good or Bad

To the Editor: My sister and I have been trying to find a sanatorium, to which we might go, where surgery and medicine are not advocated, but where physiotherapy treatments are scientifically administered; that is, massage, spinal manipulations, special diets and rest. We have been in correspondence with several institutions of this type, but they make such broad claims as to the beneficial results one could obtain by coming to their institution that we do not know which one would be the best, and we do not want to be fooled again. We are wondering if you could help us out.

I. G., New York

Answer: We know of no sanatorium which we could recommend that does not advise surgery or drugs when they are necessary. It would be most unwise to send any patient to such an institution. The most important asset of any sanatorium for the treatment of the sick is a staff of thoroughly competent, skilled and conscientious physicians, who are able to make accurate and thorough observations of the patient, a correct diagnosis, and to advise what is the best method of treatment. Often this includes methods of physical therapy, such as massage, passive movement and rest, but, in some cases, drugs may be indicated, and in other cases surgical measures are necessary. The physician in charge of the patient should be competent to determine which of these are indicated and must, if he is conscientious in the performance of his duty, advise such measures.

Any institution that advertises to cure illness by special methods and urges patients to patronize it is decidedly of the sort to be avoided.[7]

At this time physicians were loathe to advertise their services, and usually anyone who did so was considered less than professional and his treatments questionable.

Health Homes, Health Resorts, and Sanitariums

In the nineteenth century, health homes and sanitariums were very prevalent in the eastern United States, while spas, cure clinics, and resorts predominated in Europe. Health homes and the early hospitals were the first institutions that took medical care from its historical place in the home. The sick poor constituted most of patients in the few hospitals that existed prior to the turn of the century, while the wealthy typically had a variety of alternatives.

A health home was usually an inner-city facility, often a hotel-like hospital housed in a large home staffed by local practitioners, such as physicians, gymnasts, nurses, hydrotherapists, and massage specialists. Health homes typically did not accept contagious or infectious cases. More conveniently located than the more rural sanitariums, the health home was a private and often expensive retreat for the wealthy who wanted more personal care than that found in the larger and more crowded sanitariums, or at home, the traditional place of convalescence. The city homes and institutes tended to be more medically oriented toward drugs and surgery than sanitariums, which often provided a drugless therapy regime.

Other facilities provided exclusively homeopathic remedies for the treatment of all conditions. They were variously called retreats, homes for the insane, health resorts, and sanitoriums. To homeopathy was often added other natural healing methods, such as hydrotherapy, vegetarian or special diets, exercise, and plenty of fresh air, sunshine, and rest. There were also specialized institutes offering some of the most outrageous remedies, and from which more of a poor reputation was produced than real healing results. Unfortunately, massage practitioners who worked at these facilities

DR. E. P. MILLER'S

HOME OF HEALTH,

A full-page advertisement in *The New Illustrated Health Almanac* of 1873 shows a typical "home of health" found in many major cities in the United States in the late nineteenth century. The body of the text reads, in part: "This is the largest City Institution in the world devoted to the treatment of the sick by Hygienic agencies. The establishment comprises . . . the finest and best arranged Turkish Bath in the world [and] a fine Movement Room. . . . Room and board from $10.00 to $30.00 per week."

were often labeled with the same reputation as the institution for which they worked.

The major treatment facilities of the time were the health resorts and sanitariums that were typically located in rural settings with beautiful grounds. They emphasized natural healing methods and offered outdoor sports and games, an abundance of fresh air, delightful and invigorating climates, low rates, and good terms. Unlike the health homes, they welcomed those suffering from obstinate and stubborn diseases, having often begun as treatment centers for patients suffering from tuberculosis. True healing facilities, the earliest sanitariums were medical establishments staffed by physicians, nurses, and other medical specialists. The primary treatments were a combination of hydrotherapy, movement cure or gymnastics, wholesome food, fresh air, and rest. They also used therapeutic techniques, such as fasting, milk diets, fruito-vegeto cure (vegetarian or fruit diets), massage, Alpine light, violet ray and X-ray, diathermy, osteopathy, chiropractic, electrotherapy, gymnastics with and without apparatus, electronic and blood-washing treatments, and other curative methods. Massage practitioners in these facilities were at first primarily home or self-trained persons but, as these facilities broadened their programs, they began to hire trained personnel or educated personnel themselves. Administering massage was in many cases not a single occupation but a job that also entailed doing a wide variety of other tasks and applying other therapeutic modalities in these burgeoning places of health, happiness, hygiene, and business.

Over time, sanitariums evolved from purely medical establishments to natural retreats for relaxation and socializing. Although medical historians—particularly those writing about the history of hospitals in America—refer to sanitariums as quack establishments or ignore them completely, they flourished circa 1875 into the 1930s. Most were located in the northeastern and southeastern United States.

Dr. Strong's Sanitarium in Saratoga Springs, New York, was representative of the many sanitariums and health resorts built near hot springs. Established in 1855, it offered treatment and recreation, and especially promoted Turkish, Russian, Roman, sulfur, electro-thermal, and hydropathic baths, as well as the French douche.

Massage was also advertised, along with "Vacuum Treatment, Swedish Movements, Pneumatic Cabinet, Inhalations of Medicated, Compressed and Rarified Air, Electricity of various forms, Theramo-Cautery, Calisthenics, and Sun Parlor and Promenade on the roof."[8] Dr. Strong invited physicians and their families to visit the facility before recommending their patients to attend.

Another well-known sanitarium was founded by Dr. Henry Lindlahr and operated by him and his son Victor, who was also a physician as well as being an osteopath. Lindlahr Sanitarium was located in Elmhurst, Illinois, near Chicago. Like most sanitarium facilities of this era, Lindlahr advertised its methods as being "thoroughly scientific systems of rational therapeutics." The sanitariums usually put together their own mixture of treatments into "a thoroughly eclectic system comprising the best in all of them,"[9] and nearly all espoused the "healing powers of Nature" as the ultimate health authority. One interesting brochure put it this way: "We have long urged, what some of the foremost medical men are now beginning to perceive, that there is no way of vicarious atonement for the violation of the laws of health—that only through obedience to these laws can health be regained."[10]

Some sanitariums published their own textbooks on the cure systems they'd developed. In addition to various books, the Lindlahr's published *America's Foremost Nature Cure Magazine, Radiant Health,* every three months. At one time their staff was nearly two hundred strong, with many notable persons such as Bernarr Macfadden, George Bernard Shaw, Sir Henry Lunn, and W. H. Anderschou offering their expertise. Exaggerated claims from their promotional literature, such as the statement: "Indeed it may be taken as an established rule that if we can not help you no one else can,"[11] have drawn criticism from medical historians:

In the Lindlahr brochure there is a section devoted to illustrating the necessity of their extensive diagnostic methods and giving examples of actual cases. One reads, "Another 'sciatica' which had vainly passed through the hands of 17 doctors. The lady had been drugged, serumized, massaged, manipulated, treated hydropathically, electrically and almost every other way to no purpose. Our incisive investigation revealed what the others had failed to observe—a broken femur."[12]

John Harvey Kellogg and the Battle Creek Sanitarium

Perhaps the most famous and successful sanitarium of the nineteenth century was the Battle Creek Sanitarium and Hospital Training School for Nurses. Originally named the Western Health Reform Institute in Battle Creek, the sanitarium was established in 1866 by Adventist church leader Prophetess Ellen White. Her vision for the facility came from two sources. During the first years of the 1860s she had visions showing her the health benefits of the water-cure treatments and of

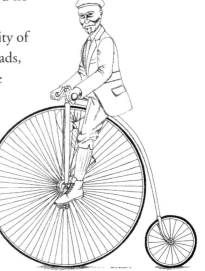

John Harvey Kellogg often rode a bicycle around the Battle Creek Sanitarium grounds. The story is that on some mornings John would be riding his bicycle while giving dictation to his brother as his brother ran alongside. Art by José Micaller, courtesy of *Massage Magazine.*

137

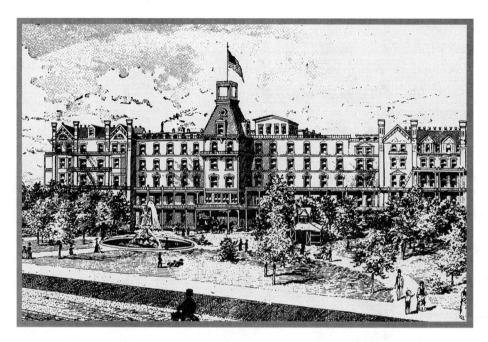

eating two meatless meals a day. A few years later she took her ailing husband to Dansville, New York, where Dr. James Jackson operated a health spa. Both their health conditions were greatly improved by the hydrotherapy, rest, sunshine, and controlled diet. This experience led Ellen White to another vision of an institution not only for Adventists, but one where anyone could be treated and taught to take care of themselves.

During the next decade the institute grew, popularizing its whole person healing methods aimed at the patient's spirit, body, and mind. Treatment included a nonalcoholic, nonsmoking, vegetarian diet, along with rest and sunshine, and sometimes drugs. Self-care was taught to patients as well. At that time the idea of a natural cure was quite revolutionary—even through the end of the Civil War, the normal course of medical practice included bloodletting, leeches, alcohol-based tonics, and high-risk surgeries usually performed by so-called physicians with little or no formal education. But at the Western Health Reform Institute all this was changed. In a publication by the Historical Society of Battle Creek we learn about their staff training. "The first nurses at the Institute were Adventist farm women who volunteered their time to do everything from chopping wood to administering massages. The Whites soon recognized the need for more thoroughly trained staff as well as for more professional administration."[13]

The parents of John Harvey Kellogg were friends of the Whites and were some of the earliest contributors to the new institute. Their son was in medical school when the Whites realized the needs of the institute. Having long-term goals, the Whites subsidized Kellogg's medical education, only to have him refuse their offer to be medical director of the institute upon his graduation because he wanted to write and do research. But he accepted their offer a year later, after spending time in Europe studying healing methods, and for the next sixty-seven years he was medical director of the facility. Kellogg made sweeping reforms to the institute, changing its name to the Battle Creek Medical and Surgical Sanitarium. It later became popularly known as "the San." At the time, *sanitarium* was a new word, altered from the original *sanitorium* by Kellogg, but today the two words are synonymous. He also changed the name of the monthly magazine of the institute from *Health Reformer* to *Good Health.*

Kellogg made improvements in the water cure and many other treatments, hired a professionally trained staff, and added surgical treatments. For reasons unclear, Kellogg seldom let it be known that the hospital accepted many charity cases into its care: nearly every history of the institute generally states that they did not accept charity cases but were only available to those with financial means and social or political status. However, not only was Kellogg generous in treating those without

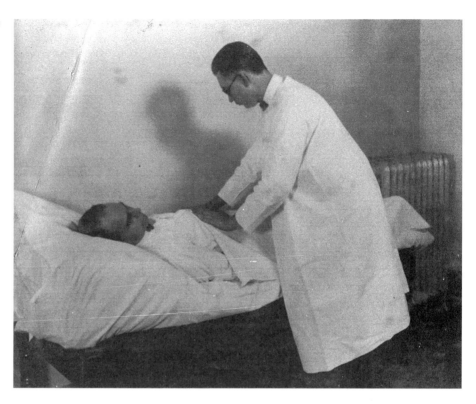

A physician administering abdominal massage to a patient at the Battle Creek Sanitarium. Note that the doctor is working upon sheets laid over the patient's midsection, not on his bare skin. Courtesy of Duff Stoltz, archives of the Battle Creek Sanitarium.

means, but he also created a nutritional program for undernourished children and their mothers in the community. Yet he was (unfairly) criticized for only serving wealthy and influential clients. One critic claims Kellogg wanted nothing to do with seriously ill patients, only "tired businessmen, sufferers from dyspepsia . . . and neurotics." But such harsh criticism seems misplaced considering the long history, vast clientele, and wide array of methods offered by the Battle Creek Sanitarium. Kellogg was merely a shrewd businessman who realized "the San" would benefit from having rich and influential patients to serve as magnets to draw others. Dr. Kellogg wanted to attract famous and wealthy patrons from around the world, and he did. Among many of those who came were Henry Ford, John D. Rockefeller, and Harvey Firestone.

During his tenure at the sanitarium Dr. Kellogg was an innovator in the fields of diet, exercise, hygiene, hydrotherapy, light therapy, and massage. Swedish massage was one of the many treatment modalities offered, and nurses in the sanitarium who performed massage were required to receive professional training in massage. Later Dr. Kellogg offered his own courses for massage and many other modalities used at the sanitarium.

The training school for nurses was established in 1883. "The Sanitarium nurse must not only understand the dressing of wounds, the putting on of bandages and splints, and the general care and handling of sick people, but must be skilled in massage, and thoroughly familiar with all the principles and methods of hydrotherapy— a subject by itself, and one of the most important branches of scientific medicine. . . . Massage, Manual and Mechanical Swedish Movements . . . must be studied and

John Harvey Kellogg on the history of massage

The masthead from the December 1887 issue of Kellogg's Battle Creek Sanitarium publication, *Good Health*. The issue featured an article on massage.

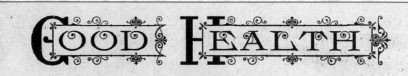

GOOD HEALTH

A JOURNAL OF HYGIENE.

MENS SANA IN CORPORE SANO.

Volume XXII.   BATTLE CREEK, MICH., DECEMBER, 1887.   Number 12.

MASSAGE.

SYSTEMATIC rubbing of the body or of diseased portions of it has been practiced from time immemorial, and among widely separated nations, in various parts of the world.

Alexander gathered at the royal tent the best Indian doctors, and proclaimed to the army that all who had been bitten must come there to be cured. These Indian doctors were in great repute. Illness was of un-

In the December 1887 issue of Kellogg's Battle Creek Sanitarium publication, *Good Health*, is an article entitled "Massage." The article states: "Systematic rubbing of the body or of diseased portions of it has been practiced from time immemorial, and among widely separated nations, in various parts of the world. In modern times this method of treatment is known as 'massage.'" The article goes on to quote an English writer who has translated "a German work on the history of massage, which will doubtless interest our readers. . . . In England a process of somewhat the same character is known as shampooing. It seems certain that massage was practiced by the Indians and the Chinese many centuries before the birth of our Saviour. It was combined with hygienic gymnastics . . . when Alexander the Great penetrated as far as India, in the year 337 B.C., his soldiers suffered much from the bites of serpents, for which no cure was known by the Greeks. Alexander gathered at the royal tent the best Indian doctors, and proclaimed to the army that all who had been bitten must come there to be cured. These Indian doctors were in great repute. . . . All who were sick resorted to the wise men, or Brahmans, who cured them by wonderful or, as they professed, supernatural means. It has been ascertained that massage and shampooing were among the remedies employed by them.

"The 'Law of Manou' prescribed diet, washing, baths, rubbing and anointing with oil, as religious exercises. . . . The gymnastic exercises of the Indians consist (1) of wrestling, (2) of what we would call boxing, (3) stick or sword exercise. They also practice movements for rendering the limbs supple, and manipulations of various sorts. Before the Indians begin their exercises, they cower on the earth, and by turns rub each other with mud from the delta of the Ganges. . . . All the muscles of their bodies are pressed and kneaded."

practiced until the technique of many hundreds of different applications has been learned."[14] Dr. Kellogg provided training for nurses to take care of themselves so that, as he said, "they may be in every way fitted for the arduous duties of the work which awaits them." The training program lasted three years, and all nurses at the Battle Creek Sanitarium were required to take six months of postgraduate courses in massage and related subjects.

A typical day at the sanitarium included morning gymnastics followed by prayer

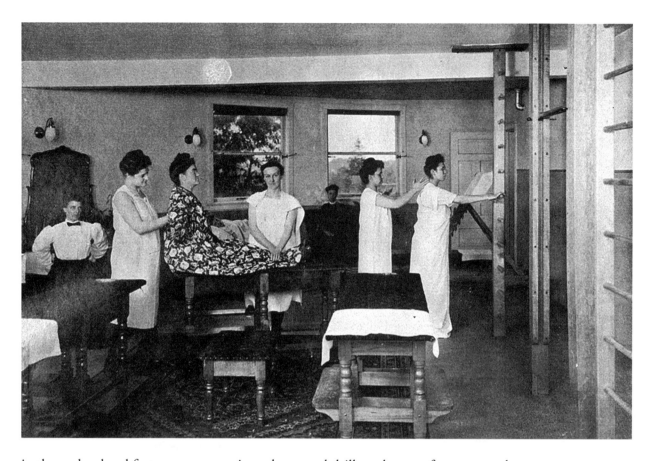

in the parlor, breakfast, more gymnasium classes and drills and games for some, and then dinner at noon. More gymnastics after lunch, prayer in the midafternoon, a presupper lecture, supper, and then more exercises, perhaps with Indian clubs or marching drills. A patient could swim or get a massage, bath, or other treatment depending upon his or her diagnosis and treatment plan. A massage session was listed under "special treatments" and cost $2 to $3. Colon massage and general massage were offered. Many of the exercise periods were performed to music, reportedly an innovation of Dr. Kellogg. The facility flourished until the depression began taking away most of the wealthy clients. The Battle Creek Sanitarium closed in 1938. Dr. Kellogg lived until 1942, when at the age of 91 he died of pneumonia.

Perhaps of all the physicians who wrote about massage in the late nineteenth century Kellogg was the most eccentric. He wrote a great number of articles and pamphlets as well as several books, and any idea he put forth in his books received wide circulation among the general public. His book has outlasted most others, even though most of his contemporaries who wrote about massage don't mention Kellogg or his work. Interestingly, some of the literature from the Battle Creek Sanitarium is displayed in the Museum of Questionable Medical Devices, located in Minneapolis, Minnesota. One of the items in the museum is a poster of the women's treatment area shown on here.

The women's treatment area at the Battle Creek Sanitarium. Like many sanitariums of the period, treatment facilities were separated by gender. Courtesy of Duff Stoltz, Archives of the Battle Creek Sanitarium.

MASSAGE IN

NINETEENTH-CENTURY

ALTERNATIVE THERAPEUTIC

CULTURES

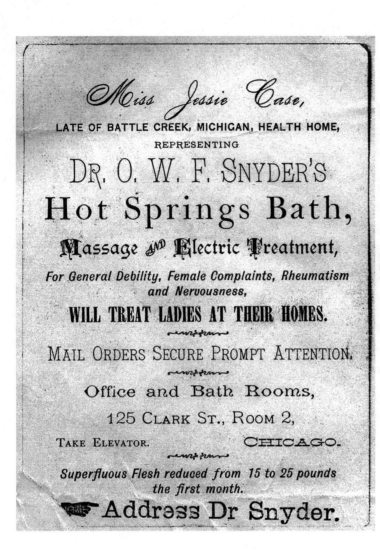

Spas and Hot Springs

Human beings have always placed a high value on natural spring water, both cold and hot. Many ancient settlements were established near springs and the water was often revered. The settlements were often named after religious deities, such as the city of Bath in England that was called Aquae Sulis by the Romans in honor of the goddess Sul Minerva. The baths there had been used long before the Romans arrived in the first century C.E. Whether the water was sulfur, carbonated, or plain, most natural springs were eventually developed into baths and then into spas.

Historically, massage has been closely associated with almost every facility that utilizes natural or domestic water in its therapeutic regimes. According to Jadi Campbell, "Information about spa treatments was dispersed mainly through military adventures and colonization. By the early 1800s French soldiers had brought massement ("rubbing the skin") back from Turkey to the court of Napoleon I, and Turkish baths suddenly appeared in Europe. Factory owners in Bradford, Barnsley, Sheffield, Leeds, Rotherham and Rochdale all provided Turkish baths for their workers. Turkish baths were even used at hospitals for the mentally ill."[15]

In the eighteenth century in both the United States and Europe, the spa began to reclaim its ancient place in human life. Like Karlovy Vary, better known as Karlsbad—a grand and famous spa in the former Czech Republic that the king of Bohemia, Karl IV, named after himself in 1347—the spas were established at sites that had been well known and used for centuries. By the nineteenth century spas were being well used by the wealthy and the elite. During the mid-1800s Sebastian Kneipp (1821–1897) developed Kneippism—holistic medicine emphasizing hydrotherapy. A priest, Kneipp treated patients for decades with his methods, and in 1890 established "the Central Kneipp Association, which made hydrotherapy famous worldwide."[16] During World War I spas were used as nursing stations in Europe, and in England wounded and shell-shocked soldiers were sent to spas to recuperate before being sent back to the front lines.

In nineteenth century England and in the southern regions of mainland Europe, spas were more popular than sanitariums. Sanitariums and health institutes focused

Miss Jessie Case, a former employee at the Battle Creek Sanitarium, advertises for services by a Dr. Snyder and herself. The date of this advertisement is 1865, as evidenced by the term "Health Home" when referring to the Battle Creek facility. Advertisement from *Chicago Daily News*, 1865.

primarily on healing the sick and feeble, while spas—serving mainly the affluent—aimed to please their clientele while offering them similar remedial means, including massage. The spas of Europe and the United States afforded healing in a relaxed and natural environment, which was

not so much medically oriented as it was aimed at relieving the new stresses of a world caught up in expansion and enormous growth. Many were located near hot springs or other waters that were considered to have healing qualities, or on the shores of lakes, such as Becks Hot Springs at the Great Salt Lake, Carson Hot Springs in the woods near Vancouver, Washington, or the Original Bath House in Mt. Clemens, Michigan. Competition eventually became quite fierce among the many mineral spring resorts and spas that sprang up during this time.

The healing waters were the true draw of these plush facilities, and massage was only a part of the wide menu of services offered, albeit an enjoyable and therapeutic one. Even so, the spas that grew out of the growing affluence and leisure time of the upper classes provided many opportunities for massage practitioners to hone their skills.

Over time spas evolved from facilities oriented primarily to curing the ill, catering to mostly wealthy and royal clientele, to places where common folks could rest and relax in a country setting. Treatments moved from rigorous regimes of exercise and very limited diets to games and sports and elaborate dining and drinking. Just like the Greek and Roman baths, the spas of the eighteenth and nineteenth centuries were places of culture, healing, public discourse, and the arts. Many sported spacious grand hotels, parks, concert halls, and facilities for gambling and drinking. Not since Greco-Roman times were spas enjoyed with such enthusiasm and by so many people. Most photographs of spas taken during the last quarter of the nineteenth century depict people gaily dressed, frolicking in the warm waters or sitting under an umbrella sipping sarsaparilla or lemonade on a sloping emerald green lawn, with a white Victorian-style resort house in the background.

Typical of any area rich in mineral springs, the Mt. Clemens area on the Clinton River in Michigan sported as many as a dozen spas at its peak in the late nineteenth

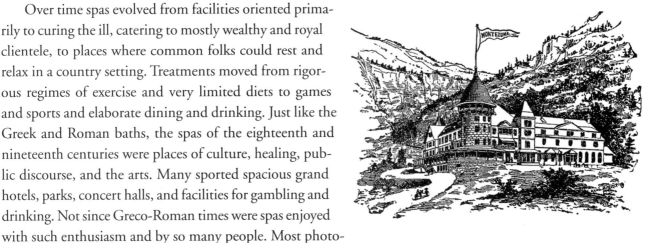

An advertisement for healing spring water available by mail from the 1869 edition of *Peterson's Ladies National Magazine.* Selling spring water was a new kind of business, driven by poor water quality in the cities and by the unbridled claims made for healing qualities of any new product.

The Las Vegas Hot Springs, located in New Mexico, about 40 hours from Chicago by train. This graphic accompanied an advertisement in the December 1891 edition of the *Medical Advance,* published in Chicago.

century. Among the most noteworthy were the Arethusa, Fountain, Colonial, Media, Park, St. Joseph, and the Plaza. Mt. Clemens became so popular it was known by some reports as the "Bath City of America." One entrepreneur bottled the famous water and sold it as "Clementine" water. An article about the Mt. Clemens baths describes the massage services offered at the baths in the early 1900s: "After a luxurious soak, the bather would undergo a vigorous massage, then be wrapped in heated over-sized towels and sent off to a lounge area, or solarium, to relax or nap."[17]

As early as 1865, hot springs facilities were being developed in the western United States, both in cities and remote areas. The facilities in cities such as San Francisco, Seattle, Portland, Denver, and Santa Fe were usually fashioned after those in the East, while those in remote areas of Utah, Montana, Wyoming, New Mexico, Oregon, and California were at first crude log structures or shanty hotels. The hot springs were first discovered by Native American peoples, who used them without building any permanent structures around them, but the white man, without regard for the Native American peoples or their cultures, built more and more elaborate structures at many hot springs throughout the United States and Canada. The spas of Europe during this time were mostly rebuilt upon the ruins of ancient facilities, but in the new frontier territories of the western United States and Canada, new buildings were established where only pristine forest or desert plains had existed before. Two of the oldest western United States hot spring developments were Wilbur Hot Springs and Harbin Hot Springs, both in northern California. In western Canada, Harrison Hot Springs, Fairmont, and many others were discovered in the late nineteenth century. Typical of hot springs in the western region, access was usually by horse or stagecoach. A log guest house or hotel was erected, and weary travelers often stopped by for a good-home cooked meal and a hot bath. Massage was added as the facilities grew to accommodate wealthy landowners, hunters, and tourists.

Most spas and hot springs advertised the healing qualities of their waters and were usually endorsed by a physician of some renown who recommended their special waters, touted for their ability to help cure diseases. Over time, the focus on the healing qualities of the water gave way to casinos, tourist attractions, and an extravagant range of treatments for body, mind, and spirit. The popularity of the spas and hot springs eventually attracted some establishments for gambling and prostitution near the end of the century.

Bathhouses

In the ever-expanding cities of the United States, spas often took the form of Turkish bathhouses. Robert King, writing about his hometown of Chicago, tells us that in the last decade of the nineteenth century and well into the twentieth there were public bathhouses and massage parlors in neighborhoods of that city. Evidently, because tubs and showers were a luxury only afforded by the wealthy, the bath houses emerged to serve the hygienic needs of the city's citizens. "The first free bath in Chicago," King tells us, "hardly more than a primitive group shower, opened in January of 1894. By 1910 more than 50 bathhouses were flourishing in the city, averaging some 30,000 patrons a year."[18] King's description of a Turkish bath reveals the ancient quality of these establishments. "Based on the original Greek and Roman baths and purification temples, many of the original Chicago bathhouses featured columns, fountains, cold baths, sleeping rooms, and circular pools. The classiest bathhouses also featured the Turkish steam bath, the oven fueled sauna, sometimes a gymnasium, and a private room where patrons received rubdowns, usually from a masseur or rubber, a designation only marginally different from the shampoos at the Turkish baths in England."[19] Massage was an essential part of the popular Turkish bath experience, such as at the Fleischman Baths in New York City, where mostly male practitioners worked on an exclusively male clientele.

However, massage practitioners working in spas, bathhouses, and Turkish bath facilities were much derided by those in the medical community who wrote about massage. The training for massage practitioners in such facilities was much less substantial than that required for those who worked in sanitariums or hospitals, as most were trained only within the bath facility itself. The city baths employed large numbers of European immigrants for cheap wages; the massage practitioners were often Irish or German women who had learned massage from their mothers or grandmothers or at a spa or health institute in their homeland.

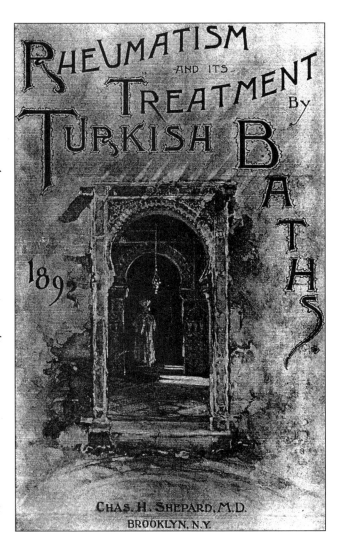

Charles A. Shepard, M.D., advertising his Turkish baths for treatment of rheumatism in the midtown facility of Brooklyn, New York (1892). From the journal *Medical Advance*, January 1892.

Public Baths: The Link Between Massage and Prostitution

The connection between massage and prostitution that continues even today began in ancient times, largely due to the association between massage and public baths. In the Roman empire the baths gradually transformed from civic institutions into citadels of debauchery. Toward the end of the Roman empire bathing became a social institution of immense proportions, which eventually deteriorated into "a cult of sensuality." Massage was an established part of the ancient public baths, and it was a part of the growing historic relationship between bathing and prostitution as well. Massage became associated with decadence and sensuality because it was being used in the baths no longer as a strictly therapeutic and relaxation tool, but one from which pleasures of the flesh were enjoyed. William Sanger, a noted historian on the subject, writes this:

> As early as the Augustan era [Rome around the time Jesus Christ was born] . . . the baths were regarded as little better than houses of prostitution under a respectable name. . . . In the early Roman baths, darkness, or, at best, a faint twilight reigned; and, besides, not only were the sexes separated, but old and young men were not allowed to bathe together. But after Sylla's [sic] wars [82 B.C.E.], though there were separate *sudaria* and *tepidaria* for the sexes, they could meet freely in the corridors and chambers, and any immorality short of actual prostitution could take place. . . . At a later period, cells were attached to the bath-houses, and young men and women kept on the premises, partly as bath attendants and partly as prostitutes. After the bath, the bathers, male and female, were rubbed down, kneaded, and anointed by these attendants. It would appear that women submitted to have this indecent service performed for them by men, and that health was not always the object sought, even by the Roman matrons.[20]

Reportedly emperor Elagabalus, who reigned from 218 to 222 C.E., gave a scolding lecture to male and female prostitutes rounded up from the local houses of prostitution and the baths. The growing decadence of the baths continued to draw sharp criticism, especially as more citizens and leaders began subscribing to the Christian doctrine.

Nearly every history of prostitution refers to the bathhouses of every age as centers of sensual enjoyment. Consider this terse statement by one medical historian: "Wine was prescribed as freely as massage, diet, and rest."[21] During the period from circa 476 to 1492 C.E., bathhouses could be found in nearly every city in western Europe. One author goes so far as to assert that every public bathhouse in the Middle Ages was a brothel.[22]

As in Europe, the institution of bathing also degenerated in the United States and other countries. For centuries in Japan the Yoshiwara (red light) district included many bathhouses, staffed by women called "shampooers" (a term that once meant one who does massage), that were considered low-class brothels. In the late nineteenth and early twentieth century the public baths in the cities of the United States came under the influence of corrupt public officials, and prostitutes were hired to offer more than massage services.

As cities started clamping down on parlor houses—the first brothels in the United States—and other locations where prostitutes plied their trade, such as saloons, restaurants, and hotels with sleeping rooms, prostitution was forced into "a hide-and-seek" game with authorities. Massage parlors arose from the bathhouses to serve as legal fronts for the continuation of prostitution. Eventually scandal arose, and the newspapers began calling the baths and certain massage parlors "dens of vice." About this same time there were also scandals associating massage and prostitution going on in New York, Philadelphia, and London.[23] Prostitutes fronting as masseuses were also common in Paris, and openly advertised their services in local newspapers. However, in 1926, Paris officials cracked down on this unseemly practice and forbid such advertising. This led to the separation of massage from prostitution in Paris, as prostitutes were housed in clubs and special houses and massage became regulated by professional associations and supervised by government officials.[24]

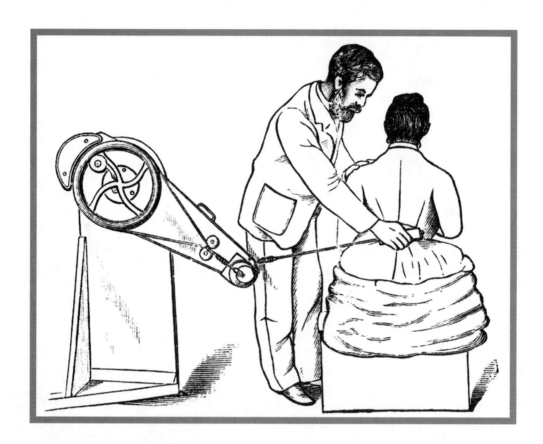

The first mechanical "vibrator," a portable device invented in 1886. The instrument was operated by manually cranking a handle attached to a large wheel, causing a camshaft to vibrate a cable. An end piece on the cable was applied to the patient. From *A Manual of Instruction for Giving Swedish Movement and Massage Treatment* by Hartvig Nissen (Philadelphia and London, 1889).

9 Massage Tools and Mediums

Manual Massage Devices

At the Freer Gallery of Art at the Smithsonian Museum of History, there is an object purported to be the oldest massage tool ever discovered. Although the obvious candidate for this distinction is the human hand, the object is identified as a Neolithic jade ritual blade from the Longshan culture of China, dating back to the Shang dynasty (circa 2000–1500 B.C.E.). "Scholars have suggested that it was a ritual healing tool related to massage stones—smooth stones that were heated and placed on tired muscles."[1] Despite the respectability of the source for this claim, staves or *strigils* are known to have been used to scrape oils from the body after anointing or massage in the cultures of Mesopotamia and Egypt more than a thousand years before the Shang dynasty.

The Byzantine physician Oribasius, born in 325 C.E., served as palace physician to the Roman emperor Julian. He saved many of the ancient writings of Greek and Roman origin that include references to massage implements and techniques. Quoting from Oribasius, Kamenetz tells us that "massage was administered in ancient times either with bare hands, with pieces of cloth of various textures, or with instruments. . . . Rough cloth was used to produce warmth; it drew blood to the treated area. The instruments were mostly long and thin, made of bone, wood, or metal. Staves, or ferules, were straight; strigils were curved. . . . The ferule was probably used for tapping."[2] The strigil would have been used to remove excess oils after the bath and after massage, as well as to clean the skin of its dead epithelial layer.

"Among the ancients," says nineteenth-century physician Reveille Parise, "the fact was generally recognized that friction with the strigil over the skin constituted a very appropriate means of maintaining the strength."[3] N. Dally, a French author of the nineteenth century, wrote that during the time of the first Olympic games (776 B.C.E.) strigils were used "for removing the oil before exercise, especially since it

Mechanical massage may be advantageously used as a substitute for a number of the procedures of manual massage. I have, however, found no device quite equal to the human hand, for the administration of kneading movements. Shaking and vibratory movements, on the other hand, may be applied more efficiently by apparatus than by hand in cases requiring vigorous and prolonged application.

—John Harvey Kellogg, M.D.,
The Art of Massage (1895)

149

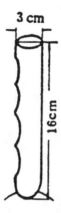

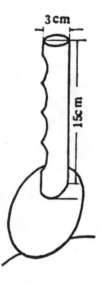

This image shows a "fingertip club" with a flattened tip held in one hand and the end placed on the area to be worked. The tool is moved in a rotary motion to knead the underlying muscles with gentle pressure, gradually moving to stronger pressure.

This "palm-of-hand club" can be used with one or two hands and is applied in a kneading fashion on the muscles for the purpose of relieving muscle or bone pain.

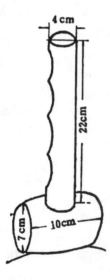

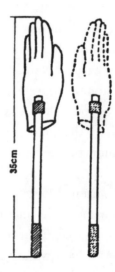

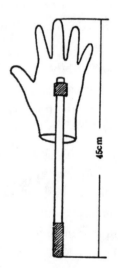

This "short club" is used on broad muscles over a large area and is helpful in treating muscular pain in the torso and limbs.

The chopping club is used for chopping or tapotement movements, using the edge of the hand for treating spasms in the back or limbs. Two chopping clubs can be used simultaneously.

This "patting club" is used for tapotement of large areas of the body, such as the back or abdomen and chest areas, for stiffness, indigestion, and congestion. Two clubs can be used simultaneously.

Five types of Chinese massage clubs are shown above. Of the more than a dozen books on the subject of Chinese massage, only the 1993 Pacific View Press book *Chinese Bodywork* includes photos and descriptions of these unusual tools. The book shows a total of thirteen Chinese massage clubs. From *Chinese Bodywork*, Berkeley, California, 1993.

collected the dust of the arena during the exercise period. In the baths, the rubbers used the strigil to scrape the skin following inunction" (a process of applying ointments to the body).[4] Dally believed the strigil originated in India; the geographer Strabo remarks that during the time of Alexander the Great, circa 300 B.C.E., the Indians used friction a great deal. "In the way of exercise," writes Strabo, "they think most highly of rubbing; and they polish their bodies smooth by ebony staves, and in other ways."[5]

Throughout history and in prehistoric shamanic/priestly traditions, various items have been used as tools for flagellation, including twigs, with or without leaves, and green nettles. Flagellation has been used after baths or sweat bath procedures for medical purposes, such as "against atrophy and emaciation," and, as Kamenetz adds, "for its erotogenic effects."[6]

According to William Murrell, a British physician, the ancient Chinese massage system utilized a variety of devices, including massage stones not unlike those still used today in spas around the world. The stones, usually jade, marble, or other dense stones, are either heated or chilled. They are placed on the patient to achieve a penetrating effect from the heat or cold, or they are used as manual massage tools to rub a specific area. A bundle of swan's feathers, lightly tied together, was used for tapotement. Numerous "massage clubs," such as "Finger Club . . . Palm-of-Hand Clubs . . . Arm Clubs . . . Elbow Clubs . . . Chopping Club . . . Patting Club" were used as substitutes for the arm, and to "supplement the therapist's physical strength."[7] Although modern clubs are made of plastic or rubber, older versions were fashioned from bamboo and mulberry wood. The wooden needle was also used as a substitute for the fingers in applying deep pressure.

Another device used by the Chinese is what they call a bat, constructed of lead wire, cotton, and rolls of bandage material. The lead wire is wound around the cotton to form a "bat," then the bandage material is wrapped around that.

The Chinese also used devices made from stone in a shape reminiscent of the brass knuckles used by gangsters for hundreds of years. But these stone knuckles were made for healing, not hurting. A jade pair in my collection were handcrafted in China an estimated one thousand years ago, according to experts who have examined them. This device is not cold like some stones and provides smooth movement when rubbed over the body. A modern manual massage tool, the Index Knobber II, is shaped much like the jade knuckles but with a protruding knob on one end.

At the Bishop Museum in Hawaii several artifacts of Hawaiian lomi-lomi massage are found. In the past, two devices—the Laau lomi-lomi and bath rubbers—were

A Chinese wooden needle, used instead of the fingers to dig into the body's pressure points.

Below: A Chinese bat, a portable tool for massage replacing the fist or hand to pat on the limb or body. From *The Home Hand-book of Domestic Hygiene and Rational Medicine* by John Harvey Kellogg, M.D. (London, 1899).

151

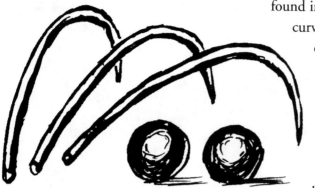

found in nearly every Hawaiian's home. The Laau lomi-lomi are curved sticks used in self-massage to work or scratch the back, or to apply pressure upon specific points. Lomi-lomi sticks, carved from the branch of the guava tree, are still available in some specialty shops in Hawaii. Commercial models, such as the Backnobber, Theracane, and Body Back Buddy are readily available. These are not only used by some practitioners but are also sold widely to the general public. The bath rubbers are balls of lava that were used before soap was brought to the Hawaiian Islands to clean the skin after a lomi-lomi session.

Hawaiian Laau lomi-lomi sticks are curved wooden sticks used for self-massage of the back, or for applying to specific pressure points. Originally the balls were lava rock used to clean or scrape the skin after a lomi-lomi session. From *Lomi-Lomi Hawaiian Massage* by Paul A. Lawrence (San Anselmo, 1980).

The Hawaiians also used "walking sticks" to support and balance themselves so that they could do a "walking massage" upon their subject. While walking up and down upon the prone person, they would control the pressure and keep their balance by the use of sticks or bars secured at the sides of the area. Or they would secure a single bar, usually bamboo, above their head so they could hold it while walking on the person.

A number of more sophisticated massage "instruments" were developed in Europe and the United States during the eighteenth century. The skin was rubbed with a flesh-brush, or with gloves made of hair or coarse woolen yarn. A very popular product called the "Carved Horse Hair Flesh Brush" was made by the J. J. Adams Company of Brooklyn, New York. The brush was about sixteen inches in length with a cut handle at one end, the body of the brush curved to accommodate various parts of the body when used. The label printed on the beautifully carved wooden handle reads, "The Friction by this Brush is produced by the ends of the hair—being more effectual than the Strap or Mitten, and much preferred for pleasantness, as it does not retain particles from the surface of the skin."

A British officer, Admiral Henry, decided to craft handmade mechanical devices when physicians could give him no relief for a broken thighbone that did not heal properly. Believing that the blood needed to be in good circulation and that the tendons and nerves required stimulation for them to be healthy, the admiral began fashioning instruments at his home in Rolvenden to assist these processes. The first instruments were made of wood, but when they proved too harsh for the skin, he boiled bones to remove the "grease," then smoothed and shaped them with a file. The bones came from the ribs of cattle, chosen primarily because of their naturally bent shape.

Walter Johnson provides an account of how Admiral Henry came to use the "instruments," and why. The account is taken from Sir John Sinclair's book, *Code of Health and Longevity.*

It was in the year 1787 that he was accidentally led to apply the wooden tools to his knees, ancles [*sic*], and insteps, which were all much swelled and hard, owing to the rheumatism, and very painful when touched; and though the operation was slightly done, yet he found considerable benefit from it. This gave him more confidence in the success of his plan, and induced him afterwards to try larger and stronger instruments, and to apply them with more force. To strengthen the feet, Admiral Henry was accustomed to tread the one over the other with the shoes off; and he also used the hammer, with a piece of cork, covered by leather at the end of it, for the soles; and the bone instruments to move the tendons. His feet thus became perfectly sound and well. By the same instruments, he greatly strengthened his heels, and the tendon achillis [*sic*], both of which require constant beating, the circulation being very sluggish in both places. The thighs cannot be too much hammered, and if it is left off, they soon feel the want of it.[8] (It is now known that stimulation of the tendons and ligaments through manipulation can aid in the repair of these tissues.)

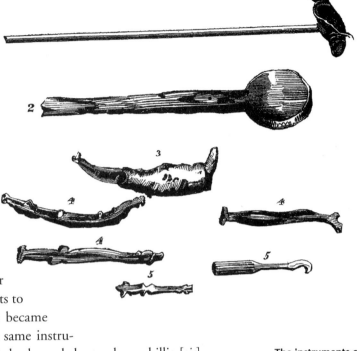

The instruments carved and used by British Admiral Henry in 1787 for self-massage: (1) a cork-head hammer covered in leather; (2) a wooden paddle for beating heels and soles of the feet; and (3, 4, 5) carved bones for rubbing various parts of the body, with knobs to work among the tendons. From *The Anatriptic Art* by Walter Johnson (London, 1866).

These kinds of descriptions go on for pages, telling how the admiral cured himself of rheumatism, gout, cataract, tic douloureux (degeneration of or pressure on the trigeminal nerve, resulting in neuralgia of that nerve), and other disorders. However, there is no mention in other literature of the period in which these instruments were invented and used by Admiral Henry. Their existence and use may not have been well known, or the treatments were so radical and painful that no one wanted to employ them. It is also possible that as self-help tools they gained no favor among medical practitioners. A number of modern manual massage tools available today are similar in design and in application concept to Admiral Henry's. One, the Hand-L, is made of stoneware and is ergonomically designed to fit the hand for comfort and ease of use.

Professor Goodno's book, *Practice of Medicine,* mentions an abdominal massage technique using a cannonball. Dr. Kellogg describes this method of massage for us.

A cannonball covered with leather is a valuable mechanical accessory in the application of abdominal massage. The ball is simply rolled upon the abdomen, following the course of the colon from right to left. A ball weighing from four to six pounds is usually employed. I have found the cannonball very useful when employed in connection with other

153

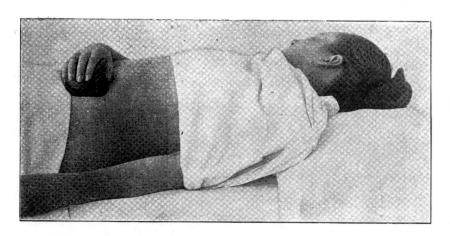

The cannonball was considered a therapeutic tool by John Harvey Kellogg, to be used either by an attendant or one's self to aid in movement of the colon. From *The Home Hand-Book of Domestic Hygiene and Rational Medicine* by John Harvey Kellogg, M.D. (London, 1899).

Appropriating the terminology of the time, in this 1904 advertisement the self-help tool known for twenty-five years as the body roller was renamed the Massage Vibrator. Competing with the new electric massage devices of the time, this device and others of similar design helped encourage self-care. Courtesy of World of Massage Museum.

Nº 1

THE MASSAGE VIBRATOR

Nº 2

PAT. APPLIED FOR.

measures of treatment. It has an advantage in that it may be employed by the patient himself. It should be used for fifteen minutes morning and evening. In the morning it may be employed just before rising, or half an hour after breakfast.[9]

A "shot-bag" massage was also employed in a similar manner.

The manufacture of handheld massage rollers began just after the Civil War in Europe and America. The first such devices had a rolling wheel or other such tool made of ivory, mounted on the ends of wooden handles. The first device called a "massage vibrator" was in fact a massage roller.

Many claims were made for the beneficial effects of massage rollers, such as the following: "As a matter of fact, there are very few disordered conditions of the system in which the massage roller will not, by equalizing the circulation and stimulating the vital functions, be a valuable factor in the treatment."[10] When used as self-care devices, rollers were proclaimed by some physicians and especially by the advertising that promoted them as serving two functions—giving the massage and getting exercise while using the device.

A variety of rollers and other implements were developed in the early twentieth century for the burgeoning field of massage as a beauty treatment. The Institute of Beauty in Paris, France, developed several porcelain devices used for giving facial massages. Elizabeth Arden manufactured several models of body rollers that were large and expensive. Helena Rubinstein & Co. distributed Valaze Face Massage Rollers that were patented in Russia in 1908. The handles are made of black bakelite and the rollers of cream-colored bakelite, a strong and lightweight special-

MASSAGE TOOLS AND MEDIUMS

formula plastic. They were used to contour the neck and facial muscles, in tune with the popularity of facial massage expressed by writers such as Carl Rosen, author of the 1906 book *The Face, Hair and Scalp.* "The object of this procedure is twofold—it develops the muscles of the face and at the same time improves the circulation."[11] These were high-quality items, probably sold throughout Europe and the United States to beauty operators doing specialized treatments in sanitariums, urban clinics, spas, and resorts.

A device sold by Dr. John Gibbs made the transition to the electric age through the use of static electricity. The "Electric Massage Roller" was a single roller mounted on a wooden handle between two metal arms. The roller is made of two copper bands and two metal bands that—when rolled with sufficient speed over the skin—generate static electricity. Gibbs claimed the device "will remove crows feet, wrinkles (premature and from age). Also, all facial blemishes,

for massage and curative purposes it has no equal."[12] This of course was a true quack device that did not remain on the market long after its introduction in 1889, even though it was widely advertised.

With the invention of commercial rubber products came a plethora of products sold primarily to the general public for self-help in administering various massage techniques. In Kellogg's 1895 book, two "muscle beaters" are shown and described briefly. "Klemm's Muscle Beater"—invented in the early 1880s by a German masseur—was made of elastic rubber tubes attached to a

The Massage Vibrator

THIS new appliance consists of revolving balls and rubber cushions ranged on a strong brass chain, having a hard wood handle at each end. It can be easily worked back and forth over any part of the body; does its work moved in any direction; it has a triple action—revolving, vibratory, and compressive. There is no chain wire, metallic or other unyielding substance exposed to lacerate the flesh of the careless operator no rubber or elastic cords to wear out.

It will be found especially useful for the back, that cannot be reached so well by the use of Dr. Forest's Massage Rollers, and for cold feet and a lack of circulation in the limbs.

Admirable for use over the entire body in the air bath, and after the cold bath, to bring on a good reaction and glow to the skin. Its use around the legs will take out soreness or stiffness after walking or other exercise.

24 Balls, (with an extra central handle), price **$2.00**
12 Balls, - - - - - **$1.25**
Sent prepaid on receipt of price.

AGENTS WANTED. We want agents everywhere for publications and appliances, including the Massage Rollers, Vibrators, etc. Liberal terms given. Address

THE HEALTH-CULTURE COMPANY,

Later in 1904 a more sophisticated form of the Massage Vibrator was released. This "appliance" featured balls rotating on a brass chain, with rubber cushions between each roller. The advertisement claims the vibrator delivers "triple action—revolving, vibratory, and compression." Courtesy of World of Massage Museum.

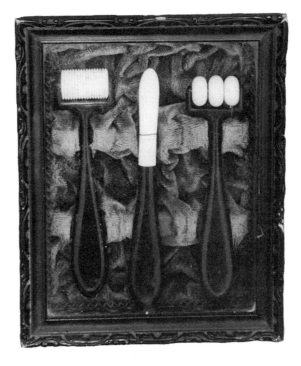

A salesman's display model of three finely made handheld massage instruments, circa 1860. The ends of each piece are of hand-carved solid ivory and the handles are ebony. These instruments were used primarily for facial massage, believed to be a beauty treatment; they were also used around joints and along tendons and ligaments in a manner similar to the instruments created by Admiral Henry. Courtesy of World of Massage Museum.

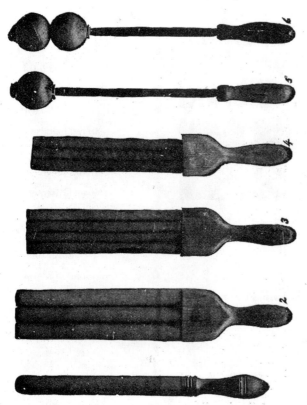

wooden handle. Kellogg claims credit for developing the second device, called the "Ball Muscle Beater," which he likes much better than Klemm's device. They were used by an operator, one in each hand, to beat upon the large muscles of the back, and are the precursors of today's massage bongers.

Rubber massage rollers came next in the long line of devices preceding electro-mechanical machines. The new line of "gum," or rubber, rollers was extolled by W. R. Latson, M.D., who wrote, "Of the many mechanical devices for the application of massage there is not one that combines the qualities of convenience, effectiveness and cheapness so fully as the massage roller."[13] Almost all rubber massage rollers produced between 1880 and 1910 conform to Latson's description of a roller that "consists of a rod, more or less flexible, upon which are mounted a number of wooden wheels about one and a half inches in diameter. Around each wheel is a rim, or buffer, of specially prepared soft rubber. . . . The rod bearing the wheels is set in a substantial handle of wood. . . . Another important feature is that the wheels turn separately and independently of each other, each in accordance with the resistance that it meets. There is no drawing or pulling of the flesh or skin, as would be the case if it were all one solid wheel. . . . In using the massage roller no lubricant is needed for the skin. It is not necessary even to expose the skin, as the roller will act as beneficially when applied to tissues thinly covered as for instance, over the underclothing. . . . With the best instruments there is an interval or space between the rubber buffers or tires of the adjoining wheels. This space allows the tissues to be crowded up between the buffers, and thus gives a slight lateral or pinching compression, as well as a direct perpendicular pressure, much as though the flesh had been gently squeezed between the fingers."[14] As a physician, Latson's association with a commercial massage-roller company is not unusual for his time. Many physicians and celebrities endorsed products then, just as they do today.

Although these devices are now considered quackery by most

Top two: Ball muscle beater from 1895—one or more rubber balls attached to a flexible rattan or whalebone handle. From W. R. Latson, Common Disorders *(New York, 1904).*

Bottom four: Klemm's Muscle Beater, invented by a German masseur, circa 1883. The device is made of rubber tubes attached to a handle. From W. R. Latson, Common Disorders *(New York, 1904).*

Using the ball beaters, circa 1895. From W. R. Latson, Common Disorders *(New York, 1904).*

MASSAGE TOOLS

AND MEDIUMS

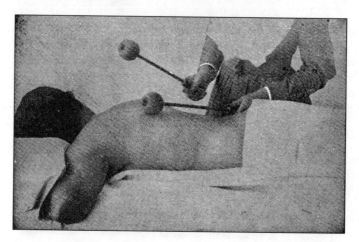

medical historians, they served an important role in bringing the possibility of self-care into the consciousness of the public. The claims for their use extended to a wide range of medical conditions, including constipation, neuralgia, and insomnia, as well as beauty treatments for such things as bust development and abdomen reduction. This description of performing a massage on oneself comes from a book entitled *Womanly Beauty in Form and Features*. "At night before retiring bathe the breasts lightly with cold water, dry carefully with a soft towel, and over a loose sack or undervest roll Dr. Forest's bust developer from underneath upwards and from the side forward, always toward the centre, throwing the chest well out while doing this. . . . When the breasts have become warm and in a glow, bathe in warm water and rub in thoroughly the Health Culture Skin Food, which is absolutely pure, containing no animal fats, and the best bust food made."[15]

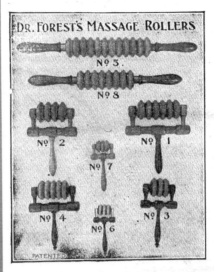

Dr. FOREST'S MASSAGE ROLLERS.

THESE rollers are coming into general use wherever massage is needed and are a cure for many of the functional disorders, as Dyspepsia, Constipation, Biliousness, Debility, Emaciation, Neuralgia, Rheumatism, Paralysis, Sleeplessness, Obesity and wherever there is a lack of a good circulation of the blood; and the developers and facial rollers are used successfully for building up the form and the prevention of wrinkles and age in the face. The rollers consist of wheels about 1½ inches in diameter; around the centre is a band or buffer of elastic rubber.

The object of the Health or Massage Roller is to make massage practical, to bring into the home the easiest and pleasantest method of Cure and Exercise. It can be used with little fatigue and entirely without exposure or even undressing, by yourself or an attendant.

No. 1, Body Roller, $2.—The best size for use over the body, and especially for indigestion, constipation, rheumatism, etc. Can also be used for reduction.
No. 2, Body Roller, $1.50.—Smaller and lighter than No. 1, for small women it is the best in size, for use over the stomach and bowels, the limbs and for cold feet.
No. 3, Scalp Roller, $1.50.—Made in fine woods, and for use over the scalp, for the preservation of the hair. Can be used also over the neck to fill it out and for the throat.
No. 4, Bust Developer, $2.50.—The best developer made. By following the plain, physiological directions given most satisfactory results can be obtained.
No. 5, Abdominal Roller, $4.—For the use of men to reduce the size of the abdomen, and over the back. The handles give a chance for a good, firm, steady pressure.
No. 6, Facial Roller, $2.50.—Made in ebony and ivory, for use over the face and neck, for preventing and removing wrinkles, and restoring its contour and form.
No. 7, Facial Roller, $1.50.—Like No. 6, made in white maple. In other respects the same.
No. 8, Abdominal Roller, $3.50.—This is the same as No. 5, except with the less number of wheels. Is made for the use of women, for reducing hip and abdominal measure.

THE HEALTH-CULTURE CO.,

Among the most prominent and widely advertised, Dr. Forest's massage rollers were quite popular for nearly a decade until the electric vibrator outpaced them in popularity. This advertisement claims the rollers will cure many disorders, including neuralgia, sleeplessness, and rheumatism, while helping you to reduce unwanted cellulite from your hips and thighs. This advertisement appeared in the October 1904 issue of *Physical Culture* magazine.

Although the massage roller quickly faded from prominence when the electric handheld vibrator was introduced in 1901, massage rollers did not disappear. They took a second seat to the new electric devices but are still with us today. Today we find hundreds of gadgets of this sort that are manually operated, run on batteries, or get their power from electrical wall outlets.

Home bathtubs seem de rigueur to us today, but prior to the late nineteenth century they were not so common. For those who lived outside of large cities, where public baths were available, a bathtub at home was the next best thing. Around 1891 the first folding bath cabinets for home bathing became available. They eventually became very popular in home-based massage practices, the style of practice that predominated in the lay massage business for one hundred years, from 1890 through 1990. In the 1920s, practitioners who practiced massage out of their homes generally replaced their bathtubs with steam cabinets.

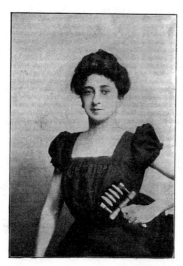

Roller massage for bust development.

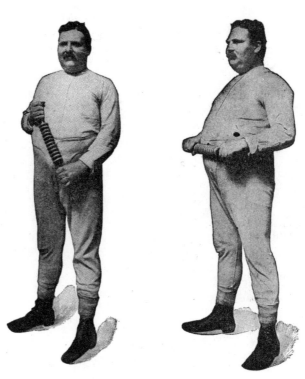

Roller massage for abdomen reduction

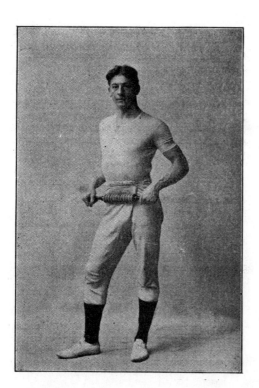

Roller massage "for the purpose of stimulating pneumo gastric centre [the solar plexus], as well as increasing the activity of the colon."

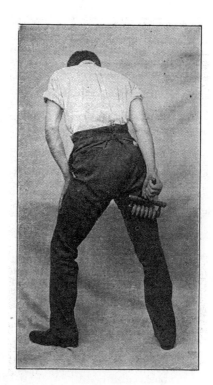

Roller treatment for crural neuralgia, or sciatica as we know it today.

Some of the conditions that the promotional literature for massage rollers promised to address included rheumatism, dyspepsia, constipation, insomnia, and obesity. From W. R. Latson, *Common Disorders* (New York, 1904).

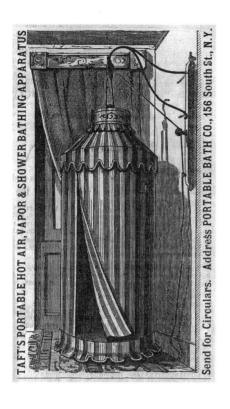

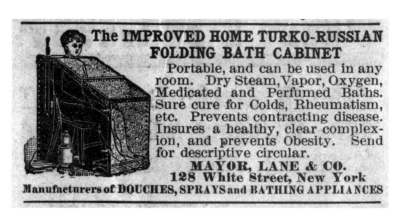

Mechanical Massage Devices

The first mechanical devices associated with massage—if they could really be called mechanical—were the ropes, swings, hanging bars, and dumbbell weights used in the exercise and movement cure systems of the late eighteenth and early nineteenth centuries. But true mechanical massage apparatuses—designed specifically to replace or augment the human hand—did not appear until the middle of the nineteenth century. Vibration was the first stroke imitated by machine; the idea was to provide slower and more regular movements with the machine than those obtainable by a massage operator. First came hand-cranked devices operated on mechanical concepts similar to a hand drill. The simple two-gear system transferred manual energy to the end of the device and then to the body with which it was in contact. This method provided much more power and penetration than the human hand could deliver. Developed in Germany circa 1855, the Macurator Blood Circulator was the simplest of these first manufactured massagers. The Macurator delivered a high variable frequency pounding effect on the body that resembled a vibration effect if it was cranked fast enough.

In the United States and England the VeeDee was the next level of hand-cranked massagers. This device was more sophisticated, even though it utilized the same drill-like principles to deliver its vibration to the body. An extra apparatus was attached to the end of the VeeDee to accentuate the vibration and provide more horizontal movement to the body, thus creating the first true vibrator. The extra apparatus is a small adjustable flywheel that can be calibrated to provide more or less vibration. The VeeDee, unlike its predecessor the Macurator, came in a variety of sizes and shapes

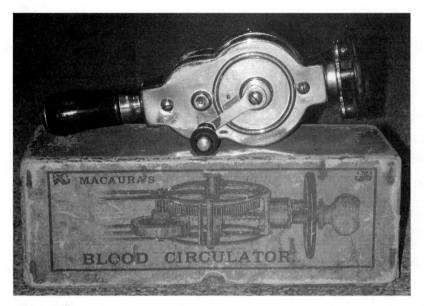

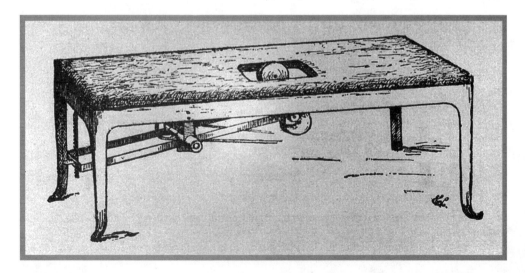

and with a number of attachments.

Dr. Zander, a Swedish physician and director of his own institute in Stockholm (Medico-Mechanical Institute), gained widespread fame at the end of the nineteenth century because of his application of steam power to mechano-therapy. Only a few of Zander's more than seventy steam-powered devices were massage machines. They were primarily used for active, assistive, and resistive exercises. Zander's devices were so popular, and their application to the gymnastic movement so widely accepted, that Zander Institutes were opened throughout Europe and the United States. George Taylor, M.D., is credited with being the first American to create a steam and foot/hand-crank device circa 1880. Taylor's "Manipulator" simply turned a wheel that pushed a rod that created a movement on a handle or padded surface. The patient would either hold on to the handle and receive the vibration or oscillations, or sit or stand against the padded surface to receive the movement from the machine. Dr. Taylor explains, "The natural rate of motion of the voluntary muscles is considerably greater than is that of the involuntary which preside over the movements of the abdomen and its contents. The respiratory and the peristaltic movements are slower than those of the hand. It follows that motions, natural for the hand of a massage operator, do not so apply to visceral parts as to merge with and assist those of the latter. The imparted motion will not agree as to time with the pre-existing motion. This disagreement does not exist in case of the mechanical processes."[16] Taylor is saying the application of the human hand to volun-

The Macurator Blood Circulator. Photograph courtesy of World of Massage Museum.

A mechanical massage table from 1887 designed for kneading the abdominal region to facilitate digestion. G. H. Taylor, *Massage* (New York, 1887).

160

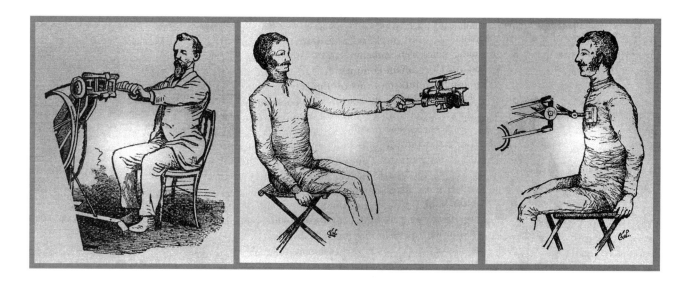

tary muscles, such as those used in locomotion, can be properly calibrated to coincide with the rhythm and rate of those muscles, but that the hand cannot be calibrated to coincide with the slower-moving muscles of the internal organs, such as the colon and diaphragm, whereas mechanical devices can. These kinds of devices faded entirely from use after the power of electricity became available.

In 1889 Hartvig Nissen presented a new invention called "the Vibrator" in his book, *A Manual of Instruction For Giving Swedish Movement and Massage Treatment.* Invented by Mr. J. W. Osborne, Nissen claimed it was made especially for his institute and that, by 1889, he'd been using it with success for three years.[17] However, as illustrated above Dr. Taylor utilized such mechanical devices; Dr. Kellogg was also using them in the sanitarium at Battle Creek as early as 1888.

Most medical applications of these new approaches to massage were applied to diseases particular to women. As early as the 1820s, physicians (most notably in France) were curing hysteria in women with vibration induced by water, the hands, or horseback riding. The advent of mechanical methods of applying vibration improved the success of this therapeutic practice. Rachel Maines reports that physicians have failed in large part in writing about the connection between vibratory massage and the cure of hysteria as they relate to sexual issues, except to say that vibratory massage was a common cure for hysteria. Maines provides detailed descriptions of these treatments.

> Massage was indicated for a broad spectrum of disorders in both sexes but was thought to be especially effective for women's complaints. Some of these were local to the pelvic area, such as dysmenorrhea, amenorrhea, leucorrhea and vagismus, and others more general in character, including obesity, headaches, debility, sleeplessness, menopause, nervousness, nymphomania, and neurasthenia, chlorosis (greensickness) and, hysteria, for which it was a traditional remedy. . . . For all of these disorders . . . physical therapy in the form of massage was recommended from at least the mid-eighteenth century through the first quarter of the

Left and center: Vibration machines from 1887. The user would receive either percussion or vibration depending upon how the handle was held. Similar devices were used for the feet as well.

Right: As with other such devices, the amount of pressure applied to this vibration machine determined the kind of motor-energy transferred to the patient. Light pressure produced percussion while heavy pressure resulted in vibration. From George Taylor, M.D., *Massage* (New York, 1887).

161

twentieth. . . . Hydrotherapy and manual massage were both well-known gynecological treatments in the nineteenth century. . . . Extant accounts of patient behavior under the douche include screaming, wild sobbing, uncontrollable laughter, and even occasional lapses of consciousness. Manual massage of the pelvis and vulva . . . was apparently common but controversial treatment.[18]

Maines later states that "massage to orgasm of female patients [for hysteria particularly] was a staple of medical practice among some (but certainly not all) Western physicians from the time of Hippocrates until the 1920s."[19] However, mechanotherapy's popularity within medicine was short lived, since massage was too labor intensive for physicians to continue its use.

Between 1870 and 1885 the first devices purporting to be "electric" were advertised for sale. With electricity being available in only a few homes, the entrepreneurial spirit of the promotion of electricity was way ahead of its application. Hence we find many devices being offered for sale using the word *electric* in some form or another, yet no electricity was used in their operation. Dr. Scott's Electric Flesh Brush may be one of the first of these promotional devices. The advertisement for this product makes outrageous claims made on its behalf. "Astonishing Cures!" the text reads.

"Royalty, members of her Majesty's Government, and many professional gentlemen who have tested the power of the brush are unanimous in its praise, and its therapeutic value cannot be disputed, having the approval of numerous medical men. Constructed upon scientific principles, the result of twelve years' study and practice. It is thoroughly and permanently charged with an 'Electric' force which produces remarkable cures. It generally gives relief in five to seven minutes, and feeling attending its use. Always doing good, it cannot harm. . . . [It] is a beautiful flesh brush (wet or dry), elegantly carved and lasting for years. Its power can always be tested by a silver compass which accompanies each Brush. Our Dr. Scott's Electric Hair Brush having met with the same appreciation here, which its excellent merits secured for it in England; we now introduce to the American public his Electric Flesh Brush, confident that it will soon find its way into every household."

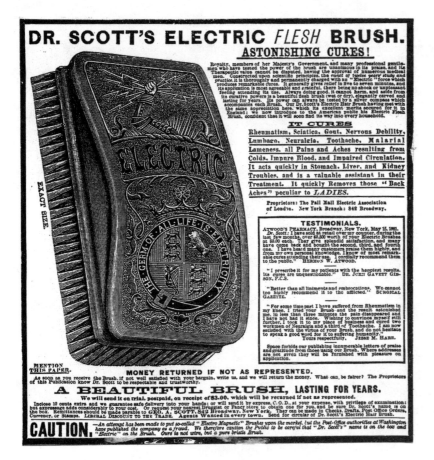

Dr. Scott's Electric Flesh Brush advertisement as it appeared in a newspaper in New York City in 1883. This is one of several models of brushes by Dr. Scott. Courtesy of World of Massage Museum.

The bristles of the actual brush are made of horsehair, and the so-called electrical qualities of the brush, proven by a compass that comes with the brush, are activated by a magnetic bar placed within the handle of the brush. Dr. Scott's Brush—widely advertised throughout the United States and England—is considered a quack medical device by most modern historians of the subject.

In addition to other ads from Dr. Scott's product line, The Pall Mall Electric Association of London, England, a division of the C. B. Harness Company, advertised the "Electricpatent Socks." Evidently, the heat of the body was thought to induce "Thermo-Electricity" from perspiration, which created a galvanic current. Actually, the socks contained small magnets. It would be another fifty years before magnetic therapy was to rise once again, but this time it came out of Japan in the form of the Nikken Company, which provides magnetic products to the market today.

Electrical Massage

Electrical power became available through a series of steps in the 1800s. The first battery was developed in 1800 by Italian physicist Alessandro Volta (1745–1827). Twenty years later, French physicist Andre-Marie Ampere (1775–1836) created the first opposing electrical current running through wires. In 1831 Joseph Henry (1797–1878) invented the first electric motor. Then, in 1867, a French inventor would build the first alternating and direct current generators, paving the way for the first electric generating station, built in London in 1880 by Thomas Edison to provide electric power for streetlights. As with so many other areas of human endeavor, massage also utilized the new resource.

Most applications of electricity in the field of massage came well after the Civil War, even though European physicians were experimenting with it during the two decades before the war to stimulate muscles in the hopes of treating atrophy. In an article from *Electric Quarterly,* Rachel Maines reports: "Vibratory massage as a medical treatment developed from two parallel and related traditions, that of electrotherapeutics and that of massage or physical therapy." The field of electrotherapy consisted of "galvanism, faradism and franklinism."[20] Electrical massage consisted of manipulating muscles with rollers, shakers, and vibrating devices.

The first attempts at electrical massage were either battery-powered devices or those operated by foot or hand mechanisms moving a wheel or friction belt. One of the first battery powered massage devices was the Swedish vibrator. This little device was made of solid brass attached to a wooden handle. Etched into the sides of the brass body are images of lightning bolts indicating the electrical character of the device. The action of the detachable head was unlike most other vibrators that came before or after this device. When plugged into a dry-cell battery the operating head moved up and down to create a rubbing sensation when applied to the body. Several shapes of heads were available, but the most commonly used was the round bakelite head. In 1902 the first commercially available vibrators began being marketed for home use.

Many massage advocates of the late nineteenth century objected to electro-mechanical massage because it attempted to do away with the use of the hands and omitted the most important element of massage treatment—human contact. Some inventive Europeans attempted to overcome this criticism and yet extend the capabilities of the hands by inventing "sponge electrodes" and "glove electrodes," but these devices only decreased the manipulator's sense of touch. The next phase brought "arm electrodes," which have the appearance of two bracelets that can be tightened around each wrist by means of a lock or screw. The wire going to the two arm electrodes splits in two, bringing either positive or negative charges to both hands, while the other electrode, which was of a larger size and easily bent, was adaptable to different parts of the body. The hands and fingers could continue to work their magic, electrified, if you will, but not interfere with one's sense of touch. The arm electrodes were used with batteries and are reported to have produced very agreeable sensations. Nevertheless they did not last long, even in the fad product environment so prevalent between 1885 and 1906 in Europe and the United States.

In 1906 President Theodore Roosevelt signed the Federal Pure Food and Drug Act in response to the plethora of unfounded claims made by patent medicines and quack healing practices. Claims for cures of nearly every disease or disorder, from baldness to cancer, were being advertised in newspapers, magazines, catalogs, and even painted on the sides of barns. These claims extended into the realm of newly invented electrical devices, including vibrators.

In a chapter of photographs in *The Art of Massage,* John Harvey Kellogg depicted many types of mechanical apparatus, most of which were operated by electric motors. Dr. Kellogg shows rooms full of such equipment, some large and some small, which he called "appliances." Kellogg claims credit for having invented some of the devices, giving credit to a few colleague-inventors as well (Taylor, Zander, and Klemm) but never mentioning Nissen, Osborne, or others. However, archives from several sources show that such things as the mechanical tables and gymnastic machines were in use, albeit in more rudimentary forms, years before Dr. Kellogg had his machines built.

Among the devices used at the sanitarium by Dr. Kellogg and his staff were a vibrating chair, vibrating platform, and vibrating bar, a device for providing endwise and lateral vibration of the feet and legs, rotary vibration of the legs and arms, vibration of the trunk, a nerve percuter, and an apparatus for kneading the abdomen similar to the one used by Dr. Taylor, but more elaborate. Also used was an apparatus for kneading the arms and legs and rolling the trunk. Dr. Kellogg even created a large beltlike device to provide friction to the bottoms of the feet, similar to a giant, slow-moving belt sander. He devised several tilting tables, one specifically for bending the pelvis, and a large apparatus designed to provide artificial respiration.

Dr. Kellogg claims he invented the "nerve-percuter, or vibrator," which he describes as having "a metallic chamber in which a mass of soft iron is made to play to and fro with considerable force by means of an alternating electrical current passing through a coil of wire which constitutes a part of the chamber. The blows struck by the oscillating mass of iron are communicated to the portion of the body under treatment by a brass rod terminating in a knob."[21]

One of the most popular devices of this period was thought to help reduce fat around the waist, perhaps in response to the first Hershey Bar sold in 1894 or the first pizzeria opening in New York City in 1895. Aside from the hand vibrators popular from this time to our own today, the "vibrating machine" shown here, with the belt attachment fixed around the lady's waist, was the most popular electro-mechanical device of its time.

It is not possible to list all of the electro-massage devices offered to physicians and the general public during the latter two decades of the nineteenth century. But one more from 1899 provides a representative example of a "magic box" touting the winning combination of massage and electricity. An advertisement in an 1899 *McClure's Magazine* depicts the Vibratile Electric Massage, a device aimed at giving tapotement from "a delicate tap to a decisive blow."

Dr. Taylor points out that devices such as mechanically powered vibrators were not meant to replace the human hand. In fact, he says, this idea is "radically erroneous." "The two methods," he explains, "do not in reality cover the same ground. . . . So far from being substitutes for, they are helps to each other, both being employed in the remedial treatment of the same individuals, to comply with separate and distinctly differing indications."[22] Dr. Kellogg took a little different view of mechanical devices as replacements for the human hand.

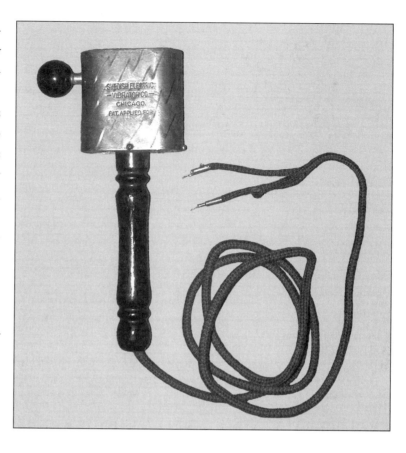

The Swedish vibrator, a battery-powered device circa 1875 made of solid brass attached to a wooden handle. Courtesy of World of Massage Museum.

> Mechanical massage . . . more commonly termed Swedish movements . . . may be advantageously used as a substitute for a number of the procedures of manual massage. I have, however, found no device quite equal to the human hand, for the administration of kneading movements. Shaking and vibratory movements, on the other hand, may be applied more efficiently by apparatus than by hand in cases requiring vigorous and prolonged application, for the reason that much more vigorous, rapid, and uniform movements can be executed by machinery than by the hand, and the movement may be continued as long as necessary;

MASSAGE TOOLS

AND MEDIUMS

whereas these movements are exceedingly trying to the masseur, and cannot be maintained, at best, for more than a few minutes continuously.[23]

Emil Kleen provided his point of view on the subject of mechanical versus manual massage.

> Generally speaking, massage as a whole is performed best by hand, and no instruments exist or can ever be produced with which one can, even approximately, perform the various manipulations that go to a massage seance as well as by the hands. . . . But it cannot be denied that in some cases one may with advantage make use of instruments. Certain forms of tapotement and especially vibrations are performed much more smoothly, quickly, and strongly by means of instruments than by hand.[24]

Taylor's, Kellogg's, and Kleen's remarks represent the general sentiments of their time about mechanical massage, but as the portable electric vibrator became readily available around 1902, the human hand was largely replaced by these instruments of technology in the medical practice. Physical therapy started with manual treatments but ended with the famous shake-and-bake treatments utilizing machine vibration and heat packs.

Dr. Kellogg's "Vibrating Machine," circa 1895. This particular device is not shown in Kellogg's *The Art of Massage* but was used extensively at the Battle Creek Sanitarium in Michigan. Photo courtesy of Duff Stoltz, Archives of the Battle Creek Sanitarium.

Faradic massage was quite popular within the new field of physiotherapy during the 1920s in America and Europe. Its roots go back to the battery-operated electric shock devices used by so-called quack physicians of the late nineteenth century. Electrical stimulation of muscle tissue comprises a variety of treatment modalities that have been around since the 1880s and that continue being used today as weight reducers, muscle relaxers, and anti-spasm devices. The "sponge electrodes" and "glove electrodes" mentioned earlier were a part of this technology. The violet-ray and sinusoidal current machines were also well developed within the physiotherapy field. Some models of faradic, galvanic, and violet-ray devices were sold to the general public from about 1890 to 1930. (Violet-ray treatment is still being taught at a few massage schools today.) A few such devices are illustrated here. In the growing field of physiotherapy, later called physical therapy, these devices were soon replaced by TENS (transcutaneous electrical nerve stimulator) units, diathermy, and ultrasound.

To finish our discussion of massage devices, let's discuss massage tables. In the World of Massage Museum (WOMM) there is a display of massage tables dated in range from 1000 B.C.E. to 1998 C.E. The term *massage table* is less than one hundred years in use, arriving sometime during the late 1920s. Prior to that devices used for massage were called *couches.* The first so-called massage tables were used during the time of the Greeks and Romans and were marble slabs called *plinths.* These were used in the great gymnasiums and the solariums for hydrotherapy treatments, cleaning, and scraping or defoliation procedures, as well as for massage.

The next generation of massage tables were the doctor's examination table. These were usually made of solid oak, had various adjustments available, and were a multiuse device, among which massage was just one of its uses. These tables are often found depicted in the books about massage written during the second half of the nineteenth century. The padding on these exam tables was made of horsehair, and the tables were covered with rough leather. Horsehair was the most widely used because it was resistant to insect damage, whereas cotton was not.

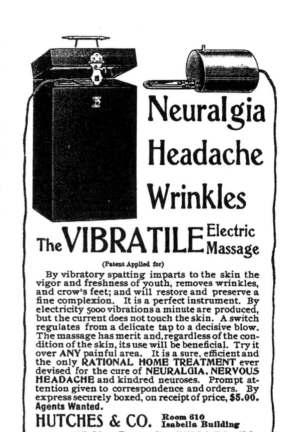

The VIBRATILE Electric Massage

Neuralgia
Headache
Wrinkles

(Patent Applied for)

By vibratory spatting imparts to the skin the vigor and freshness of youth, removes wrinkles, and crow's feet; and will restore and preserve a fine complexion. It is a perfect instrument. By electricity 5000 vibrations a minute are produced, but the current does not touch the skin. A switch regulates from a delicate tap to a decisive blow. The massage has merit and, regardless of the condition of the skin, its use will be beneficial. Try it over ANY painful area. It is a sure, efficient and the only RATIONAL HOME TREATMENT ever devised for the cure of NEURALGIA, NERVOUS HEADACHE and kindred neuroses. Prompt attention given to correspondence and orders. By express securely boxed, on receipt of price, $5.00. Agents Wanted.

HUTCHES & CO. Room 610 Isabella Building
48 Van Buren St. CHICAGO, ILL.

An advertisement for the Vibratile Electric Massage in the March 1899 issue of *McClure's Magazine.* The advertisement claimed that "the massage has merit and, regardless of the condition of the skin, its use will be beneficial."

The *massage couch* was a term used for massage tables that were truly pieces of furniture. These were in vogue during the Victorian era of the late nineteenth century; they were usually stuffed with horsehair and were upholstered with velvet or similar material. They were quite cushy in their comfort compared to the doctor's exam table and were fashionably colored in bright reds or yellows.

Between 1900 and 1925 electric vibrating tables were manufactured for use primarily in the sanitariums or doctor's office. These were solid wood with no cushions except those that might be added for a bony person's relative comfort. The first portable massage table was invented around 1930 and was made of a wooden frame with metal or wooden legs. A stationary massage table used after World War I was made from common woods, with simple padding under a vinyl covering. Neither the first portable nor the first stationary massage tables contained face holes.

The face hole cut into the head of a stationary or portable table appeared sometime during the late 1940s. Portable massage tables of this period were quite sophisticated in their design and quality, especially those that had mechanisms to unfold the legs and fold them back again as the table was opened and closed. The table presented by George Downing in his 1960s book, *The Massage Book,* was a homemade model

167

Massage and electro-magnetic appliances

The turn of the twentieth century saw a rush to apply mechanical inventions to many ends, including replacing human hands as the instruments of massage. The early body rollers of Dr. Forest, the hand-crank Macurator Blood Circulator, and the drill-action VeeDee Vibrator were eventually pushed aside by larger apparatuses, such as Dr. Taylor's vibration machine.

With the harnessing of electricity came the rush to ascribe electrical qualities to nearly everything that could be sold as a self-help device. Dr. Scott's Electric Hair Brush and the Electric Belt are fine examples of how the magnetic craze was surreptitiously combined with the rush for electricity; magnets were embedded into devices that were then passed off as having electric power. Dr. Gibb's Electric Massage Roller produced nothing more than static electricity when applied to the body. Dr. Butler's "Electro-Massage Instrument" was another magnetic device advertised under the winning banner of electricity. The diseases "successfully treated" with this device, according to an advertisement from 1888, are too numerous to mention, but the heading for each category gives an idea of the claims made. "Diseases of the Brain and Nervous

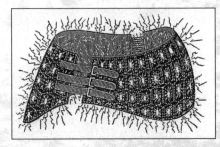

The Electric Belt, as shown in an advertisement in *Ladies' Home Journal,* 1891. Magnets embedded in the belt supposedly gave it electric power. The ad states that the belt cures many diseases "in five minutes." Courtesy of World of Massage Museum.

System . . . Respiratory System . . . Digestive System . . . Eye and Ear . . . Cutaneous (Skin) and Blood Diseases . . . Urinary and Genital System . . . and General Diseases such as Spinal . . . Rheumatism . . . Hip . . . Gout . . . Malaria . . . Bad Circulation . . . Writer's Cramp . . . Paralysis . . . Stiff Neck . . . Lumbago . . . General Ill-health . . . Obesity." Just the mere association of electricity with massage was enough to conjure up a product for sale.

The *McLure's Magazine* advertisement from 1898 shown here is one of the most profoundly outrageous selling hypes you'll ever see for a massage roller. Among the many massage roller advertisements of the time, this one can be found in the Museum of Questionable Medical Devices, located in Minneapolis, Minnesota. There were no laws prohibiting false and misleading advertising at this time, and obviously none concerning quoting newspapers. (This ad attributes five newspapers with endorsing the product.) Public outcry forced Congress to pass the Food and Drug Act of 1906, prohibiting the shipment of many of these kinds of products across state lines; Congress later added regulations prohibiting misleading curative claims.

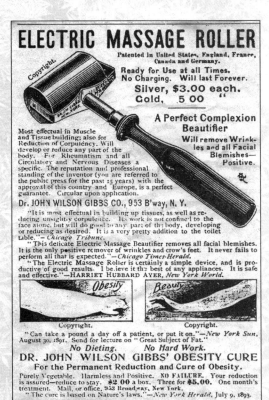

An ad for the Electric Massage Roller from *McClure's Magazine,* 1898. This is one of the most profoundly outrageous advertisements you'll ever see for a massage roller; the device merely created static electricity when rolled over the skin. Courtesy of World of Massage Museum.

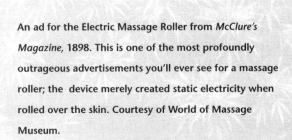

copied by many practitioners for the next decade until the 1970s, when commercially manufactured tables became more readily available. The Battlecreek Company manufactured the first lightweight massage table with their introduction of the aluminum folding portable table in the 1950s. The face cradle of today that attaches to the end of the massage table was first introduced in the 1980s. The first tables were almost entirely made of wood and vinyl-covered foam padding. Current models are ergonomically designed of special alloy tubing and multilayered padding and come in a variety of colors and styles. Specialty tables, such as those designed for working on pregnant women, doing special bodywork that requires an extrawide tabletop or tables that will also fold down to lie flat on the ground for Asian therapies, are among the numerous options available in today's market.

Quite a number of the devices sold in the late twentieth century were merely reinvented versions of those we find created many years earlier. The one-thousand-year-old Chinese jade massage knuckle is similar to the wide array of exotic stone tools made from marble and jade today. The ancient Polynesian lomi-lomi sticks evolved from the simple curved

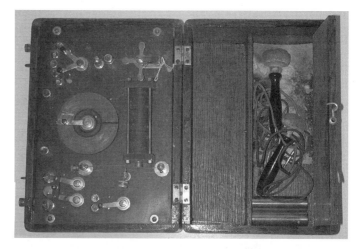

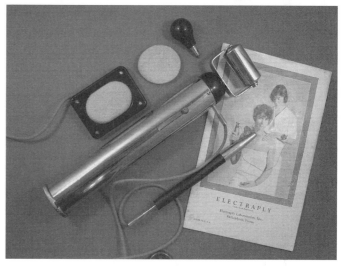

branch of a guava tree to S-shaped devices that can be folded up to fit inside a suitcase, some of which include knobs protruding like smaller branches along their curvature. The instruments carved from bone and wood by Admiral Henry in 1787 are now seen in the form of the wood Knobbler, the ceramic Hand-L, and similar devices made of plastic or stone. A handheld device called the "vibrator" was a string of wooden beads with a handle at both ends advertised in the late nineteenth century and now a common massage device sold in stores everywhere. The Ball Muscle Beaters depicted in Dr. Kellogg's 1895 book are now widely known as "bongers."

The earliest form of vibration therapy goes back to Greek and Roman eras, when patients were swung on swings, rhythmically rocked on horses, or shaken in wagons with uneven wheels moving over stone roadways. Swinging, horseback riding, and wagon riding can also be found as vibratory treatments used during the eighteenth and nineteenth centuries. The first hand-cranked vibrators were used by physicians to deliver percussion, vibration, and stroking movements to their patients for treatment of neuralgia and constipation.

The invention of Victorian vibrators using dry-cell batteries was the precursor to the modern alkaline-battery-powered vibrator. Modern medical vibrators, such as the

Top: Early electric shock device.
Bottom: Electric home appliance for stimulating the circulatory and nervous systems. Courtesy of World of Massage Museum.

169

G-5, are reinventions of the older percussion devices sold to doctors late in the nineteenth century, such as Dr. Macuara's Macurator. And the array of foot-massage devices found in novelty and health stores today have had their counterparts a hundred years ago in cruder forms. Today you can find a manual massage tool made of virtually any material known to man, in as many shapes, colors, and sizes as there is the imagination to create them.

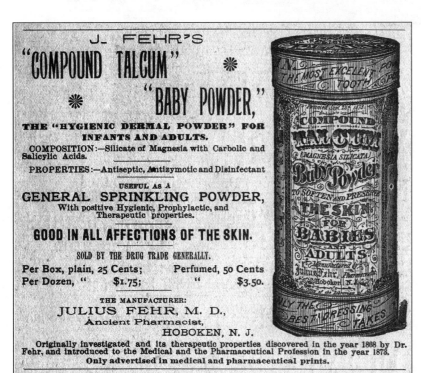

Dr. Fehr's Compound Talcum. Placed on the market in 1873, this talcum product was promoted for use as a baby powder and adult powder. Courtesy of World of Massage Museum.

Massage Mediums

The oldest lubricants used for massage were olive oil, hog fat, natural mineral water, and powders. Talcum is believed by some authorities to be the original "Egyptian dust" referred to by ancient and medieval writers as an after-bath treatment in many countries around the world. The aesthetic and healing virtues of oil have also been extolled since ancient times. Psalms refers to the "oil of gladness" and "oil to make the face shine." In Proverbs, oil is the "ointment and perfume to delight the heart." In another passage of the Bible, the prophet Isaiah refers to the "oil of joy." There are several examples of this kind of high praise for oil in Greco-Roman times as well. Johnson writes, "Plato, by the mouth of Socrates, reckons oil as only less necessary to human life than wheat and barley—not speaking of oil as an article of diet, but as applied externally; because he terms it 'assuager of pain.'"[25]

In the centuries after the fall of the Roman empire little was written about massage and even less about the mediums used for massage. However, it is most likely that the traditional mediums, such as talcum, oil, lard, and water, continued to be used. The oldest chemists and perfumeries in the United States, established in 1752, produced the Caswell-Massey Talcum products for use with massage and in the bath, still available today. Another talcum product was Dr. Fehr's Compound Talcum, a "hygienic dermal powder" said to be good for all affections of the skin or as a tooth powder or for dressing bandages. This product was primarily advertised to physicians and pharmacists.

The nineteenth century, the age of the patent medicine, produced a proliferation of mediums for massage. Many "new" and "improved" liniments were for sale, most of them coming out of the medical bag of the traveling "doctors," fast-talking, quick-

MASSAGE TOOLS

AND MEDIUMS

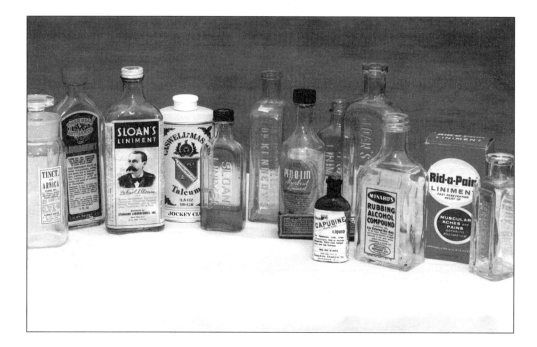

selling con men who sold primarily alcoholic beverages disguised as medicinal remedies.

One of the first liniments used by those who practiced massage was Dr. Kennedy's Rheumatic Liniment, made in Roxbury, Massachusetts. It was mass produced in plain, rectangular-shaped bottles with no label and no list of ingredients.

Minard's Liniment, out of Boston, was another pre–Civil War product. Minard's also produced a very popular rubbing alcohol compound containing 70 percent alcohol, for external use only. It was advertised for use "in the Home, Hospital, Camp and Training Quarters." Then came Larkin's Derma-Balm, out of Buffalo, New York; for headaches there was Hick's Capudine Liquid. The same liniment claimed to cure "neuralgia, sick headache, sciatic, rheumatic and periodic pains, nervous headache, sea sickness, and train nausea . . . also for . . . colds, grippe and nervousness from use of tobacco." Hick's Capudine was especially marketed to immigrant populations; the folded brochure contained in the small box with an even smaller bottle of the product was printed in English, French, Spanish, German, Italian, Polish, Scandinavian, Hungarian, and Slovak. Hicks's products were from Raleigh, North Carolina.

Sloan's Liniment was an early entrant into the commercial production of such products. Named after Dr. Carl Sloan, Sloan's was distributed by Standard Laboratories of Morris Plains, New Jersey. These bottles are perhaps the most prevalent in antiques and specialty stores today. Many had no labels, only being identified by the words, "Sloan's Liniment" raised on the glass bottle's surface. This indicates a product with a well-known name identity. The ingredients of Sloan's Liniment were "extract of Capsicum (Cayenne Pepper), Methyl Salicylate, Oil of Camphor, Turpentine, Oil of Pine." Most bottles with labels also provided directions for "Veterinary Uses" besides the usual "Directions." Rubbing Sloan's liniments into the skin was not advised. Sloan's liniments were meant to be "patted" on the skin and were supposed to cause skin irritation if rubbed in.

Pen-O-Lin was an "Absorbent Liniment," advertised as "Excellent as a rubdown for trainers and athletes." The directions for Pen-O-Lin read, "For sore muscular sprains rub the affected part three or four times a day with a small quantity of Pen-O-Lin. When used as a rub-down for athletes add 1 part of Pen-O-Lin to 16 parts water." It was also advised for treating ringworm and for relief of small insect bites. It was likely it was the acetone in it that was helpful for these last two suggested uses. From St. Louis, Missouri, the Pfeiffer Company produced Rid-a-Pain Liniment. This product was promoted as a "deeper penetrating, more effective and non-staining and greaseless" liniment. The directions read, in part, "Massage gently into affected muscles or joints. Gentle rubbing may be applied if skin is not too sensitive." Ben-Gay ointment for sore muscles was invented in 1898 by a French pharmacist, Jules Bengue, and Vick's VapoRub was invented in 1905 by a North Carolina druggist, Lunsford Richardson.

Tigerhead Antiseptic Liniment contained 65 percent alcohol and was promoted for use as a "fast temporary relief of minor discomforts, aches, and pains due to over-exertion, exposure, or fatigue. For temporary relief of aches and pains of arthritis or rheumatism." It was also recommended for relieving nonpoisonous insect stings. The Lucky Heart Company out of Memphis, Tennessee, produced the Tigerhead Antiseptic Liniment beginning about 1923, and it was on the market at least thirty-five years.

Tincture of arnica, containing about 50 percent alcohol, was used for bruises, sprains, rheumatism, and other painful afflictions. Tinctures usually were sold in more elaborate bottles, with fancy tops and glass stoppers. These were used by physicians more than the other liniment-type products.

In London during the late 1880s a series of advertisements placed in magazines and newspapers provided a graphic appeal aimed directly at those who engaged in a variety of athletic activities. "Elliman's Universal Embrocation" was indeed, according to its very creative advertising, a liniment for universal applications. In addition to the "universal" liniment just mentioned, there were the "Royal" embrocations. Of the six ads in my collection, the four shown here feature women. The two featuring men depict them playing polo and driving a coach, around which are many men and women riding on horseback, side-saddle style.

Elliman's Embrocation brings to light another historic marker in the history of massage. These advertisements, alongside those for the Pompeian Massage Cream, represent a concerted effort at selling traditionally male products to women: liniments. These campaigns were at their zenith during the height of the woman's suffrage movement, obviously by design to capture a newly emerging customer—women. Not only was Elliman aiming its advertising at women. They also created a new name for an old product, changing *liniment* to *embrocation,* a word with a much more feminine appeal.

"Mother's Friend" was a liniment advertised in a small booklet entitled *Motherhood.* It was specifically marketed to pregnant and nursing mothers in the 1890s by the Bradfield Regulator Company of Atlanta, Georgia. For morning sickness, Mother's Friend is directed for use as follows: "Pour a few drops on a soft cloth, or on the bare hand, and rub gently over the pit of the stomach for five or ten minutes. The liniment's very penetrat-

172

MASSAGE TOOLS

AND MEDIUMS

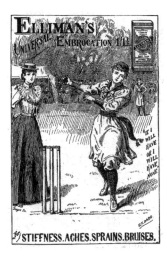
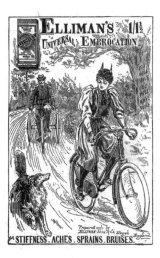
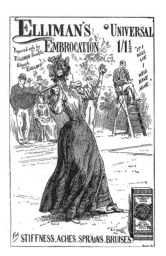

Elliman's Universal and Royal Embrocation was a liniment not only for men and women, as depicted engaging in a variety of social and athletic activities, but for horses, cattle, goats, sheep, and dogs as well. Obviously, using Elliman's Liniment meant you could participate in all these activities with style and grace while leading the pack. From the *Illustrated London News*, 1895

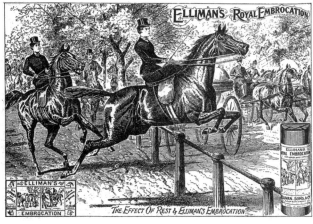

ing and will quickly be absorbed. Repeat in half an hour if necessary." Care for the breasts of a mother-to-be should start with good hygiene, and then, "Rub the whole breasts thoroughly but gently with Mother's Friend for five or ten minutes, letting it penetrate . . . and continue once or twice a day until the very hour of labor. After the birth of the child, it may be advisable . . . to continue the use of the liniment for many days until the milk is freely flowing." They also advise "rubbing gently" to allay the pains of pregnancy in the abdomen and colon. To prevent miscarriage, "The abdomen and breasts should be thoroughly rubbed every day according to direction." These recommendations were based on advice from the company's advising physician.

Pompeian Massage Cream was one of the most widely advertised products in America for nearly fifty years, beginning in the late 1800s. This cream was advertised in many ways, but most often as a night cream to eliminate wrinkles and dry skin. It was not just a product for women; many of the advertisements were directed at men, particularly those visiting the local barbershop.

The Pompeian cream was an advanced solution based on an older type of facial cream called "rolling massage cream." The rolling creams were widely used by barbers and beauty salon operators from about 1880 to 1920, when it was replaced by other products, such as the Pompeian cream, which was absorbed into the skin through rubbing instead of brushed or wiped off as the rolling creams were removed.

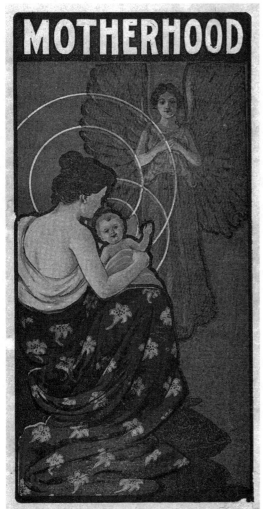

MOTHERHOOD

The cover of a promotional booklet from 1898 advertising a liniment called Mother's Friend used for expectant, laboring, and new mothers and their babies. Frequent "rubbing" was recommended to apply the penetrating liniment.

A number of nineteenth-century physicians and Nurse Mary McMillan recommended using no lubricant at all in giving a massage treatment. James B. Mennell, M.D., writing in 1886, advises "The massage should be 'dry,' that is without the use of oil, or liniments, or ointments of any kind."[26] They felt it prevented the hands from properly sensing the "finer" tissues beneath them, and they asserted that lubricants prevented the proper "drag" necessary to achieve desired effects of the massage. They also pointed out that, in some cases, adverse reactions occurred. However, in 1892, Dr. Kleen affirmed the need for lubricants. "Most masseurs make use of some lubricant to make the patient's skin soft and smooth. This is often a necessity, especially for firm effleurage, as otherwise one causes pain by dragging the hairs of the skin, and may irritate the glands of the skin and so cause acne or boils. . . . Different skin lubricants may be used; glycerene [sic], vaseline, lanoline, lard, 'cold cream,' olive oil, cocoa butter, etc."[27] Of the possible lubricants named by Kleen, he claims that glycerin and vaseline irritate the skin; liquid oils are "troublesome" to handle; and that cocoa butter is a fine lubricant, but its odor is offensive. He recommended lard as the best overall lubricant, although talc was another positive choice, and comfortable for the patient. Liniments were not usually commented on by those writing about massage during his time. It seems they were used more by athletic trainers, athletes, and ordinary citizens, much as one might use aspirin, Tylenol, or Tiger Balm today.

During the second half of the twentieth century, lubricants used for massage ranged widely. Several nursing texts recommended using no lubricant at all, but most practitioners utilized some form of lubricant when working on the naked skin.

Powders in the form of talc or cornstarch-based powders were widely used for several decades, especially in Europe, but died out sometime during the 1950s. Powders are sometimes used today as a replacement for oils when conditions of the client merits.

Massage creams, popular at the beginning of the twentieth century, died out for a time and have come back in specialized forms during the last quarter of the century. Most early creams were petroleum-based products; those used today are more often vegetable based to better prevent reaction from contact with the skin. Creams employed today are primarily used with techniques that require a heavy drag across the skin, such as a deep-tissue technique or myofacial modality.

Mineral oil was a very common lubricant for well over fifty years, but is rarely used today because of its toxicity. Many of us have heard of the "alcohol rub" used for decades in exercise clubs. Alcohol is no longer used in the massage trade as a lubricant. And the liniments of yesteryear used during the nineteenth century and early twentieth century are all things of the past. Today in their place we find products

MASSAGE TOOLS

AND MEDIUMS

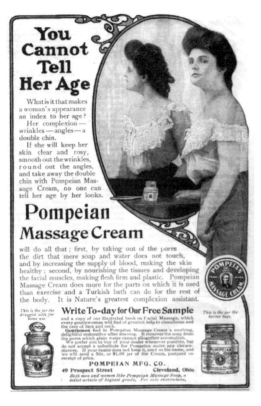

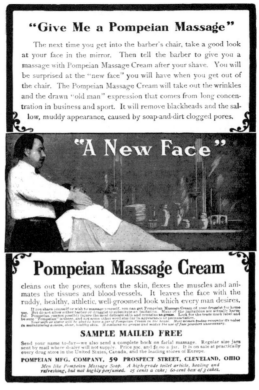

such as "Sports Rub," "BioFreeze," and "Tiger Balm" being used as specialized rubbing compounds for small areas, whereas the old-time liniments were used over a broader area of the body. There may be no antique equivalent to the modern gels and waxes found today being used by practitioners who need a controlled and high degree of drag when working on the body.

Common oils used in ancient times, such as olive, grape seed, and almond oil, were widely utilized by practitioners working out of their homes or with small storefront practices for most of the twentieth century. Commercial lubricants that included filtered or blended oils came on the scene during the 1960s and became widely available from 1970 onward. Today's lubricants are oil based or water based, and some contain scents and essential oils. Most practitioners today utilize a filtered oil purchased from a major massage-industry producer, such as Biotone, but in the 1990s a few small companies began selling their products to a worldwide audience, competing directly with the larger, more established firms. The addition of essential oils into the base of a common oil is quite popular, but essential oils are not ordinarily used directly on the client's skin. Most practitioners who do massage for a living today use some kind of commercially manufactured oil.

Noting the advice given and promises made for using any of the products mentioned here, let us not forget the assertion made earlier by Dr. Graham regarding the application of massage and external measures, that "every substance capable of being rubbed on the human body has had wonderful virtues ascribed to it, and it must be that which is common to them all that does the good—namely, the rubbing."[28]

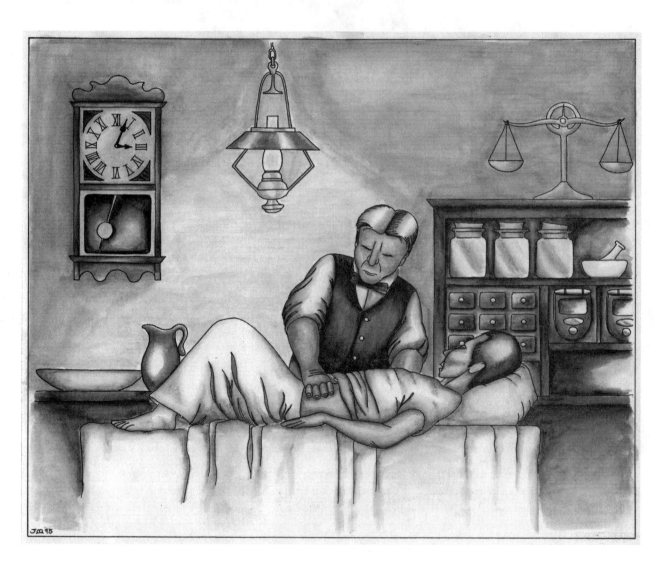

Abdominal massage being performed by a physician in the late 1800s in the United States. This "séance" is taking place in the physician's home office. Courtesy of *Massage Magazine*.

10 The Evolution of Massage Technique

Early Massage Techniques

As discussed earlier in this text, the first written descriptions of massage technique are found in the writings of Hippocrates. In his treatise entitled *On the Articulations*, Hippocrates writes, "Friction can relax, brace, incarnate, attenuate: hard braces, soft relaxes, much attenuates, and moderate thickens."[1] In other words, applying friction with hard pressure strengthens tissues and with soft pressure relaxes them; a lot of friction weakens or thins tissues and moderate friction can add substance to tissues. This succinct principle was followed and elaborated upon for centuries after Hippocrates. Exploring the effects of combining the variations of pressure and frequency is a pursuit that has occupied practitioners ever since.

Nearly five hundred years after Hippocrates, Galen, considered one of the greatest admirers and followers of Hippocratic medical practice, provides us with even more detail on the techniques of medical rubbing. In discussing the preparation of an athlete for exercise by warming his body, Galen describes the massage technique he administers.

> It is necessary to warm the whole body moderately by rubbing it with muslin and then with oil. For I do not recommend the immediate use of oil before the skin has been warmed and the pores dilated and, in a word, the body prepared to receive the oil. For this purpose generally a few strokes of the hands are sufficient, gentle and moderately swift, having as objective to warm the body apart from rubbing it. . . . Apply oil and rub with the bare hands, which are midway between hard and soft.[2]

This is the technique of applying friction for two purposes; to serve as a pre-exercise

It is almost impossible to teach the art of massage by written or verbal description. It is very much as if one were trying to make a pianoforte player by describing how it is done without recourse to the instrument.

—William Murrell, M.D., *Massage as a Mode of Treatment* (1886)

warm-up and to open the pores of the skin to help absorption of the oils considered valuable at this time. The massage techniques are, again, pressure and frequency.

More detailed descriptions of Hippocratic massage technique come from a chapter in Galen's book *Hygiene* entitled "Techniques and Varieties of Massage." "Now in the preparatory rubbing before exercise, having as its objective to soften the body, the median quality between hard and soft should prevail, and everything else should be maintained in that accordance." He then goes on to explain the effects of these techniques, using the same concept as expressed by Hippocrates: "that the body is constricted by hard rubbing, relaxed by soft, thinned by much rubbing, and thickened by moderate."[3] Galen discusses for an entire chapter what other physicians of his time wrote about these techniques and their effects, but in the end concludes that they say nothing more or less than Hippocrates himself on the subject.

About the time Hippocrates and his colleagues were developing their medical practices, the Asians were improving on the primitive forms of their healing arts. With its origin in ancient China thought to be nearly five thousand years ago, "The amma massage method [used throughout Asia] grew from the simple habit of pressing or rubbing numbed or chilled hands and feet with the fingers and palms of the hands."[4] Zhang Tao, commenting on the Chinese roots of massage technique, says, "In the Ming dynasty [1368–1641], the name was finally switched to 'Tuina.'"[5] Tuina consists of more than one hundred distinct hand techniques. A few examples are the palm press, thumb press, palm rub and thumb rub, palm-heel rub or press, flat-palm push method, rolling cylinder, single-finger dig, thumb kneading, and palm rub-roll. The single-finger dig technique is described as pressing the tip of the thumb or middle finger into the flesh. Using either digit, the technique is aided by support of the digging finger by the other fingers around it, such as holding the middle finger tightly between the index finger and thumb when applying pressure. Tuina techniques are almost exclusively described by the parts of the hand, forearm, and elbow, applied to the patient on what are called *tsubo,* or vital points. These points are usually the painful spots on muscles; it is in these areas that the amma or tuina massage focuses with a combination of pressure and rubbing techniques.

Every writer on massage asserts that India has a long history of massage, even though there is controversy about its origins and little description of technique from the ancient writings. However, we do have several sources from the nineteenth century that provide hints about the Indian technique of *tshampua,* or shampooing. Taylor describes it this way. "Extended on a seat, the operator manipulates his members, as he would knead dough for bread. He then strikes him lightly with the side of the hand, applies perfume and friction, and terminates by cracking the joints of the fingers, toes, and neck."[6] In a discussion about baldness Latson mentions "dry shampooing" as a form of scalp massage. "Among the local methods the most important measures are shampooing, brushing, manipulation with the hands (dry shampooing), pulling and massage."[7] He describes the technique of dry shampooing as "manipulation [of the scalp] with the finger tips."

THE EVOLUTION OF

MASSAGE TECHNIQUE

Graham gives us a look at ancient Egyptian techniques seen through the eyes of a sixteenth-century writer. "Alpinus, 1553–1617 A.D. . . . says that frictions . . . are in use amongst the Egyptians. The person is extended horizontally; then he is malaxated, manipulated, or kneaded, and pressed . . . upon the various parts of the body with the hands of the operator. Passive motion is then given to the different articulations."[8] "Friction" consisted of stroking or effleurage, while "malaxated, manipulated, or kneaded" refer to squeezing and pressing techniques we now know as petrissage. The pressing technique was probably some kind of compression used in conjunction with the other manipulations. The passive motions referred to in the last sentence are what we now call range-of-motion movements.

No further descriptions of technique are available from the ancients except that they referred to other techniques, such as flagellation, percussion, vibration, and slapping. The most detail we get from any description is about the amount of pressure to use, the frequency of the movements or treatments, and where to apply them. Nearly all the ancient accounts focus on the benefits derived from these techniques without giving adequate descriptions of how to perform them. Most of the historical writing about massage techniques dates from the nineteenth century, when books about massage proliferated.

Nineteenth-century Massage Technique

In the literature on massage from the nineteenth century the technique represented is varied. Some writers gave very little specific direction, while others give in-depth descriptions and illustrations. Because terminology was not consistent the same technique might not be easily recognizable between various writers. Techniques and movements (mobilization and therapeutic exercise, for example) were grouped differently by individual writers. Movements that we now think of as elements of physical therapy sometimes played a larger role than kneading or other such techniques in a massage session, depending on the practitioner.

The few physicians who embraced massage used it more as a method for restoring health than as a method for preserving it. Active and passive movements were prescribed for specific conditions and only the injured or affected portion of the body might be treated. A general massage might be given as a restorative to the whole system but not as a preventive measure against future problems. Many of the techniques were applied quickly and frequently. Vigorous treatments given two and three times a day were not unusual when administered by a medical practitioner or under his supervision.

In 1877 Douglas Graham, M.D., wrote an article for the *New York Medical Record* entitled "The Treatment of Sprains by Massage" in which he expressed the following:

> Massage may be used very early after an injury, within the first 24 hours.
> The skin over the affected part should be anointed with oil to protect it,

for it is the deeper tissues that are particularly to be affected by kneading. The thumbs and fingers are then to be applied with steady and firm pressure, their force being graduated according to the tenderness of the part, so as through the skin to rub and knead, and roll the deeper tissues, diffusing the exudations present, stimulating the languid circulation, and exciting the absorbents. The manipulations should be begun beyond the margins of the tumefied [swelling] and painful spots, which should be gradually approached. The soothing effect of the rubbing, when patiently and delicately applied, is such that soon pressure and movement over the points of chief injury are readily tolerated. By massage a more speedy relief from pain and swelling and an earlier restoration of the function of the part can be secured in many cases than by any other method. It is particularly of value in the treatment of contusions, distortions, and sprains of joints and their sequelae. Sprains recover in one-third the usual time under this treatment.[9]

Addressing medical students and nurses, Axel V. Grafstrom, a Swedish physician practicing in New York, wrote a small book entitled *A Text Book of Mechano-Therapy (Massage and Medical Gymnastics)* that provides illustrations of massage technique worth noting. He describes two kinds of kneading—palmar and digital—and provides an illustration only for the latter form. "Kneading usually follows friction," writes Grafstrom. "It consists of manipulations of either a single muscle or a group of muscles. It is applied differently to different parts of the body. When several muscles are treated simultaneously the palmar surfaces of both hands are employed *(palmar kneading),* and in treating a single muscle or the intestines the fingers and thumb of each hand are used, while in the treatment of glands and nerves the finger-tips only are used *(digital kneading).*"[10]

Grafstrom also describes two varieties of friction—palmar and digital—but with some interesting additional information: "All friction should be done directly on the patient's skin, without the intervention of any coverings, and should invariably begin at the periphery and go toward the center; that is, in the same direction as the venous circulation."[11] The word *coverings* refers to lubricants and clothing or draping material to stand between the operator's hands and the skin of the patient. His technique is clearly Hippocratic as he recommends rubbing up, not down.

Dr. Graham, writing in 1890, provides a look at the "Aix douche-massage." Normally used in conjunction with dietary treatments for diabetes, the Aix douche-massage was originally developed in France around the latter part of the 1880s at the Aix-les-Bains, a well-known mineral springs spa in France. The technique was used at the Carlsbad Baths, the Brides and Vichy spas, and others.

The simultaneous use of massage while the patients are being douched is the characteristic mode of treatment of diabetes at Aix-les-Bains. The hydrosulphurated thermal waters of Aix are too feebly mineralized to be employed in any other way than externally, which is thought to favor

THE EVOLUTION OF

MASSAGE TECHNIQUE

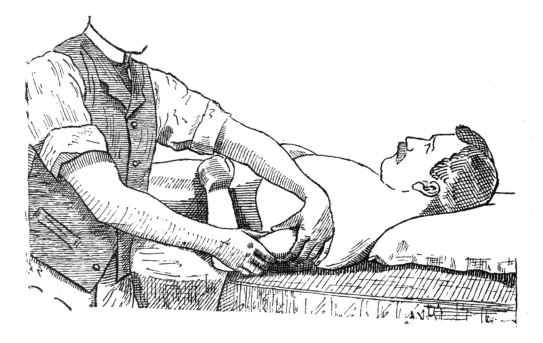

Digital kneading of the bicep area.

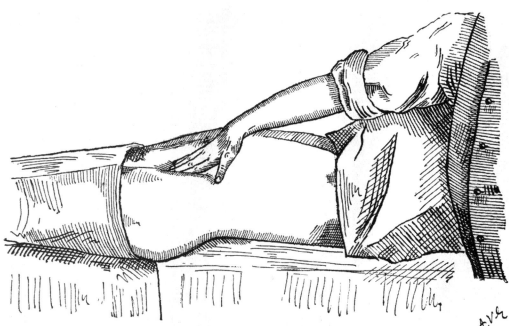

Deep digital kneading of the descending colon. From Axel V. Grafstrom's *Textbook of Mechano-Therapy* (Philadelphia, 1898).

the absorption of sulphuretted hydrogen by the skin. Dr. Forestier has treated seven cases of saccharine diabetes in fat people by means of the douche-massage with the result that there has been in all a great decrease in the glycosuria. The douche-massage was given while the patients were sitting or lying by two masseurs, one of whom took the limbs, the other the trunk, each directing a jet of water from a nozzle under his arm, douching and masse'eing [*sic*] at the same time for ten or fifteen minutes daily, the water being at from 37° to 40° Centigrade (about 100° F.).[12]

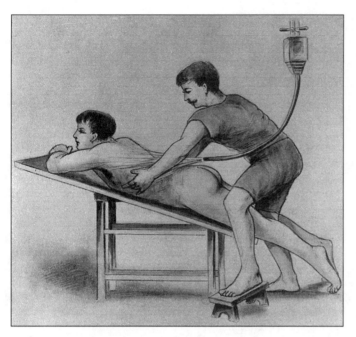

The Aix douche-massage developed at a mineral springs spa in France and used at European medical spas in the later two decades of the nineteenth century. Dr. Graham describes the massage as being given by two masseurs simultaneously. From *Manual Therapeutics* by Douglas Graham, M.D. (1902).

The "douching" method applies high-pressure water streams or sprays externally upon the body. This method is still used today but with more sophisticated equipment. It is not used outside the spa setting and probably never was.

In another passage from his book discussing modes of applying massage, Graham writes: "Friction or *effleurage* may be spoken of as circular and rectilinear; the latter may be vertical or parallel to the long axis of a limb; or horizontal, transversal, or at right angles to the long axis."[13] This description is very similar to that of Galen noted above. Graham goes on to offer his own innovation.

A slight deviation from the method ordinarily recommended in doing straight-line friction I have found to be more advantageous; for though in almost every case the upward strokes of the friction should be the stronger so as to aid the venous and lymph currents, yet the returning or downward movement may with benefit lightly graze the surface, imparting a soothing influence, without being so vigorous as to retard the circulation pushed along by the upward stroke, and thus a saving of time and effort will be gained.[14]

This latter remark is strikingly similar to the description given by Hippocrates earlier.

It is important to clarify the use of the word *friction* in the quoted passages of Hippocrates, Galen, and Graham; they are not referring to the techniques known today as friction. Friction in contemporary applications consists of two types. The first is done by placing a hand on the skin and moving the superficial skin over the underlying tissues without moving the hand on the surface of the skin. This method is referred to in ancient writings by the term *deep friction's* [*sic*], and was a squeezing or kneading technique. The second type is a technique consistent throughout history, that of rubbing the hands or a cloth in quick, rapid motion across the surface of the skin to create heat. It is clear that *friction* as used by the ancients, and by nineteenth- and early-twentieth-century physicians, is massage because of the various movement directions, pressures, and such that their writings describe.

First published in German in 1898 and translated into English in 1909, Robert Ziegenspeck's *Massage Treatment in Diseases of Women* includes the following: "Massage of the pelvic organs is employed almost exclusively in the form of circular rubbings, only in special cases, as in the process called 'malning' (painting), and to be described hereafter, in the form of stroking movements. In principle there is really only a slight difference between gynecological massage and general massage as used on other parts of the body, because in making circular rubbings we do not press equally upon all parts, but increase the pressure at one place of the periphery of the circle and possibly in the direction of the venous and lymphatic circulation."[15] *Malning* is the Swedish word for "painting," a technique that is administered in certain kinds of peritonitis located in the pelvic area and is similar to the strokes used in painting, being applied in one direction only.[16]

A rare piece of advertising found in a Chicago newspaper from 1892 alludes to another technique specific to women, but gives no description of the method used nor any of the scientific or practical theory behind it. Practitioner Lucille Young offered a special massage technique to develop firmness and plumpness of the bust. (It is interesting to note that this is the only nineteenth-century advertisement found by this author that was placed by a female practitioner.)

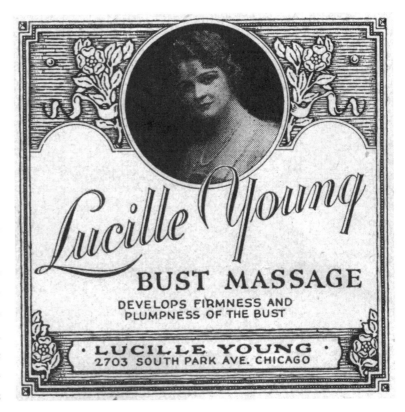

A Chicago newspaper advertisement from 1892 for Lucille Young's bust massage, a technique of unknown origin and methodology. The ad suggests that massage was used for cosmetic purposes at this early date. Courtesy of World of Massage Museum.

Kellogg writes about shampooing as performed in Japan during the nineteenth century. This description was given to him by a friend who had "personal experience with Japanese massage, which was administered to him by a first-class manipulator. . . . The shampooer sat in Japanese fashion at the side of the patient, as the latter lay on a futon . . . on the floor, and began operations on the arm; then took the back and the back of the neck, afterward the head . . . and ended with the legs. On the arms, back, back of the neck, and legs, he used sometimes the tips of his fingers, sometimes the palms or the backs of his hands, sometimes his knuckles, sometimes his fists. The movements consisted of pinching, slapping, stroking, rubbing, knuckling, kneading, thumping, drawing in the hand, and snapping the knuckles. . . . On the head he used gentle tapping, a little pounding with the knuckles, stroking with both hands, holding the head tight for a moment, grasping it with one hand and stroking it with the other. . . . He is to be criticised, however, for one serious fault in his operations—that of shampooing down, instead of up. A portion of the good done is thus neutralized, one object of scientific massage being to help back toward the center the blood which is lingering in the superficial veins."[17]

This description coincides with our knowledge of Asian massage techniques of today that utilize various parts of the hands for applying the technique, and the variety of movements corresponds to those we find in other descriptions of ancient practice that are still used today. Most interesting is Kellogg's response to his friend's criticism about rubbing down, not up. He writes, "I do not agree with my friend's criticism of the mode of manipulation employed by the Japanese masseur, who seems to have

THE EVOLUTION OF

MASSAGE TECHNIQUE

been more skilled than most of our own manipulators, since he was apparently aware of the fact that the limbs should be rubbed down, rather than up, for the relief of the condition of feverishness and irritation from which his patient was suffering."[18] Kellogg knew that in cases of fever, massaging up, or with the venous flow toward the core of the body, could increase the overall body temperature, thus increasing the fever. For this reason he recommended ending with centrifugal massage, or rubbing down in all pulmonary cases. This is a classic Hippocratic principle—rub down the limbs in case of fever, not up. It is one of the few exceptions to rubbing up, or toward the heart and with the venous flow. This simple remark by Kellogg demonstrates the lineage of technique from Hippocrates to Kellogg, more than two thousand years apart. Today we no longer hear of "rubbing up" or "rubbing down" in the teaching of technique. Instead, students are taught to massage with the venous and lymphatic flow, which is the same as rubbing up practiced by the ancient Greek physicians.

Kellogg wrote extensively on the techniques used in massage. He provided such a complete breakdown of massage technique that his book *The Art of Massage* is still being used in a few massage schools in America today. In 1895 Kellogg was the first to present contraindications for massage under the heading "Rules Relating to Massage." These included rules for good health, personal hygiene, qualities and care of the hands, personal appearance, and others. A few examples of contraindications are interesting to note.

28. When it is desired to stimulate the skin to a high degree by friction, lubricants should be avoided.

29. Some authorities recommend that the parts should be shaved before the application of massage, but this is rarely necessary.

30. The amount of massage administered must be suited to each case and to the mode of application.

31. Do not recommend massage for everything.

32. General massage should never be given in cases of fever. Local applications should not be made to parts which are the seat of acute inflammation.

33. Fleshy persons do not bear massage well, for the reason that the manipulations set free a large amount of waste matter and imperfectly oxidized products which, absorbed into the system, produce the same effect as excessive exercise—effects resembling those of consecutive or secondary fatigue, to which fleshy persons are very liable. Fleshy persons often complain of languor, lassitude, and lameness after massage, and the tissues are very easily bruised because of the weak circulation and on account of the excessive amount of adipose tissue.

34. Massage is contra-indicated in nearly all forms of skin disease, except in the thickened condition of the skin left behind by chronic eczema. It is also contra-indicated in cases of apoplexy and in the early stages of neuritis, when excessive irritability still exists, and should never be administered to abscesses, tumors, or tubercular joints.[19]

Among the texts written during the late nineteenth century Dr. Kellogg's is perhaps the most interesting to read, although there is much information that is inaccurate and unsubstantiated, a criticism that has been laid upon Dr. Kellogg regarding a number of his eccentric therapies. Bob McCoy, proprietor of the Museum of Questionable Medical Devices, labels Kellogg one of the great American quacks. Even so, *The Art of Massage* is still obtainable, and well worth reading.

From a 1909 book about German home medical treatments we find an interesting array of techniques. The illustration here shows two forms of abdominal massage, kneading the calf, gown rubbing, and two types of gymnastic exercises for treating asthma. Note that in the gown rubbing drawing the person being rubbed is standing in a large tub. The tub is there to catch water that drips off the gown because the operator is using water on her hands during the procedure.

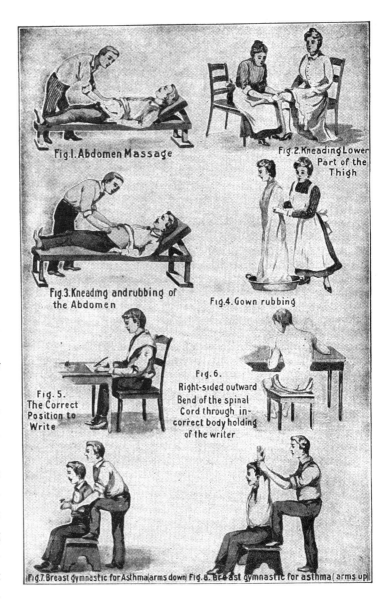

Fig. 1. Abdomen Massage

Fig. 2. Kneading Lower Part of the Thigh

Fig. 3. Kneading and rubbing of the Abdomen

Fig. 4. Gown rubbing

Fig. 5. The Correct Position to Write

Fig. 6. Right-sided outward Bend of the spinal Cord through incorrect body holding of the writer

Fig. 7. Breast gymnastic for Asthma (arms down)

Fig. 8. Breast gymnastic for asthma (arms up)

German massage and exercise "home medical treatments." From *The Cottage Physician*, Introduction by George W. Post, M.D. (Springfield, Mass., 1908).

George Abbott, a physician in Portland, Oregon, wrote about massage in the early twentieth century. His book, *Technique of Hydrotherapy and Swedish Massage,* explains that the Turkish shampoo is a method of exfoliation. "The shampoo proper is preceded by manipulations and heavy friction to loosen the outer epidermis (so-called dead skin)."[20] By "shampoo proper" Abbott is referring to a "sweating bath, such as the Turkish, the Russian, or the electric light bath." The procedure goes like this: heat the patient with sweat bath or by having him lie on a warmed slab. Give him rapid, full-body frictions on both sides of the body and then lather him up and wash him thoroughly before rinsing him with cool water. The frictions were usually given by hand, dipping the hands into a container of warm water or using a "friction mitt."

Nurse Mary McMillan taught massage techniques in cases of dislocation and fracture, methods derived from her work in European and American military hospitals during and after World War I. The use of massage in fractures usually entailed manipulation of the adjoining musculature primarily to reduce atrophy that could result from the area being immobilized. In the case of fractures of bones that cannot be immobilized, such as the collarbone, ribs, or sternum (all moved by simple respiration), massage was used to assist in the formation of "exuberant callus," and often Swedish movements were utilized along with massage. A so-called tenth commandment in the treatment of fractures reads: "Passive motions are useless, unless the fractures are near a joint. Make passive and active motions when the tendon sheaths are inflamed."[21] In dislocations, massage was frequently used to strengthen muscles. Swedish movements usually followed treatment in these cases. These joint and inflammation techniques were not taught much in lay massage schools from the 1930s through the 1970s because, without medical prescription, dislocations and fractures were considered contraindications to massage, likely due in large part to liability issues. Today these methods are much more common in lay practice.

The Evolution of Swedish Massage Technique

George Taylor, a New York physician, wrote numerous books, four of which are relevant to our topic. *An Exposition of the Swedish Movement-Cure,* first published in 1860, was published again in 1885 under the title *Health by Exercise Showing What Exercises to Take.* In 1887 he published *Massage: Principles and Practices of Remedial Treatment by Imparted Motion,* and in 1888 a new and enlarged edition of *Health by Exercise* with the subtitle *The Movement Cure* was published. The 1860 text does not contain a chapter on massage, and unlike almost every other text on massage during this time, Taylor's 1887 book—which was all about massage—contains no illustrations to support his descriptions of how to perform the various techniques.

The subject of massage was not covered in Taylor's first book, but he gave it seven chapters in the next two editions. He explains the passive movements of the Swedish gymnastic system originally developed by Peter Ling earlier in the century.

> The division of movements into *active* and *passive* relates to the sources whence the moving power is derived. The motion of riding, for instance, is *passive,* if the body be supported. So also are the *clappings, knockings, strokings, kneadings, pullings, shakings, vibratings,* etc., of the duplicated [passive] movements, because both the motion and will that gives it energy are derived from another person.[22]

Most of Taylor's book, however, focuses on the proper position of the patient in performing the active exercises.

Prior to giving explicit directions on how to perform each movement, Taylor provides a lengthy overview of the principles of technique for all the Swedish gymnastic movements. The manner of the movements includes both a mechanical and a mental

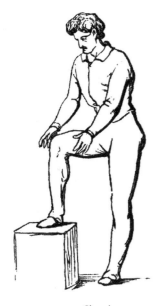
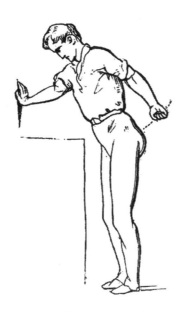
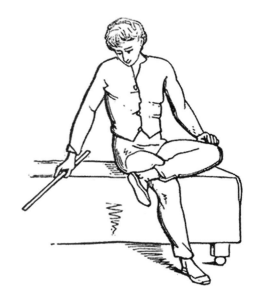

Clapping   Chine knocking—a form of vibration   Foot percussion

element. The mechanical manner is the "correct posture" of the limb being moved and "the prescribed line" for that particular limb or joint, or the limits of its range of motion. The mental aspect consists of the operator's intention in the case of passive movements, and the patient's internal participation in the case of active movements. Next there is the rhythm, exertion, or pressure; the number of repetitions; the proper order in which they are performed; the relationship of the diseased part to the movement being performed; and finally, the region of the body upon which the exercises are done.

Despite his elucidation of these principles of technique Taylor gives very little attention to describing the passive movements of "clappings, knockings, strokings, kneadings, pullings, shakings, vibratings, etc." In fact, he gives no descriptions in his 1860 text for the techniques of stroking, kneading, pulling, and shaking. Why these descriptions are omitted among dozens of the active movements might be explained by the following passage. "But the employment of duplicated [passive] movements, it must be confessed, is attended with difficulties that will prevent their general use as a medical resource. An ordinary course of medical instruction does not confer the necessary qualifications for their successful application; the tact necessary to prescribe and apply them properly is only acquired by long and patient practice, and the labor is excessively severe."[23]

This extraordinary statement by Dr. Taylor may be considered a pivotal point in the history of massage. It might explain some of the reasons why massage was not separated from the gymnastic movement, and why Kleen, thirty-two years later, would be fighting to have them separated. But Taylor preceded Kellogg and Kleen in presenting massage as a stand-alone therapy, writing chapters on massage separate from the passive movement manipulations contained in the gymnastic exercise and movement systems covered in the rest of his book.

Three examples of passive movements from the Swedish gymnastic system. According to the author, special training and "long and patient practice" was required to master these movements. From *Health by Exercise: Showing What Exercises to Take* by George H. Taylor (New York, 1885).

Mathias Roth in 1851 wrote extensively about the passive movements, or "single movements," within Ling's Swedish gymnastics. In describing squeezing and pressing movements, Roth emphasized their role in effecting the change of circulation in a local area. "The pressing and squeezing movements produce, according to their greater or less intensity, a local effect."[24] This technique consisted of holding pressure on a local area by one operator; or two operators each pushing the same body part toward one another to derive pressure. The idea was to press the area to remove or lessen the blood; when the pressure was removed, blood would come rushing back. Today this technique, called ischemic compression, is used widely in massage applied in sports.

Professor Hartvig Nissen gives us an illustrative look at massage techniques from the nineteenth century in his 1889 book, *A Manual of Instruction for Giving Swedish Movement and Massage Treatment.* He describes "passive movements" thus:

> Centripetal stroking, pressing, kneading, circular friction, and vibratory friction are all to be given from the tip of the fingers toward the shoulder. Grasp the patient's finger with your thumb and two first fingers, and make a firm pressing and stroking movement upward toward the hand; at the same time let your fingers glide in a circular way round the patient's finger, describing the motions of a screw. Let your fingers glide easily back to the starting-point (the tip of the patient's finger), and repeat the motions fifteen to twenty times on each finger.[25]

Nissen's technique of working the arm while always moving the bloodflow toward the heart continues today. His method of working the fingers, however, is found much less often. Instead of working the fingers toward the heart, or proximally, most practitioners work the fingers distally, pulling as they twist and press the fingers with the "motions of a screw."

Nineteenth-century manual massage techniques, a la Hartvig Nissen

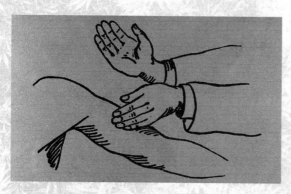

Percussion
Percussion—is performed with the edge of the extended fingers, which are kept loose, and with a quick motion of the wrist-joint the fingers are flung *across* the muscles from the shoulder toward the hand.

From the mid-1880s until just before World War II, Hartvig Nissen was a force unto himself in the field of massage within medicine. Nissen taught massage at Harvard University summer school, Johns Hopkins University, and Wellesley College, and served for a time as director of the Swedish Health Institute in Washington, D.C. These drawings from his first book, *A Manual for Instruction for Giving Swedish Movement and Masssage Treatment* (1889), represent classic examples of Swedish massage technique. Although Nissen claimed that the drawings and text in this book were not the result of his life's work but were "written on the authority of others," he continued to use these representations and text in his teaching and his writings, through his last published book in 1932.

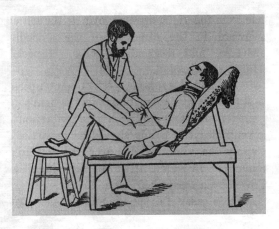

Stomach Kneading

Stomach Kneading—Stomach friction is made with both hands all over the abdomen from the middle and out to the sides several times, followed with an upward stroke with the one hand on the right side and over to the left in the direction of the ascending and transverse colon, and then a downward stroke with the other hand on the left side in the direction of the descending colon. Repeated four to eight times.

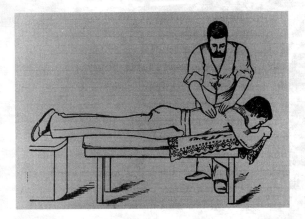

Back Kneading

Back Kneading—Back kneading, vibration, and friction is applied from the base of the skull downward, and from the spinal column outward to the sides, all over the back. A very good movement in connection with these is to put the heel of the hands on the spinal column at the neck and apply a rapid shaking movement, letting the one hand slowly glide downward to the end of the spine.

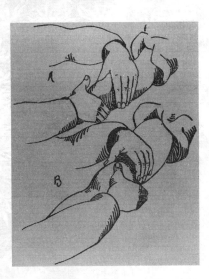

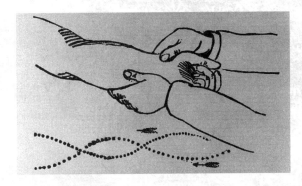

Circular Friction

Circulation Friction—Grasp the hand with both of yours, and make upward pushing movements, constantly moving the hands and fingers in a circular direction, thereby making a sideways friction together with the upward stroke.

Kneading

Kneading—Knead the muscles from the fingers toward the elbow by picking up each group of muscles with the one hand, and when releasing the grasp make an upward pressure with the other hand (kneading).

Muscle Rolling

Muscle Rolling—Grasping the limb with the palms of both hands, and making a quick, alternate pushing-and-pulling motion, and gradually gliding downward from the shoulder, the muscles of the arm will be rolled against each other, whereby the circulation of the blood is very much increased. Repeated three to five times.

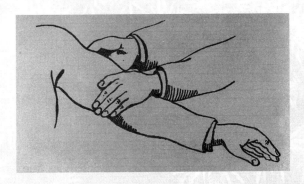

The Swedish physician Emil Kleen may have been the first to publish drawings of the massage manipulations we now know of as Swedish movements. His book, *Handbook of Massage* (1888) predates Nissen (1889), Kellogg (1895), and others in using French terms to describe the four basic massage strokes. The term *vibration* was added to complete the five basic strokes used in today's Swedish massage system. From Emil Kleen, M.D., *Handbook of Massage* (Philadelphia, 1892).

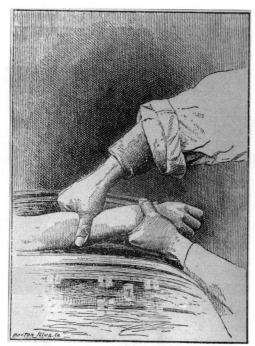

Effleurage

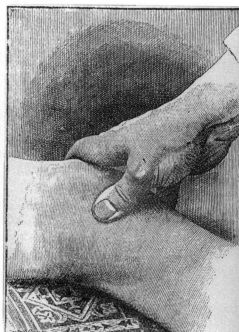

Friction's

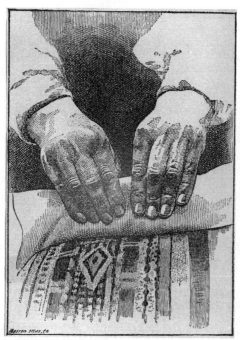

Petrissage

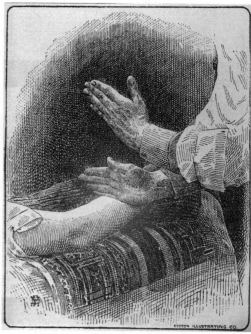

Tapotement

In 1892 Dr. Kleen described the four basic strokes that have come to be known as Swedish massage.

The manipulations employed in massage have been classified in a variety of ways. The Mezger school, and a considerable number of German masseurs, arrange them in four classes, which are designated by the French terms—(1) effleurage=stroking, (2) friction's=rubbing, (3) petrissage= squeezing, and (4) tapotement=striking.[26]

In a footnote he adds, "This is surely the most rational and the simplest classification, and no massage manipulation can be conceived that cannot be assigned to one of these four classes. . . . To add a division of 'passive movements' is to invade the domain of gymnastics."[27] Kleen is true to his task by keeping the distinct manipulations of massage separate from the passive movements of the gymnastic exercise and movement systems.

It is most interesting that the development of Swedish scientific massage, so prevalent from 1928 to 1978 and taught in nearly all the massage schools in America during that time, never gave Kleen credit for his staunch position on the four basic strokes and the separation of them from gymnastics. To this original list of four, vibration has been added to become the fifth basic stroke in the Swedish Massage system.

Dr. Kellogg was a staunch supporter of Peter Ling's system of medical gymnastics and of Ling's successor, T. J. Hartelus. M.D., who directed the Royal Central Gymnastic Institute from 1865 until 1890. Kellogg's descriptions and photos of the traditional Swedish massage are nearly the same as most others we might see except that he provides a variety of applications, such as palmar kneading, digital kneading, deep vibration, shaking, digital vibration, lateral vibration, knuckle vibration, and so on.

From the Hahnemann Medical College in Philadelphia, Pennsylvania, Richard Haehl, M.D., a little known but earnest advocate of massage, wrote a small book of instruction in 1898 entitled *Massage: Its History, Technique and Therapeutic Uses.* Dr. Haehl describes "massage `a friction" as "The finger tips of one hand held at right angles to the axis of the limb, rub across and across in narrow ellipses, while the fingers of the other hand stroke parallel to the axis of the limb."[28] He adds a new stroke under the heading of effleurage called "cog-crasp-manipulation." The fingers of both hands being flexed, the right thumb surrounded by the fingers of the left hand. The stroking is applied with the dorsal surface and by the angles formed through the flexion between the phalangeal joints. This kind of effleurage is mainly used on the back and buttocks, occasionally on the posterior surface of thighs and legs. It is really a manipulation midway between effleurage and massage `a friction."[29]

Haehl also describes another new technique named "tapotement `a l`air comprime" (with compressed air) as being frequently used in abdominal massage. It consists of percussion of the part being massaged with hollow hands, so that the latter really forms an air cushion when reaching the surface: "Another form of tapotement is the punctuating, also frequently used in abdominal massage. The tips of the fingers alternately press upon the abdominal wall and enter the abdomen as deep as possible, without, however, giving pain to the patient."[30] Both of these methods are used today in some form. Tapotement `a l `air comprime is now called "cupping," and is used more on the back than on the abdomen. The use of the fingertips in the "punctuating" tapotement technique has been replaced by the palm of the hand; instead of alternately pressing the abdomen, the movements are more circular and conform to the direction of fluids moving through the colon.

A description of the general massage techniques used by Weir Mitchell as part of his rest cure is instructive. In 1877 Dr. Haehl describes Mitchell's general massage (with period spelling of body parts).

> The masseur begins with a massage of the feet. The interosii muscles are carefully treated by effleurage and massage 'a friction. Every joint of the phalanges should be bent and extended a number of times. Next, attention is paid to the malleoli which are manipulated by massage 'a friction; the ankle joints should be bent and extended several times. The leg at first is treated by a light effleurage, gradually, however, becoming more powerful and entering the deeper lying tissues, as though it would be the intention of the masseur to empty the veins and lymphatics. Special care should be taken to the inside of the thighs. Following this we give petrissage in order to manipulate the different groups of muscles, especially the glutii and adductors. The same treatment is carefully extended to back and arms, to chest and abdomen. The skin of the patient here as in all massage manipulations should be bare, so that the individual structures can easily be felt and thoroughly manipulated. In order to prevent chilling of the patient it is advisable to cover all but one part, undergoing manipulations. Whether or not tapotement should be used in all its forms depends largely upon the strength and general condition of the patient. Individualizing is of great importance. Some authorities massage the legs, abdomen and chest early in the morning, and spine, neck and upper extremities late in the evening. Following the procedure, it is advisable to make passive motions of all the joints.[31]

The last suggestion—"make passive motions of all the joints"—refers to the joint manipulations done by the operator. Basically, these were range-of-motion movements designed to move each joint about in its fullest possible range without causing pain. Dr. Haehl considered the Swedish active, passive, and resisting movements (range of motion) a part of massage. He agrees with many of his colleagues that "massage by one of the family is without value; indeed it is almost worse than useless."

Haehl's book was specifically written for physicians, and was used in a few medical schools as an introductory text. His description of a full-body massage is strikingly similar to what Kellogg recommended in 1895, even to the detail of beginning at the feet. This description of massage written in 1898 is as close to the Swedish massage techniques that were taught and used throughout America and many other parts of the world for the next one hundred years as any description available; much of it is still the foundation of Swedish massage as we know it today.

Proliferation of Techniques in the Twentieth Century

One of the major differences in technique between the nineteenth and twentieth centuries was the rate and frequency of massage applications. As noted earlier, nineteenth-century and early-twentieth-century massage was most often applied vigorously and with speed. The strokes were done quickly, and with considerable pressure. The physician, nurse, or medical assistant often provided treatment two or three times a day. As massage moved away from medical applications the techniques changed. The focus of the lay practitioner was on making the client feel good in the barber's chair, or applying water, oil, or liniment and giving a full-body rubdown in the Turkish bath or bathhouse. As massage progressed in the twentieth century, so did the length of time devoted to a massage session, and the goal of making a client feel good became increasingly important. Massage techniques were performed much more slowly, with pressure applied more softly and usually not more often than once a week or so. In deep-tissue massage techniques the pressure might be heavy, but was usually applied with greater precision than the general massage given in earlier times.

For a number of massage practitioners operating from around 1930 until recent times, massage included manipulation of the joints. A perusal of the school catalogs available from this period does not show that manipulation, now the realm of chiropractic, was a part of the regular curriculum. In private conversations with a number of "old-timers" that are retired in the field today, who did manipulations during their career, I've discovered that they used manipulations as a natural outgrowth of their practice and had little or no formal training. The use of manipulations by a massage practitioner was not unusual during this period. However, today it would be extremely rare to find anyone still performing massage doing manipulations on his or her clients in defiance of existing laws that prohibit them from applying this kind of treatment.

Another difference between the two periods is the diversity of techniques and the conditions for which they were utilized. In the early days there were fewer techniques available, the primary ones being stroking, kneading, vibration, tapotement, and friction, the five basic Swedish Massage strokes. Variations on these techniques were mostly limited to degree of pressure and to the transition from one movement to another. But there were few techniques to choose from. Although the claims made earlier in the century for conditions benefited by massage were broad, the actual beneficial applications were limited. In later years the disease conditions treated by massage dwindled as disease became less and less the focus. Instead, specific body tissues, such as muscles, tendons, ligaments, organs, and connective tissue, became the primary focus for the application of massage techniques.

The distinctly definable techniques available at the end of the nineteenth century numbered a few dozen at most. They included the five basic Swedish massage strokes; the various range-of-motion movements; the use of water-cure methods in conjunction with massage; the mechanical applications of vibration, tapotement, and kneading; the various types of friction; cross-fiber methods; compressions; and stretch and rub techniques.

By the end of the twentieth century, the definable techniques of massage therapy numbered at least seventy-five, with a large number of other systems that included massage as a component. The proliferation of technique happened in conjunction with the human potential movement of the 1960s and 1970s, which brought new attention to the field of massage. With the fresh attention came new innovations.

From the basic five strokes of Swedish massage to the more technical neuro-muscular therapy and deep-tissue methods, massage techniques have improved as hand dexterity and the theoretical knowledge upon which they are based has been learned. The new massage-technique repertoire included techniques from the previous century, but those being defined more by their venue than by their application to a specific disease or disorder. For example, sports massage existed early in the twentieth century but the science of its application dramatically improved over the century. The actual strokes used in sports evolved into more specific and complex maneuvers specifically designed, in many cases, for a specific type of sporting activity. Previously the same techniques and protocol were applied to nearly every sport.

The use of massage in rehabilitative medicine and physical therapy has moved from the hands of the medical specialist into the hands of independent massage specialists. If massage is found in physical therapy it is almost always provided by an aide, and then only in small doses in conjunction with heat or electrical stimulation of some kind.

In the second half of the twentieth century massage applications became specific to many arenas, such as childbirth, pregnancy, geriatrics, and in-office chair massage. Techniques were tailored to aid in the reduction and management of stress, body contouring, weight loss, and general well-being. New venues developed in the latter period of the twentieth century, and massage is now seen in hospice-based programs, pediatrics wards, disaster relief operations, airports and shopping malls, cruise ships and clipper ships, and even in the nonhuman domain of animal care. Each of these specialties has created a new set of techniques, tools, and concepts to deal with their special clientele.

The following list of modern massage techniques is by no means exhaustive, but it does represent the major methods being used today. It must be noted that many of these methods are not so much specific techniques as they are the application of one or more techniques to a particular type of clientele or those who engage in specific kinds of activities or belong to particular age groups. For example, sports massage is not so much a specific technique as it is the application of a number of techniques to an athlete in a timely and systematic fashion. You would not apply cross-fiber friction techniques to an athlete the day before a competition, but you would use effleurage and perhaps light compression techniques at that time. After an event the athlete's muscles need to be flushed of acid waste and the soreness abated, and so the long, slow strokes of effleurage would be used, with some light petrissage or energy techniques added to the massage for balancing. The descriptions given for each massage technique is necessarily brief and broad.

Amma: The traditional massage of Japan, which includes techniques such as compression, stretching, and percussion.

Swedish or classic massage: The defining characteristic of Swedish massage is the presence of the five basic strokes: effleurage, petrissage, vibration, tapotement, and friction.

Esalen massage: Named after the Esalen Institute at Big Sur, California, this method of massage is very similar to Swedish massage except that it adopts a slower-moving and rythmically applied approach that focuses on nurturing the client's emotional self.

Connective tissue massage (or Bindegewbsmassage): This technique focuses on the muscular facia, the membranous tissue that lies among and between muscles.

Bindegewbsmassage is a German word meaning "connective tissue massage" sometimes used when referring to this technique.

Cyriax cross-fiber technique: A medically oriented cross-fiber technique developed by English physician James Cyriax.

Manual lymphatic drainage: A light-application technique designed to assist lymphatic fluids along the lymph vessels and toward the colon for eliminating the wastes that accumulate in lymph fluids.

Deep-muscle therapy: A therapy that works the muscle tissues with deep applications of various techniques, such as compression, petrissage, and cross-fiber.

Pfrimmer deep-muscle therapy: A regimented application of light and deep cross-fiber techniques to muscle fibers.

Infant massage: Various massage techniques, primarily Swedish massage techniques, applied to infants.

Geriatric massage: A technique similar to infant massage except that it is applied to elderly patients.

Pregnancy massage: Massage applied prior to birth of a child on the mother-to-be and during the birthing process. Pregnancy massage usually consists of Swedish massage techniques.

Sports massage: The application of a variety of massage techniques in a timely and systematic fashion.

Lomi-lomi or LomiLomi: This technique of Polynesian origin features long, flowing strokes applied with the forearms, and includes compressions and vibrations. A central feature of true Hawaiian lomi-lomi is prayer done before and after the treatment.

Medical massage: This is an example in which the name of a technique is not a specific method but the application of a variety of techniques applied to a particular setting. Medical massage generally is massage applied in a hospital setting or under a physician's supervision.

Neuromuscular therapy: This method of massage is a variety of techniques applied to specific parts of the body. Most are cross-fiber and compression techniques applied to the muscular-tendinous junctions, as well as to the belly of muscle and connective-tissue connections.

On-site, seated, or chair massage: This type of massage is used while the patron is in a seated position, but the techniques are not always massage. Often the techniques are Asian therapies such as shiatsu or acupressure.

Thai massage: Originating in Thailand, Thai massage is a combination of Swedish massage, stretching, acupressure, and movement gymnastics.

Fijian massage: There are two types of Fijian massage; the first type is similar to the Hawaiian lomi-lomi, while the second type is applied exclusively with the feet. The patron is not walked upon, but manipulated with operator's feet.

Tuina: The traditional massage of China, tuina consists of more than one hundred hand techniques. The techniques consist of pounding, pushing, shoving, vibration, tapotement, and variations of rolling movements applied with hands, knuckles, and forearms.

Russian massage or Kurashova method: Russian massage is comprised of a vast body of techniques applied to everything from sports to medical conditions. The primary technique applied in a relaxation or therapeutic setting, such as we might find in the United States, consists of heavy doses of friction and tapotement. Zhenya Kurashova is a naturalized American who brought Russian massage to this country.

Myotherapy: The prefix *myo* simply means "muscle." Myotherapy is a muscle therapy that primarily utilizes Swedish and cross-fiber techniques.

What are not massage techniques? The following is a list of the names of a number of body-therapy systems that might in some cases include massage techniques among their repertoire of tools, but are modalities commonly referred to in the massage industry as "bodywork systems." The distinguishing feature between massage and bodywork is that the former focuses primarily on the soft tissues of the body while the latter focuses primarily on the structures or functions of the body.

Bodywork methods can be educationally based, movement based, or psychologically based, but most are structurally based. Popular bodywork therapies include Alexander technique, Aston patterning, craniosacral therapy, do-in, Feldenkrais method, hakomi, Hellerwork, jin shin jyutsu, myofascial release, Ohashiatsu, Pilates method, polarity therapy, reflexology, Reiki, Rolfing, Rosen method, Rubenfeld synergy method, shiatsu, somatoemotional release, therapeutic touch, touch for health, Trager approach, trigger-point therapy, and zero-balancing technique.

Most practitioners today hold a variety of techniques in their bag of tools. For example, it is not unusual for a practitioner doing Swedish massage to incorporate energy-balancing techniques found in polarity therapy. The application of a sports massage to an athlete might include Russian, neuromuscular, and Swedish techniques. Where the Swedish methods were dominant fifty years ago, an eclectic approach of wide-ranging techniques is common with today's practitioner.

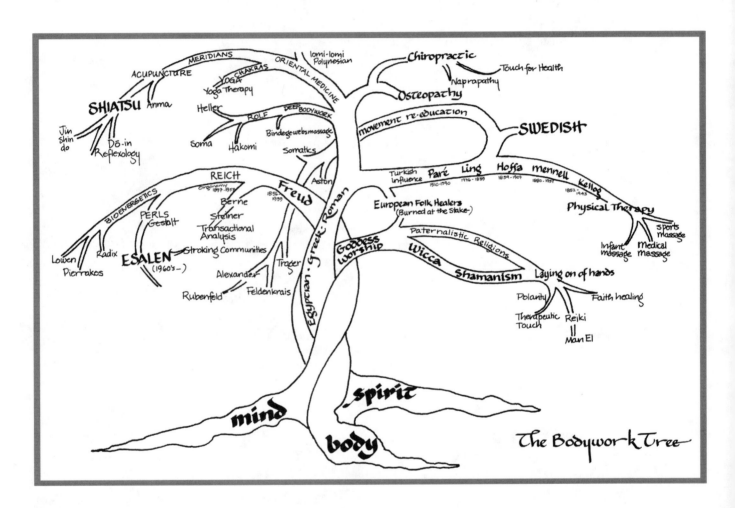

The Bodywork Tree, conceived by David Linton in the 1970s. Reproduced with kind permission of the artist, Laurene Waggoner-dow-Bradford, and the Stroking Community Network.

11 The Golden Age of Massage

Before we look at the most recent history of massage in the twentieth century, let us pause for a moment to look at the broad historical and cultural context in which present-day massage exists. The Bodywork Tree—published in 1987 by East Coast massage practitioner David Linton—offers one pathway for that viewing. The roots of the tree begin with three simple words—mind, spirit, and body—drawing our attention to the three aspects of the human being touched by the healing arts. By following each of these roots up into the tree, one journeys into the maze of alternative and complementary healing arts, also referred to as natural therapies, spiritual bodywork, or just plain massage and bodywork.

The Bodywork Tree demonstrates the evolution, complexity, and integration of these various healing arts. It also shows that some of the more technologically based Western systems of medical practice have their roots in ancient and esoteric foundations. This graphic further illustrates that all healing arts are first and foremost about the human beings who both benefit from and provide them. It shows how personalities are an integral part of alternative therapies, with a significant number of systems named after their founders. This is similar to the myriad anatomical landmarks, diseases, and remedies of Western medicine named after those who discovered them.

David Linton was not an ordinary massage practitioner. He was a member of an active organization of massage lovers called the Stroking Community. The group met regularly for the purpose of exchanging massages, sharing their love of massage, and teaching others about massage. David passed away in 1991. Unfortunately, numerous reproductions and copies of The Bodywork Tree have been published without the permission of his wife, Laurene Bradford, and the Stroking Community Network. As a piece of history, and to honor the vision of David Linton, The Bodywork Tree is presented with their permission in this book.

Who has not experienced in headaches and other pains relief from the most unartful rubbing? You receive a blow, and involuntarily rub the part. Cold will kill; the remedy is brandy and friction. The resources of this process surely deserve to be developed with as much care as that which has been bestowed upon the Materia Medica. *Here is a new method to add to the old. Wherever it can be employed, how much it is to be preferred to nauseating substances taken into the stomach.*

Personal testimony in an 1853 pamphlet on the Turkish bath, from *The Anatriptic Art* **(1866)**

Massage in the First Half of the Twentieth Century

The history of massage is coeval with that of mankind and worthy of being preserved; its mode of application can be cultivated as an art second to none that the human hand can perform, having a harp of more than a thousand strings on which to play; its range of usefulness is increasing all the time, and has long since extended into every branch of medicine, so that those who would keep pace with its developments must be well informed in all departments of the healing art.[1]

When Douglas Graham, M.D., wrote this in 1902 it was more a statement of hope than of fact. Massage had not "extended into every branch of medicine," as he wished, yet Graham was addressing doctors and nurses to convince them to pay heed to the value of massage. Herman Kamenetz perhaps describes the situation at the time more accurately when he writes, "There is probably no older analgesic than massage; yet massage, which was lauded by Hippocrates and applauded by Galen, was ignored by physicians for centuries. Since its medical reacceptance in the middle of the nineteenth century, there have been as many detractors as enthusiasts."[2]

In the first few decades of the twentieth century medicine was growing at unprecedented rates, engulfing nearly all other therapeutic measures, including what little medical massage had emerged from the movement cure systems begun by Ling a century earlier. Nearly every text written during the nineteenth century regarding massage focused primarily on the gymnastic movements. This trend continued well into the twentieth century, although the emphasis gradually began to shift in the other direction. After World War II Swedish gymnastics became much less a part of the massage texts used in American massage institutions.

The separation of massage and exercise advocated by Dr. Kleen and others eventually did take place—not because massage was given "careful, special investigation" or had become a widely accepted form of medical treatment, as he had promoted, but because gymnastics eventually became a branch of medicine known as physical therapy, while massage was left pretty much on the sidelines. Even though massage was an integral part of the initial development of physical therapy, it was quickly replaced by mechanized exercise and manipulation. With the advent of medical technology the focus of medicine changed from hands-on care to more clinically based medicine, from a small pharmacopoeia to more complex drugs, from simple surgery to more complex surgery. Medicine moved rapidly away from the hands-on, general practice that had held hope for massage becoming more widely accepted as a medical treatment for disease.

Leonard Goldstone, an English writer, says that massage began disappearing from nursing in England about 1930 and had practically vanished by 1953, as it had in the United States.[3] Goldstone's perspective is based on the declining mention of massage in medical literature and medical practice. He is accurate to say that massage within medicine suffered from a steady decline during that time. With the growth in the number of hospitals, medical colleges, and practitioners, and the enormous industrial-medical complex that they spawned, labor-intensive massage was replaced by the more efficient, but not necessarily better, methods devised from burgeoning new sciences, such as anesthesiology, pathology, and pharmacology.

Even while massage was being relegated to the lowest rung of the health care ladder, it was being taught and practiced outside medical circles—in baths, sanitariums, spas, and health resorts, and increasingly in private practice. Unlike medicine, which became more and more institutionalized, massage continued to grow as a healing art within the private sector of independent entrepreneurs. In letting massage fall from its medical bag the medical profession unknowingly nurtured the growth of massage as an independent modality. The seeds of this revolution had been planted by physicians who sought to bring massage into its own as a viable medical specialty separate from gymnastics and movement therapies, even though those same people had often sought to squelch the practice of massage outside the realm of medicine.

By the middle of the twentieth century nursing had become more specialized and separate from labor-intensive manual therapies, physical therapy had become established as an independent field, and the long leash on massage held by the medical community was gradually released. All these factors left the independent massage practitioner free to make his or her own way and, in so doing, to nurture the evolution of massage as a professional discipline among the world's other healing arts.

The Golden Age of Massage

One author in the massage trade has asserted that the period from 1880 to 1910 was the Golden Age of Massage in America.[4] It is my assertion that the Golden Age of Massage in America and around the world was the last thirty years of the twentieth century. Although massage is as old as humankind, massage began to emerge as an independent and widely used therapeutic modality in the 1950s and 1960s, fully coming into its own in the 1980s and 1990s. During those decades massage was more widely accepted, recognized, utilized, developed, marketed, and organized than at any previous period in its long history.

As technological society advanced the need for human contact also grew, and massage responded to that need, as it has done throughout the history of humankind. Massage began to be applied in more and diverse venues. Introduction of the massage chair in the 1980s gave new meaning to the phrase "have table, will travel." The publicity surrounding the use of massage in sports had a dramatic impact on the popularity of massage. Massage also became further integrated into other forms of therapy, education, and spiritual endeavors. Massage schools dramatically increased in quality and number. Professional associations and publications proliferated, generating exciting and meaningful avenues of networking, information dissemination, and political and cultural involvement. Regulation of the field increased primarily because of association initiatives, helping the business and ethics of massage to become more evident. All of these factors helped to significantly alter the public perception of massage, and the image of massage as connected to prostitution faded. The field of massage thus moved from the fringes of many other worlds to become a world unto its own over the course of the century, especially in the last third of the century—the Golden Age of Massage.

New Applications and Venues for Massage

Through most of the twentieth century the most prevalent place in which massage was offered was the home. However, in the last few decades the venues for massage expanded rapidly. Innovative and often bold entrepreneurial ventures, aided by portable massage tables and chairs, moved massage from closed rooms to the office place, sports arena, hospital, birthing room, hospice, hotel, airport, shopping mall, and even out onto the streets of American cities. In the 1970s massage provided in one's home constituted nearly 70 percent of all massage being done, whereas at the end of the century in-home massage practice constituted only about 45 to 50 percent of all types of practices.[5]

The massage chair—first introduced in 1985—and the enterprising practitioners who use it have dramatically changed massage practice. No longer are rooms, sheets, and lubricants needed to provide quality massage treatments. Getting a massage is now a public event, being offered at picture-window storefronts, the wide open spaces of shopping malls, corporate offices around the country, and even in airports. Chair massage has its own retail stores where you can get a ten- or fifteen-minute massage during lunch or after work, without having to take your clothes off. Several franchise companies have been launched that sell turn-key business packages and a full line of products associated with massage. It is interesting to note that the so-called massage chair was not invented for the use of massage techniques, but for a treatment that was more like acupressure. Living Earth Crafts manufactured the first massage chair, but its conception belonged to David Palmer. David's vision for using the chair was for delivering "kata," a set form of movements, to both the front and the back of the body. The kata form devised by Palmer is based on an Asian acupressure system that contains no massage movements. The irony is that today most practitioners utilize massage techniques with the chair, even though Palmer continues to teach his kata form of acupressure.

Around the United States businesses large and small are providing massage for their employees or allowing them access to it on company property during business hours. Boeing Corporation is one example, providing special locations where employees can get a seated chair massage during their regular break times. Teachers in some parts of the country are encouraged to purchase a chair massage during their breaks. At airports new businesses offer massage at "massage bars" designed to take the place of traditional airport drinking establishments. In 1999 one airline, Virgin Atlantic, began offering massage aboard their planes as part of a special promotion. At sporting competitions one often sees long lines of aching athletes waiting to receive their postrace rubdowns, and many professional athletic teams in baseball, basketball, football, and tennis utilize the services of massage practitioners. Massage has been a mainstay of cruise lines since they were first built and continue today as hundreds of ships cruise the earth's oceans.

The applications of massage have widened to include not only the traditional types of massage but also massage for the isolated elderly and those suffering from AIDS, cancer, and severe trauma, such as victims of rape, terrorism, and torture. These and other groups are increasingly coming under the careful touch of massage practitioners. Massage has begun being used in optimal health applications as well. The entire area of pregnancy and birth has emerged as an important and growing area of massage application. Massage practitioners are also working more with children as well as promoting the massage of newborn infants by their parents. Bonding with one's baby through loving touch with massage is now becoming widely accepted in Western culture, while in many other parts of the world it has a long and steadfast tradition.

Touch deprivation, a subject not yet discussed in this work, is one of the causes of apprehension toward massage that has been brought to the attention of the trade. The many venues where massage is now found have helped alleviate some of those fears. Recreational structured touch has taken touch directly to the lay public, not just as receivers but as givers. Playing to the rhythms of specially designed music in a structured format, participants both give and receive safe touch—often for the very first time. And practitioners who bring play back into their touch-therapy practice move outside of their usual massage session rituals to enrich and enliven themselves and their practice.

Surprisingly, a few medical schools are experimenting with teaching massage as a way to develop tactile skills and sensitivity toward patients. Massage is enjoying a revival within the ranks of the nursing profession, and more and more hospitals and hospices are creating programs to accommodate alternative healing arts practices.

There is also renewed interest and dialogue about touch in the ministry of religion. The heritage of the women of the Church in the Middle Ages lives on today as nuns (and some priests) around the world continue to minister their faith through the healing power of massage. In the book *Healing Touch: The Church's Forgotten Language* author Zach Thomas shares the results of his survey of hundreds of pastoral teaching institutions in the United States, showing that nearly half offered some instruction in healing touch.[6] In a Jesuit University in the western United States a priest uses touch to help students deal with the stress of university life. Sister Rosalind Gefre of St. Paul, Minnesota, a Catholic nun who was mistakenly arrested by city police for prostitution (because they didn't understand the difference between massage in prostitution and lawful practices) was released shortly afterward when they realized she was offering legitimate massage services. She has since established five schools teaching massage therapy as a career option.

The Continuing Relationship of Massage and the Spa

Massage and the spa share a rich and long history that is still being written. The traditions of the spa changed with the changing face of health treatments and the demand for beauty treatments. Originally most spas advertised the healing qualities of their waters, and the massage services available were seen as secondary. But in today's spa ads and promotional literature massage is emphasized. As destination, resort, day, and medical spas developed in the twentieth century, the role of massage and numerous other touch-therapy modalities increased to that of being one of the major revenue producers in nearly all spas of the world.

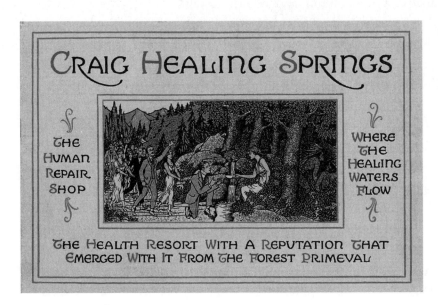

Spas and resorts are by far the largest employers of massage practitioners because these facilities present the public with very easy access to massage services. The Arizona location of Canyon Ranch Spa is the largest employer of massage practitioners in the United States today. In the small town of Calistoga, California, there are nearly a dozen spas operating. And in Europe at the Dead Sea resorts, the Vada baths near Pisa, Italy, at Baden Baden in Germany, and at many other locations in France, England, and elsewhere, spas continue to provide a place of rest, relaxation, and curative waters, where massage is available—as it has been for more than two thousand years.

Getting back to nature and taking in the healing waters was the "call of the spa" in Victorian times. Today's spas, like those of earlier times, continue to sell their special environment, their healing waters, and now their signature massage treatments. Courtesy of World of Massage Museum.

However, the legacy of disdain toward practitioners working in Turkish baths and spas that began with the physicians who promoted massage continues today as well. The spa setting has traditionally been labeled a "club rub," "flesh factory," or "meat market," implying a scene of faceless people coming through in what some describe as conveyer-belt fashion. The image is unfair, but it persists in both the massage trade and the spa world. The truth is something different because most practitioners care about their work. While it is true that spa workers see an endless array of clientele passing across their tables, so too does the private practitioner.

The spa environment is considered by most as a starting point, an easy place to get a first job and to learn by working on lots of bodies, but to be left behind as one pursues the "real" business of doing massage in private or clinical practice. This kind of attitude has crept deep into the consciousness of the trade; it lives in the schools where most practitioners get their initial training. This is unfortunate because the spa environment is much more than a place to get started. It is not only a place to learn and grow, but also a place where one can find a long-term career doing work one loves.

Massage technique has advanced in the spa, particularly in the development of therapies involving the use of water. Special showers, tanks, and sprays used while giving a massage come from the spa. The salt glow is a technique created in the spa that consists of rubbing special salts onto the body to defoliate the skin. Mud packs, herbal wraps, and a number of other techniques that involve massage all came from the spas of the world, with many now being utilized outside the spa environment.

Massage Around the World

During the years that the practice of massage prospered in the United States it also grew in many countries around the world, although less dramatically, while at the same time it faded in a few others. In Europe the historic relationship of massage with medicine has in many ways continued, even though a so-called underground of practitioners has grown up outside the medical setting. This situation is very much like that which exists in Canada. Two Canadian provinces regulate the practice of massage by designating practitioners as registered massage therapists, or RMTs. This entitles the RMT to utilize the title in advertising and receive reimbursement from the government's national health plan. One can practice massage in either of these two provinces without the RMT designation, but without the RMT designation and without reimbursement from the health plan for their services. This two-tiered system exists in some form in a number of European countries as well with massage being within the physiotherapy field of medicine and operating outside that realm without the benefits of title and insurance.

Massage in Europe has a parallel history but different timing from the history of massage in North America. For a long time during the nineteenth century, massage in Europe was advanced and utilized in medicine, in bathhouses, and in private practice, while at that time in North America massage was being introduced along the fringes of medical practice, and in bathhouses and sanitariums. The great spas of Europe were well established by the time the sanitariums in America began their rise from treatment centers for tuberculosis to destination and resort health farms. Nurses were trained in massage throughout Europe for decades before the American sanitariums began their nursing schools in the Victorian era of the late nineteenth century. It is interesting to note that Douglas Graham, M.D., traveling in Europe at the turn of the nineteenth century, could find no "general massage for its tonic and sedative effects . . . except in the most ordinary form of rubbing. In the summer of 1889" he says, "I could find no one in Amsterdam to give me general massage to rest me from the fatigue of travelling."[7] Dr. Graham does not mention anything about the spas where massage was readily available, nor about the bathhouses and hospitals where massage was universally used. He was looking for a relaxation massage in a Europe that was confined largely by the application of scientific massage.

At the beginning of the twentieth century, however, massage was a primary modality within the nursing profession in both Europe and America. The rise and fall of massage within nursing is a parallel history between the two continents that coincides with the advent of modern medical practice, educational standards, and physical therapy. In a popular 1907 English nursing text A. Hughes wrote, "A certificate in massage is held to be an almost essential qualification for a fully qualified nurse to possess. The demand for proficiency in the art of massage has raised standards in this respect very far above that mere knowledge of 'how to rub' which contented nurses not so long ago."[8] But by the 1950s massage had fallen almost completely from the nursing textbooks of Europe.

In America massage was an integral part of nursing practice during the same time period. For example, Nurse Mary McMillan, the first president of the American Physical Therapy Association (established in 1923) was one of the great proponents of massage within the nursing field. She authored several books on the subject and was instrumental in establishing the Reconstruction Department of the U.S. Army, which included massage as one of its primary modalities. But as physical therapy and nursing became increasingly caught up in the new medical model of the twentieth century, the manual therapies began falling away and were replaced with therapies that could be applied with mechanical devices, such as diathermy and ultrasound.

Professor Leonard Goldstone of South Bank University in London provides some revealing statistics that demonstrate one marker in the fall of massage from the nursing profession in England. This data is relevant to America as well. He writes:

> Of 83 references given in Beard's Massage on the mechanical and physiological effects of massage, 29 (35%) were written up to 1945, and 33 (40%) up to 1950. What this amounts to is that massage up to some 60 years ago was common. An "orthodox" medical therapy, an integral part of medical and nursing textbooks and journal articles, taught in major hospitals, widely available in hospitals and convalescent homes, and espoused to the public as a proper therapy-with nothing "complementary" or "alternative" about it.
>
> The 15th edition of *The Nurse's Dictionary* (Taylor 1936) offers a 41-word definition of massage plus cross-references to effleurage, hacking, petrissage and tapotement, as well as definitions for friction, masseur and masseuse, making a total entry of 178 words. The 30th edition in 1989 reduces massage references to 15 words, with no cross-references, plus a 17-word definition of effluerage, but omitting hacking, petrissage and tapotement. There is, however, a 28-word definition of friction, making up to 60 words on massage, compared with the 178 words in 1936.
>
> *Modern Surgery for Nurses* by F. Wilson Harlow, published in its 6th edition in 1963, has no reference to massage in the index, whilst *Medicine for Nurses* by W. Gordon Sears in its 9th edition in the same year has only 14 words on massage, largely associated with physiotherapy as a method to help relieve pain. *Modern Nursing: Theory and Practice*—perhaps the most popular text of its time refers to massage in the index to

the 1965 3rd edition, but the text cited is an entry in physiotherapy in which the word massage does not appear. For the 4th edition in 1968, there is no mention of massage in the index. A contemporary dictionary of nursing (Roper 1966) had no entries under massage, petrissage, tapotement, friction, or hacking, and an 8-word definition of effleurage. By the 1980s, major nursing textbooks (e.g. Middleton 1983 and 1986) do not refer to massage.[9]

In England today massage is integrally connected with aromatherapy, although their histories are quite different, with most practitioners working outside the medical field in private practice. Massage is seeing something of a small revival in nursing, but only as it is categorized among a broader range of so-called alternative and complementary therapies. Professor Goldstone reports that whereas massage was accepted more readily in the past century because of its long-standing tradition, it is making less progress in the modern era because the demand for research of its efficacy has increased.[10] Until such time as massage is proven as a "new" therapeutic tool, it will continue being on the fringes of medical and nursing practice in England and the rest of Europe.

Medical gymnastics, so very popular during the nineteen century in Europe, gave way gradually to the new field of physiotherapy. Because medical gymnastics was in large part a medical treatment, modern medicine sloughed it off as it did other manual therapies, such as massage and magnetics. Medical gymnastics today in Europe consists of range-of-motion exercises within the physiotherapist's domain.

In Russia the face of massage has changed as much as the country itself since the disbanding of the Soviet Union. During World War II massage was used as an element of complex rehabilitation treatment for wounded soldiers. After the war, major universities and specially formed institutes of resortology and physiotherapy studied massage and its use, and the Russian massage education system produced doctors of massage who specialized in all areas of medicine and sports.[11] Russian sports massage and the Russians' development of techniques and physiological rationale behind vibrational massage came to be well known and highly regarded around the world. Practitioners from many Soviet satellite countries and other countries were offered training in Russian massage. Coming from Cuba, Mexico, South America, Africa, the Middle East, and Asia, many of them spent years training in the USSR, eventually returning to their homeland to make a living doing massage, often in the tourist trade. But the picture at the end of the century is very different. Where there had been government research and sports venues for massage in Russia, today there is practically nothing. Doctors of massage, once respected members of the health community, now scavenge for clientele and offer massage as a part of a broader spectrum of services at high rates. As reported by massage practitioners who fled the old Soviet Union, the vast literature of Russian massage development is still locked up there.

In parts of Asia massage has continued its association with prostitution, but tourism in Thailand, Indonesia, and other Pacific Rim countries has led to considerable growth in the practice and teaching of massage. In China—where massage has never been linked with prostitution—you can get a massage in your hotel room or at the local hospital, the first for relaxation, the second for medical purposes. From personal experience of massage at a Chinese hotel and at a traditional hospital in Beijing, neither is a relaxing, soothing experience. In the hotel one is vigorously rubbed through a towel while lying uncomfortably on a small bed, and in the hospital one is rubbed with tuina techniques by a practitioner dressed in a white lab coat who performs his or her duties through the recipient's clothing, again very vigorously.

Around the turn of the twentieth century Japan's growing acceptance of Western medicine led to the adoption of policies that reduced the number of schools teaching amma massage to the blind. Dubitsky claims the reduction in massage schools, "degenerated [amma] into a pleasurable indulgence for the rich and powerful."[12] But the practice of massaging cattle for several days before they are slaughtered—a centuries-old tradition in Japan—continues. The meat from such animals is the most expensive and most desirable because it is believed that the massage renders the muscles of the animal supple and free of stress, making the meat very tender.

In Australia and New Zealand the battle continues to separate massage from the massage parlor image, and some progress is being made in that direction. Australia has attempted to organize its divergent trade groups nationwide.

Most of the African continent shows little signs of massage activity, outside of South Africa and tourist facilities in Egypt and a few other coastal countries. In the Middle East massage is done only on a same-sex basis, due to Islamic religious restrictions. In some countries, such as Kuwait and Saudi Arabia, massage practitioners and other specialists are imported to work in the clinics and hospitals.

In South America private practice is slowly increasing, especially in the many seaside resorts and health clubs. In Ecuador and Central America the indigenous people are being trained to do massage to accommodate the growing tourist trade. Today massage in Mexico is divided between the few who do it at home; the many who work the tourist locations; and the indigenous practitioners known as *massajistas* who offer relaxation and *sobadors* (males) and *sobadoras* (females) who treat to relieve pain by the native practice called *sobada*. Although their hands are highly skilled at finding tension and releasing it, the indigenous practitioners are not readily available. Massage in South and Central America is usually chosen as a career option because it is an easy way to earn money from tourists. (Reportedly there are many immigrants from Mexico now living in the United States who still practice the ancient ways of hands-on healing.) The medical community has pretty much ignored massage in their practices.

Although massage is respected in Mexico, it is not widely practiced or sought by the Mexican peoples. Therapy is usually sought only after an auto or industrial accident, for posture problems, or for other kinds of physical discomfort, seldom for relaxation or preventive maintenance.

The exchange of massage knowledge between countries was virtually nonexistent before the late twentieth century. During the nineteenth and early twentieth century it was the rare nurse or physician, and even the more rare massage practitioner, who would travel abroad from the United States to study massage in Europe, Asia, or the Pacific Rim countries. And there was little to attract other practitioners to study in the United States. That situation has now changed dramatically. The international exchange of knowledge about massage began in the 1970s and has continued to expand ever since. In Italy shiatsu is being taught by Japanese masters from America. Tuina has spread, creating a new level of educational and practical exchange in and out of China. In Germany, dentists are learning about neuromuscular therapy, a technical massage technique from Floridian Paul St. John. Lomi-lomi from Hawaii is being taught in Sweden, and Thai massage is taught in California.

Changing Points of View

The general public's perception of massage has changed considerably during the past twenty years. Shopping mall surveys this writer commissioned reveal the changing public attitude. In the early 1980s respondents would practically recoil from the interviewer when asked for their reaction to the word *massage*. Respondents were generally cautious, not forthcoming with answers, and curious to know why the question was being asked. Further questioning typically revealed that their responses were based on an image of massage as related to luxury, Roman baths, and prostitution. In a similar survey conducted only five years later, in 1988, the reaction was quite different. Instead of recoiling respondents moved forward, most asking, "Do you do massage?" and proceeding to present a shoulder, arm, or neck that needed attention. To these more enlightened respondents massage meant relaxation, relief from aches and pains, and feeling good. They wanted a massage and weren't afraid to ask for it.

What happened to change the public's reaction and perceptions toward massage in less than a decade? The answer can be found in experiences such as my own. In the early 1980s I offered free sports massage at a variety of sporting events with students from the school I began in 1980. During the period from 1978 to 1983 I also gave a number of public presentations about massage to local community groups, such as the Lions Club, Rotary, business organizations, and bicycling clubs. I always asked that any prepresentation publicity state that my talk would be on stress management or sports training assistance, depending on the group. I didn't want the audience to know the speaker was a massage therapist until I was introduced, so that I could measure their spontaneous response and because I wanted to maximize participation by not turning them away before I was able to educate them about massage therapy.

The usual audience reaction when I was introduced as a massage therapist and school owner in the community was general laughing. Laughing as a response to massage might seem odd, but I expected it. Most people were uncomfortable with the thought of massage—touching another person's body—in situations unrelated to sex or family affection. Theirs were nervous reactions to something they knew very little about. That was why I was there talking to them, to open their minds about the value and benefits of massage, to assuage their fears and to draw them in as potential clients to my clinic, and to stimulate business for all the practitioners in the community.

The answer to the question about what happened to change reactions to massage in less than a decade is that the public perception has been changed largely because practitioners have educated the public about massage. Like me, thousands of practitioners reached out to their communities, making massage a less fearful experience and generally spreading the good word about its benefits and value. Members of professional associations often led the way in involving their membership in community activities, and most massage schools instituted community outreach programs that successfully promote massage. It hasn't been a massive publicity campaign or a project generated by a huge government grant. It has been a plain old grassroots development from the bottom up—a long and slow process, but an effective one.

The Practice and Profession of Massage

Massage has endured as a reliable, easy, and useful therapy for thousands of years because all living creatures, especially humans, have an innate need to touch and be touched with care and love. But being a massage practitioner today requires much more than hands-on skills. It requires business acumen, professional ethics, and an ongoing willingness to undertake continuing education. Few practices today are limited to one or even two techniques; most practices—in whatever setting they may be found—are diverse in technique and rich in personality.

Running a massage therapy business, or working for someone else doing massage therapy, is a demanding and very personal service. To be successful a practitioner needs more than talented hands. An engaging, compassionate, and healthy attitude toward people is also essential. Above all, one must love to touch people, regardless of what they bring to the table, chair, or mat. It is at once a science and an art, but it is mostly a dedication—a practitioner who doesn't love doing it won't continue. The massage practitioner is counselor, confidant(e), therapist, and friend, but most of all he or she is an assuager of all kinds of pain. All these talents and skills, and the knowledge to apply them, play an important role in succeeding in the business of touching others for health.

Psychology is more evident in massage practice now as practitioners have become aware of their role as caregivers and facilitators, particularly when using techniques that elicit emotional responses from the client. There is far more recognition today about the power differential between client and practitioner, necessitating a better practice ethic and the need for some level of detachment from the personal lives of clients. Empathy is necessary in this type of work, but a welcome evolution to a more mature approach is underway whereby the practitioner plays the role of the empathetic listener rather than the fixer in the healing process of clients.

With all the pressures on massage practitioners today, they also must take care of themselves so that burnout due to poor body mechanics, lack of business skills, and other factors does not force many from the business who might otherwise be wonderful contributors.

The field of massage has suffered from an ongoing lack of clarity about the distinction between the profession, the trade, and the industry of massage, and about whether massage qualifies as a profession. To clear up some of the confusion I offer the following distinctions. The *massage profession* consists of those who do massage—the practitioners—while the *massage trade* comprises a greater compilation of practitioners, educators, and leaders. The *massage industry* represents those who serve the trade with products and services.

Some people still question whether the field of massage is rightfully called a profession, because it has not reached maturity compared to other recognized professions. There are no universal standards of practice for massage, and no standards of ethics or protocol other than those derived from state regulation or within trade associations. (Most practitioners do not belong to any professional organization.) In many ways the massage trade is still quite immature with much growing up to do, in part because it is perceived by many as an easy vocational choice and so attracts many new practitioners who are not oriented toward a career path. As more and more schools take on the responsibility to educate their students about massage as a career path, the changes in attitude toward massage as a career will be reflected in the professional development of the trade.

The truth is that the practice of massage is different things to different people. According to some surveys, only half of those who practice massage do so as a full-time job. Many practice massage part time to supplement other income, or simply because they love to help others get relief from their pain. Some come to it through their own healing journeys and fall in love with doing this type of work. Making money by doing massage and performing massage to give another assistance in their time of need coexist as significant factors in the profession.

The massage profession has also built a reputation for service. Early gestures of helping one's neighbors while also providing a positive experience of massage as a valuable and capable helping hand have grown into statewide and national efforts. Some of these efforts have been organized by brave individuals; most are initiated by associations, supported financially by commercial interests in the industry. Early efforts were free massages at sporting events, such as marathons, triathlons, or the Olympics. Now we see massage as a community service offered to the elderly, infirm, and disabled, provided by associations, massage schools, and a few stand-out practitioners. Massage has become a part of the relief work offered at man-made and natural disaster sites. A national organization, Massage Emergency Relief Team, was established by the American Massage Therapy Association to work closely with the American Red Cross, offering massage to relief workers during major disasters. There are also independent organizations such as this operating within their own state boundaries.

But before these disaster-relief efforts can claim their position as national organizations, they must allow a broader participation from outside their membership ranks. In the 1990s massage brought healing to those recovering from natural disasters such as hurricanes, earthquakes, floods, and fires, and to those enduring the conflicts in Ireland, to shell-shocked survivors of the drawn-out conflict in Bosnia, and to those suffering from inner revolutionary strife in Central America and Africa.

The first effort to organize the field of massage therapy nationwide in the United States came in 1988. Motivated in part by the announcement that a national certification examination was being developed, but primarily by the observation that there was a need to discuss common issues and advance the field as a whole, this writer offered to provide a forum for these purposes. The event was called Head, Heart, and Hands and comprised three meetings—one in the middle of the country, another on the East Coast, and one on the West Coast. Various other movements followed, but none have survived except those devoted to furthering an agenda of a particular organization. They basically dissolved into research granting and educational meetings, but none with a national agenda or appeal to all aspects of the trade. By the end of the century, though, there were signs once again that innovative efforts designed to unify the field of massage therapy were underfoot.

Australia held its first convention and trade show devoted to massage in 1990. Canada is also making some preliminary moves to unify across provincial borders as well, but those efforts have not borne fruit as yet. The European community has done little to bring about communication and unity among its extremely diverse elements, but they may soon follow the ways of other movements mentioned here; in 1991 an international conference was held in Lanzarote, Spain, but a second event was not scheduled. There have been attempts to organize in Korea with no success. Japan has a history of organizing its blind amma practitioners, but no contemporary organization exists.

Among the organizational developments must be included the fight against massage parlors and the associated image of massage with prostitution. The telephone directories of many countries have helped continue the legacy of connection between massage and prostitution by refusing to separate the two. Along with the Yellow Pages listings, the books, films, and other media that help perpetuate this image are now receiving criticism from activists in the trade, almost always leading to positive results.

Until 1992 trade shows featuring massage were restricted to association conventions or a select number of booths at a holistic health fairs. The world's first trade show dedicated solely to massage was the Anatriptic Arts Expo held in San Francisco in 1992. This show featured presenters from all five continents and focused on bringing together the innovators of the major techniques then in vogue. The three-day event was followed by five days of workshops. An estimated 12,000 persons attended the expo event, practitioners from around the world and across the United States and Canada as well as large numbers of the general public. (Most association conventions are lucky to have a 1,000 attendees at their annual events.) Such expos have become vanguards of educational opportunity for those seeking to fulfill continuing education requirements mandated by various states and provinces. The Anatriptic Arts Expo has been revived and is now an annual event beginning in May of 2002.

Computer software is now available to assist in managing a massage clinic and for billing insurance companies (from the few underwriters that reimburse for massage outside a state workman's compensation plan). There is even software that provides teaching aids in anatomy, physiology, technique, and other subjects. Many schools have developed their own database software to manage and coordinate student records, curriculum, and class and teacher schedules. And most schools now have a Web site on the Internet.

Schools of Massage

For education in massage, early practitioners in the United States had to rely on books and instruction or apprenticeships by immigrants from Europe, or else travel abroad, which only physicians were wont to do. Training in a formal setting was first offered in the sanitariums of the late nineteenth century. The primary purpose of this training, given predominantly to nurses, was as a means of acquiring new and qualified employees for the facilities. Individual apprenticeships were available with a few physicians who might either specialize in massage or advocate its use for their patients. But until 1906 most training was usually obtained either on the job or from lay persons who themselves had often been trained at a Turkish bath, gymnasium or gymnastic institute, European spa, or rest-cure clinic.

Andrew Taylor Still opened the American School of Osteopathy in Kirksville, Missouri, in 1892, offering some coursework in massage. However, it was an introduction for beginning osteopaths, not meant to train career-oriented massage practitioners. Interestingly, Eunice D. Ingham, the developer of reflexology, taught her specialty at this school sixty years later.

Medical gymnastics were taught at the YMCA College in Chicago and a number of other metropolitan cities. Various natural therapies, including massage, were studied at the Columbia Institute of Physio-Therapy in Washington, D.C., an institution chartered by Congress. The United States Army trained practitioners to treat the wounded of World War I and World War II. Training also went on in hospitals, clinics, and nursing schools. During the 1950s physical therapy education moved from its base in hospitals to the university where massage continued to be a part of the training but not a major component. Because physical therapists trained in the last half of the century received massage only as a few hours of elective coursework, massage was not a significant part of the practice of physical therapy, even when physical therapy became more independent of physicians in the 1980s. Today we see more and more physical therapists enrolling in massage courses to learn the lost art of hands-on therapies they now see as valuable. There was some animosity between the physical therapy field and the massage trade during the last two decades of the twentieth century and lingering feelings still exist, but the future holds promise for more cooperation between the two fields.

Meanwhile massage education moved into private schools as the practice of massage moved further away from the medical community. In 1906 the National College of Massage and Physiotherapy (later renamed the College of Swedish Massage) was established in Chicago. This school operated at least until 1942. The 1939 school catalog for the College of Swedish Massage asserts massage is a "fascinating field . . . a permanent, successful career with a splendid income, either working for someone else or as your own boss. Here is your chance to serve your fellowmen in the dignified capacity of a health builder." The Swedish Massage Institute began teaching its first class in 1916 in New York City and is still open as the Swedish Institute today. From that point on there was a slow but steady stream of schools opening around the country. Older schools still in business include the Institute for Natural Health, established in 1947, the Bancroft School of Massage Therapy, established in 1950, the Central Ohio School of Massage, established in 1964, and the Heartwood Institute, established in 1968.

The number of massage schools in the world increased dramatically in the past century. From none devoted solely to training in massage therapy at the end of the nineteenth century to more than 1,600 worldwide at the end of the twentieth century, one can see the proliferation of schools in only one hundred years. The great majority of those schools were established in the last quarter of the century, after the 1970s. In the United States alone at the end of the century there were more than one thousand schools devoted primarily to training in massage therapy, and more than three hundred more with curriculums that included massage therapy as one of its major training modalities. For several decades community colleges have offered unaccredited courses in massage within their adult education coursework, and a growing number of them are now offering accredited programs.

Massage education is now big business, with some schools operating in large institution-like facilities. The Boulder College of Massage Therapy, the National Holistic Institute, and the Swedish Institute in New York are examples of schools with large facilities, permanent staff, and diverse curriculums. In the last five years of the twentieth century establishment of multiple campuses by the same school became a trend, while the sale of schools also increased. One corporate organization purchased nine different massage-school campuses in the eastern seaboard region. Alongside the massage schools we've also seen the advancement of retreat centers that offer-full course training in massage. Many of these are in rural locations, but some are within the walls of community colleges and holistic health centers and institutes.

School graduations range from a low of a half dozen students to those in excess of one hundred students per session. The average training session is six months to a year, depending on whether a student attends full time or part time. In the United States the average program is about 500 hours, but is now starting to grow to about 650 classroom hours. Some schools are increasing their core programs to 1,000 hours or more, but this is a slow movement. Canada has a two-year minimum program in two provinces expressed as a 2,300-hour requirement, which may be raised soon to 2,600 or 3,000 hours.

Although thousands of students are graduated from these schools each year, estimates are that nearly half are not doing massage one year after graduation. The drop-out rate is likely due to the variety of reasons people attend massage school. It is not always as a career option, rather serving to augment another career choice or just to fulfill a desire to learn how to do massage. Many are also ill prepared for the demands of being in business for themselves or for acquiring a job in an unusual field of endeavor.

In Europe schools of massage have emerged much more slowly than in the United States. In England there are about a dozen schools, including the Northern Institute of Massage, which was founded in 1924. In England and Australia there are a number of institutes—colleges or universities of holistic health—teaching a wide-ranging curriculum, with some courses in massage. Australia and New Zealand claim at least twenty massage schools between them, while Thailand, Hong Kong, and China also provide formal school education in their indigenous techniques. Italy, Germany, France, and other European mainland countries have massage or related specialty schools, and Austria has one of the most famous schools devoted strictly to the Dr. Vodder Method of Lymphatic Drainage. Spain, too, has several schools, with sports massage and applications in the orthopedic area being very popular. Fewer schools exist in the Scandinavian countries.

Massage practitioners in the United States differ quite a bit from those in many other countries when it comes to their learning habits. Typically, American practitioners are not so much interested in the theory behind a specific technique as they are in how to do it. For example, those attending a seminar on massage techniques in Australia will gladly sit through a half-day of instruction on the theory behind a technique and be satisfied with a few hours of practical demonstration and practice. In contrast, American practitioners won't sit long listening to a lecture about the theory of a technique; they'd much rather get their hands into action practicing it. Most practitioners in America are interested in the application of specific techniques to specific conditions, research results concerning the efficacy of massage, help in developing their business, and self-care techniques designed to help them take care of themselves or to help their clients help themselves between sessions. Learning as many techniques as possible is the trend of continuing education today.

School owners have often been association leaders and members of regulatory boards. As such they have become very involved in the political and legal aspects of massage. National certification of massage practitioners has been a hotbed of controversy ever since its inception in 1988 by the AMTA. This is a subject of considerable complexity and goes to the heart of commercial and private interests as well as professional concerns in the trade. Accreditation and curriculum development are growing issues, being given little coverage in most trade journals except to praise them, but they will be of increasing concern in the future as competition continues to heat up and research further validates the efficacy of massage.

Accreditation of curriculum has moved from complete self-credentialing (termed "certified" from 1930 to 1970) to "curriculum-approved" schools from 1970 until about 1987, to present-day credentialing from outside agencies. Whether a school is in a state that has statewide regulation or not, it may seek accreditation of its massage curriculum from such agencies as the state's trade school accrediting agency or from several national organizations, such as the Accrediting Commission of Career Schools and Colleges of Technology (ACCSCT). These types of organizations not only assess curriculum but also assess facilities and administrative operations.

The issues surrounding the accreditation of schools and their curricula center on two general areas. The first is the choice of accrediting agency. With several of the leading massage associations having their own accrediting agencies, schools must decide whether to choose between these or the more established and respected outside agencies. In some cases this is a matter of loyalty to a long tradition of relationship between the school and the association. The availability of student loans and the conditions of offering them is another related issue schools must consider.

Associations on the Rise

The world's first association of massage practitioners—the Society of Trained Masseuses—was established in 1894 in England by five female nurses. In 1900 the Society changed its name to the Incorporated Society of Trained Masseuses. Another change of name and focus occurred in 1920 as it became the Chartered Society of Massage and Medical Gymnastics, with five thousand members. Finally in 1943 the name was once again altered to the Chartered Society of Physiotherapy, reflecting the changing role of its members.

The next formation of practitioners was the Society of Physical Therapeutists headquartered in Chicago. Established in 1918, it was limited to "those holding the degree of Doctor of Medicine." The next year the London and Counties Society of Physiologists (LCSP) was formed; it included masseurs and masseuses who practiced "remedial massage." The LCSP was for a long time limited to members in England, but since the 1980s has expanded to include a chapter in Canada, with members also joining from Ireland, Australia, Tasmania, New Zealand, and the United States. In 1921 the International Society of Medical Hydrology was formed in England as a professional and political organization aimed toward legitimizing spa medicine, of which massage was a part. This organization no longer functions. A government-recognized massage organization in Great Britain seems an eventual reality. A nationwide study was conducted in 1996 as a first step toward this goal, but thus far there remains no national standards of practice or nationwide organization representing massage interests.

During the 1920s several state organizations formed in the United States. In 1943 what is known today as the American Massage Therapy Association (AMTA) formed, eventually becoming the largest massage organization in the world in the 1990s. During the last two decades of the twentieth century several other international organizations were formed, such as the Associated Bodywork and Massage Professionals (ABMP), the International Massage Association (IMA), and International Myomassethics Federation (IMF). Today there are well over fifty organizations worldwide. There has been increasing involvement by professional associations in the area of public policy, research funding, grants, and participation in the health care reform movement. There was a time when the ABMP was at opposite poles from the AMTA on legislative matters, but today, with new leadership in both organizations, they seem to be moving closer in their support of legislative efforts in various states.

Numerous associations have formed as splinter groups of more established organizations. The International Myomassethics Federation was formed in the early 1970s by several former female AMTA members who felt the AMTA lacked heart. IMF membership rose to more than 1,200 at one time, but today is around 750.

The ABMP was established by another disgruntled female AMTA member. The ABMP was the first for-profit trade organization, formed primarily to sell professional liability insurance. Earlier in the century trade associations promoted a specific kind of therapeutic technique, such as Swedish scientific massage. Today several focus on selling professional liability insurance at a lower rate than their competition, while their members are much more esoteric in their use of techniques. Associations are the primary providers of professional liability insurance for practitioners, and most of those who join a massage association do so for the insurance coverage, generating a lot of revenue for the organization. Although no commercial efforts were made to provide insurance prior to the last decade of the twentieth century, such ventures were readily successful because they produced less expensive insurance premiums with less involvement of members in the association's activities, a desirable benefit for many.

An anti-AMTA boycott was launched in the late 1980s by an Oklahoma practitioner and school owner to protest the association's involvement in legislative matters. He claimed they sought to put him out of business as well. The boycott did little to change the direction of AMTA leadership but was in some respects a magnet for others who didn't like the large association's methods in the pursuit of regulation by state government. However, the AMTA does not hold an exclusive claim to having disgruntled members. Several state organizations have been formed by former members of state associations for similar reasons, and there have been national boycotts against several organizations.

In Canada school-affiliated associations operate under the guise or approval of the provincial government, with the government giving the school the authority to establish standards and credential practitioners. Unification of the Canadian associations has been attempted, but no substantive progress has yet been made.

In Australia there are nearly a dozen organizations; unification of them was begun in the early 1990s but is yet to be completed. Many of these organizations are affiliated with schools. And New Zealand associations, few and sparsely populated like the country within which they operate, have been fighting massage parlors and adverse Yellow Pages advertising for several years. There are no known associations operating in Africa, except beauty-oriented massage associations in South Africa, and none are known in South America and Mexico. In Asia there are two organizations affiliated with specific techniques, such as Thai massage and tuina massage in China, but these, like those in New Zealand, Africa, and the European countries, have little if any international contact. There has been an attempt to form an association in South Korea but the organizer quickly found that massage practitioners there were not interested in joining a professional association with an ethical standard. In many of the Pacific Rim countries, such as Bali, no organizations exist.

Rush to Regulate

The first regulatory statute related to massage in the United States was instituted in Ohio in 1915. During the next fifty years few other states would take on regulating massage. By 1939 only four other states had passed legislation concerning massage—Florida, Pennsylvania, Wisconsin, and Minnesota. But in the second half of the century the trend was completely reversed. While in 1985 there were only ten states with any kind of statewide regulation of massage practitioners or establishments, by the end of the century there were twenty-eight plus the District of Columbia. There is a national movement to establish massage regulation in every state in the United States, but it does not advance forward without some resistance.

The need to regulate is a hot topic of discussion within some quarters of the massage trade. Nearly every existing massage regulation in the United States, Canada, Australia, New Zealand, and in some countries in Europe was originally designed to control prostitution. Upon that foundation was built most of the current regulation that controls massage practitioners and establishments. In those states and provinces without statewide regulation, county and municipal authorities usually have statutes that exist to control prostitution, unless changed by the efforts of interested practitioners or their associations. In a number of states practitioners are still required to have their fingerprints taken in order to get a business license to practice massage. And in some areas cross-gender massage is illegal.

It has only been because of the work of ardent practitioners and associations that any kind of practitioner-based laws have been established, either replacing the old laws or supplementing them with added provisions. In 1999 a new kind of regulation was introduced in the Minnesota state legislature. The bill, commonly called the Freedom of Access law, was designed to create a living document to be used by the practitioner in cooperation with their client/patient. Its purpose is to provide the patient with information about what to expect from the session while also being a mutual agreement between them so that the patient might take more responsibility for his or her health care. Organization to pass similar laws in several other states is now underway.

The major issues surrounding government regulation of massage are the protection of the public from harm; educational standards and scope of practice; approval or credibility; coalitions for or against regulation; and the effects of including non-massage modalities in the law. Legislatures do not generally initiate legislation to establish massage regulation. Rather, it is trade interests—particularly associations or sometimes an individual—who find a sponsor to introduce a bill.

Most every state legislature is legally mandated to pass laws to protect the public from harm. Sometimes the harm may be real, having already occurred, and in other cases it may only be a potential threat or implication of harm. There has been no proof submitted to any state that demonstrates that massage is actually harmful to the public or is potentially harmful enough to need the state to regulate its practices and so protect the public from its abuses.

Legislatures are not mandated to pass laws to aggrandize a special interest group or provide credentials that would give that group public credibility, although that is often what occurs when a group is regulated by state law. This is the case with the massage trade. During the last two decades of the twentieth century unprecedented efforts were made by leaders in the massage trade to obtain state regulation over the practice of massage. In my opinion these efforts are in the main an attempt to gain credibility for massage rather than protect the public from harm. Many people in the massage trade don't want the government interfering with their freedom to do business. On the other side there are those who see regulation as a sign of professional development and credibility.

Some have argued that state regulation of massage provides an avenue of reprieve for grievances against the public—practitioners who violate the law have a state agency to answer to. However, a professional ethics board or other trade-related body can just as easily handle such issues. State regulation of massage is merely a way to gain state sanction for title protection so that a few practitioners can feel good about having a state credential hanging on their office wall. Instead of protecting the public from harm, state regulation protects persons working under that state's law from being freely infringed upon in the marketplace by those coming in from outside the state to practice. And state regulatory boards provide leaders in a state with the opportunity to establish small monopolies for schools and seminars. State regulation has also been used as a means of obtaining professional credibility in a cultural and health-field environment that sees massage as a form of relaxation, luxury, stress management, sensory delight, or as a ruse for sexual favors.

Aside from these issues, it has been the inclusion of other forms of manual therapies that has lit a fire under the regulatory pot that is often boiling with controversy. Rolfing, reflexology, shiatsu, and Reiki therapies are considered "bodywork" rather than massage because they don't utilize the basic strokes of massage known as Swedish massage—effleurage, petrissage, vibration, friction, and tapotement—and, more importantly, because each of them comes from a different healing arts perspective. Generally the focus of the work is applied to specific body tissues rather than the entire body, as with most forms of massage. Rolfing, formally called structural integration, focuses on the fascia so as to align the structural posture of the body, and the techniques applied are nothing like those used in traditional massage. Shiatsu is literally "finger pressure," and does not utilize any of the basic strokes of massage. And in Reiki—hotly contested in several states currently—the practitioner most often doesn't touch the body at all, primarily performing a prayer or channeling work. The Alexandar technique and Feldenkrais method—each of which utilizes no massage techniques—focus on re-education of the central nervous system as it relates to body movement and posture.

I believe a disservice was done to these and dozens of other modalities that are not massage therapy when the national certification movement, early in its development as part of the AMTA, added the term "bodywork" to the end of its name as the National Certification Board for Therapeutic Massage and Bodywork. Many of the states with statewide regulation have adopted the NCBTMB examination. Since this time the battle has been ongoing to exclude the many forms of bodywork from the heavy hand of state massage regulation. Today several Internet chat groups maintain their opposition to government regulation of massage therapy in any form. But the major associations, along with many school owners who are often association leaders, continue to seek state regulation throughout the country.

Rumors have recently circulated that a national regulation will be sought, perhaps by means of a Congressional effort, but it remains to be seen whether the case can continue to be made in the face of increasing opposition to regulation within the profession. Although the efforts to get laws made seem to have fostered divisiveness, monopolies, vested interests, and a false sense of acceptance, many see regulation as a positive career move for the trade. This may be why the trend continues.

Little regulation exists in other countries except Canada, where only three provinces regulate massage on a strict provincial-wide basis, but there are moves to increase that number as well. The provincial governments have given authority to the associations, usually connected with schools, to regulate themselves. Australia has some regulations that are not standardized and are usually intended to control prostitution.

Proving Massage

During the late 1970s and early 1980s Dr. Janet F. Quinn, a Ph.D. nurse, researched a number of areas related to massage therapy. One of her findings indicated "that an average decrease in state anxiety of 17% can be expected when TT (Therapeutic Touch) is used by hospitalized cardiovascular patients."[17] Dr. Quinn has continued her research and published numerous of her findings. However, therapeutic touch is not usually considered massage because in its practice the hands rarely touch the patient.

Even so, Quinn's work must be mentioned because it was an early effort to bring attention to the field of alternative therapies that includes massage.

Tiffany Field, Ph.D., at the University of Miami Medical School Department of Pediatrics, conducted studies during the late 1970s and early 1980s into the benefits of touch for premature babies. Her studies were widely publicized in the trade. The Touch Research Institute is the first of its kind and was originally funded by the Johnson & Johnson Corporation; the institute's research is an ongoing project gaining increasing attention from outside the massage trade. Many of Dr. Field's studies conducted during the 1990s included massage practitioners. Dr. Field and her team have utilized massage and other modalities in their research and continue their efforts into the new millennium. Reports of this ongoing research are published regularly in TRI's newsletter, *TouchPoints*.

Several of the larger trade organizations, such as the American Massage Therapy Association and the International Myomassethics Federation, have established research funds and support other research projects. These are sometimes conducted in conjunction with educational institutions, massage schools, or as part of the National Institutes of Health program of study and research in the field of complementary and alternative medicine.

Attempts to validate massage by other than scientific research have also been made. Anecdotal claims for the benefits of massage have been around for decades. From the 1950s through the mid-1980s, lists of benefits were prevalent within the trade. These lists comprise the major claims made regarding the benefits of massage prior to substantive modern research. Current research has yet to substantiate most of these earlier claims.

The benefits of massage have been categorized as "physical," "emotional," and "mental." Here are a few examples taken from 1984 promotional literature of the AMTA.

Physical benefits: Deep relaxation and stress reduction. Relief of muscle tension and stiffness. Reduced muscle spasms. Greater joint flexibility and range of motion, reduced blood pressure, improved posture, disease prevention and health maintenance.

Emotional benefits: Enhanced self-image, reduced levels of anxiety, and increased awareness of the mind/body connection, and greater ease of emotional expression.

Mental benefits: Relaxed state of alertness, reduced mental stress (a calmer mind), greater ability to monitor and respond to stress signals, and increased capacity for clearer thinking.

In 1992 the *New England Journal of Medicine* published the results of the nation's first study indicating alternative therapy usage. The study showed that millions of

Americans were spending billions of dollars on alternative therapies, out of their pocket and not reimbursed by insurance, without seeking the advice of their primary care physicians. They were visiting alternative care practitioners for many of the very same ailments for which they might otherwise have seen a doctor. This study had an enormous impact on managed care, HMOs, the National Institutes of Health, and within the alternative community. New books were written explaining what these alternative therapies were and how they might be helpful. Conferences were held for years to educate the medical community about them and how to integrate them into their field of experience and service. New research was spawned to seek validation of these "new" therapies. The impact of this study has yet to be completely felt and the potentials it has rendered visible continue to be realized. A follow-up study was conducted in 1998 confirming that the trend toward alternative therapies was continuing and had grown significantly since the 1992 survey. Both of these studies also revealed that the top four alternative therapies of choice were chiropractic, biofeedback or stress management techniques, massage therapy, and homeopathy.

That same year the *Journal of the American Medical Association* published the results of another study conducted in the United States and abroad that asked why patients use alternative medicine. The term *alternative medicine* was broadly defined to include any form of therapy not included within the Western medical model. Interestingly, the study did not reveal that consumers sought out alternative therapies because they were unhappy with their primary care physician or with the medical establishment in general, a claim often made by those in the alternative therapy community. The answer was that they use alternative therapies primarily because these therapies are more "congruent with their own values, beliefs, and philosophical orientations toward health."[14]

This study was conducted because there was a perception that medical doctors had lost touch with their patients, a fairly common public perception. At Harvard University Medical School an experiment was conducted on medical students that was designed to increase their sensitivity to patients by literally putting them back in touch with them. Third-year medical students were required to take a basic course in practical massage with the hope that they might better appreciate the value of tactile contact with their patients. Not only were they required to receive massages during their training; they were required to give massages as well, the idea being that by experiencing personal contact of this kind they might become better doctors, more in touch, literally, with their patients.

Massage in the Media

Media influence on massage prior to the late twentieth century was nonexistent except in the form of books and a few pamphlets. Over the years, along with credible messages about massage, there have been reports of scandals from bathhouses to massage parlors, each a part of the history of massage and events that have helped to shape its present condition, the attitude of the public toward it, and the mental state of those who do massage for a living. Newspapers reported on the first bathhouse scandals in England and Chicago, and we can find scattered stories about massage parlors in American newspapers, especially those located near military bases.

In the last two decades of the twentieth century, though, magazines and newspapers increased their coverage of the entire alternative healing arts field that includes massage therapy. Articles about massage have been featured in the *Wall Street Journal*, *Time* and *Life* magazines, and nearly every major paper in the country. Most major magazines carry an article about massage at least once a year. These articles have fostered a more positive image of massage and have helped it to become more legitimate as a therapeutic tool rather than a tainted element of prostitution and vice. Massage has risen to become one of the relaxation icons of the advertising world, with its simple yet powerful message found in many quarters of world cultures, especially Western cultures so rich in advertising.

Books on massage began to proliferate in the 1960s and 1970s. In the two decades that followed, the number of specialty books on massage substantially increased. Today books about massage fill several shelves at the bookstore, often having their own section.

Prior to the 1950s magazines covering the subject of massage did not exist, though several health-related magazines occasionally published articles on the subject of massage. The first "magazine" about massage was not really a magazine but more of a booklet published by an association to promote the affairs of the association rather than to advance the field of massage in general. The first commercial publication devoted solely to reporting on the field of massage therapy was *Massage Magazine*. This publication has successfully chronicled massage since 1985. Its influence has also been significant in providing the first independent medium communicating the business, art, science, and news of massage to a worldwide audience. The first journalists to report on the massage trade and industry did so for *Massage Magazine* readers.

Most associations throughout the world now publish some sort of journal that not only provides their members with information about the organization's activities but also—following the lead of *Massage Magazine*—publishes relevant and timely articles on the business aspects of massage, technique development, and other issues important to the professional practitioner. Several of them specialize in soft tissue or other technical aspects of the broadening field of massage and bodywork. Numerous attempts to establish competing commercial publications have been made in the past decade, but none have survived.

Massage in the movies and on television has enjoyed a long career. Since the days of silent movies massage has found its way on to the silver screen. Charlie Chaplin—in the movie *The Mutual Cure* released by 20th Century Fox in 1917—is shown sitting on a bench waiting for his turn on the marble massage table while in front of him a large, burley man is giving massage to someone else. While the image of massage sometimes has been presented as funny or poignant, it often has been mistreated.

In a number of the James Bond movies Sean Connery is seen getting a massage from a beautiful woman, but the massage is poorly done and often sexually suggestive.

Some television depictions of massage have been favorable. When they aren't the massage trade complains, sometimes effectively altering its media representation. The *Seinfeld* show was criticized for its portrayal of massage as sexual, having nothing to do with therapy or relaxation. And on the show *Friends* one of the main characters often talks about her massage clients to anyone who will listen, giving the impression that all the gossip heard on the table is publicly displayed by therapists. Because her character is something of a flake, it also suggests that massage therapists are too. In a film released in 1999 a major film star portrayed a blind massage therapist that included a number of scenes accurately depicting the personal closeness found in many sessions but—unfortunately for the image of massage—ended up being a sexual relationship, something that is strictly against professional ethics in the trade. In many ways the media reflects the culture's experience; unfortunately that image often errs more on the side of negativity than on the healing connection. Improving the image of massage is a matter of education and experience—education so that each practitioner understands the importance of presenting a positive image for the greater good of the field and many positive experiences for those who are massaged.

Many famous people receive massage from all parts of the world, and they have been used to uplift the image of massage. However, the traditional image gleaned from this association has been that massage was just for the rich and famous, a myth that has stuck for years. That myth is fading as more and more people experience the benefits of massage.

The introduction of the massage chair in 1985 and on-site corporate massage in the 1990s spawned yet another round of media coverage, not in advertising copy but in article text. And a new kind of promotion emerged in the last dozen years of the twentieth century that can best be described as "planted" articles fostered by associations. These articles usually offer information about the value of massage, a major sporting event where massage was offered, a disaster relief effort that included massage, or a profile of a noteworthy practitioner. The name and contact information of a major massage association then appears at the end of the article. This kind of promotion is not new in the media but it is certainly new in the massage trade, indicating both the growing sophistication of leadership in the field and the self-serving interests of large groups vying for national attention.

The trade media in the later quarter of the century provided a new means of reaching practitioners like never before. Many new companies have emerged because of the new media opportunities for reaching wider audiences with their products and services. The trade media has also provided unprecedented networking and access to information for practitioners and educators about what's going on within the trade in terms of its regulation, education, politics, and many other related subjects. New leaders and unknown authors have arisen out of these publications and a new industry of media coverage for massage therapy is now both competitive and profitable.

The number of Web sites related to massage continues to grow. Chat lines among practitioners are always busy. In fact the Internet seems to have afforded more opportunity for communication, commerce, and the passing of information and resources not only within the trade but from outside of it as well. Where referral services for practitioners struggled to exist before, the Internet has provided consumer access never before possible.

The first novel written with a theme using massage is *The Hundredth Monkey Conspiracy*, written by me. There are now a number of books published that tell the inside story of this intimate and powerful healing art, but the vision expressed in *The Hundredth Monkey Conspiracy* is one that most practitioners share. That vision is for a future filled with massage for everyone who lives on this planet. Bringing us closer together through the medium of touch, all practitioners know from experience, is a dynamic movement that underscores the human condition. Healing touch is not for profit, not for credibility, not for material attention of any sort. Healing touch performed by a caring professional is all about bringing peace of mind, body, and spirit to the suffering of all people.

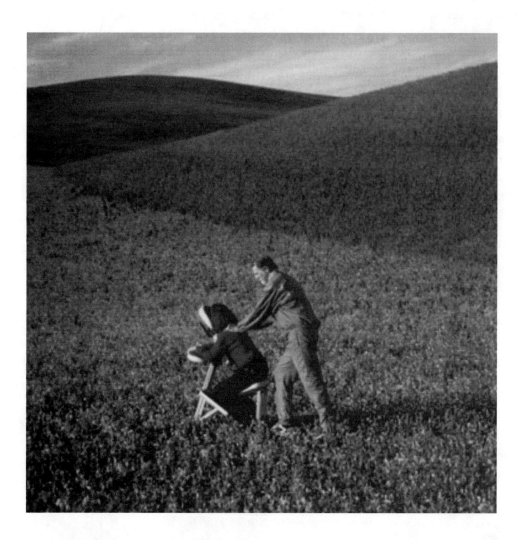

The future of massage is limited only by our imaginations as we ask ourselves and one another the question: How we can help bring relief to a suffering world? Our answers to this question in practice, in creatively applying traditions and methods developed through history, provide the continuity that is the living future of massage. This future is an open playing field, yet to be discovered and populated. Photograph by Jonah Sutherland, courtesy of *Massage Magazine.*

EPILOGUE The Future of Massage in the New Millennium

The new millennium bodes well for all aspects of the field of massage, including the growth and refinement of techniques, schools, and associations. It especially offers unprecedented opportunities for the practitioners of tomorrow—the new century is an open playing field for their enjoyment and success. As business, education, science, the arts, and social activities become more global, massage is also becoming more global. The opportunities for applying the caring and skillful hands of a massage practitioner are limited only by our imaginations, only by the creative means by which we find to apply our hands.

Trends developing in the last decade of the twentieth century will become the norm in the new millennium. The major trends now being seen include increasing the hours of education; expanding the scope of practice to include more modalities and better training in the psychological aspects of the work; further impact of state regulation and national certification on entry-level education at massage schools and continuing education units for practitioners; an expanding number of massage courses offered at community colleges and universities; a growing number of degree programs within massage institutions; massage emergency response teams that extend beyond the borders of individual states or organizations; and advanced integration of massage into the broader scope of bodywork and allied healing arts.

The number of training hours at massage schools has slowly increased over the past seventy-five years. Since the 1970s massage practitioner certification programs have required an average of 500 in-class hours. In the past five years, though, there has been an upward shift in hours required for certification, initiated by schools, regulatory boards, and accrediting organizations.

Five years ago it was rare to find a school that offered a 1,000-hour program; today there are several dozen. State regulatory boards, of which there are now thirty, have slowly begun to move away from the older 500-hour level to 650, 750, and even 1,000 hours of required training. The Commission on Massage Therapy Accreditation

Massage is the sharing of touch—hands or body, on head, hands or feet. And yet massage goes farther than skin-deep, deeper even than muscles and bones—a good, caring massage penetrates right to the depth of your being.

—**George Downing,** *The Book of Massage* (1984)

(COMTA), an organization that has grown out of the American Massage Therapy Association (AMTA), recently raised their requirements from 500 to 650 hours.

The trend toward more hours of training will continue, but the battleground feeding this trend will be occupied by those who want more hours because they want greater access to working within the national health care system versus those practitioners who don't aspire to working in medical settings and thus want less hours of training. While we may see a return to competency-based apprenticeships, it is more likely that the additional training needed to enter the medical scene will be manifested by more schools developing teaching clinics. Those schools that already offer this type of experiential training will increase student time in the clinics.

Curriculum has changed significantly during the past fifty years, moving from the so-called scientific Swedish massage to a more diversified menu. Anatomy and physiology are still mainstays in the curriculum, but trainings in adjunct modalities such as hydrotherapy has gradually fallen to minimal levels, displaced by pathology and an ever-increasing range of technique courses. Asian therapies, such as shiatsu, are increasingly a part of the core curriculum, mainly because the National Certification Board for Therapeutic Massage and Bodywork (NCBTMB) examinations cover that modality (despite the fact a small percentage of practitioners utilize shiatsu in their overall practice).

The future will bring what are now considered fringe or obscure techniques into wider use, and will encourage the development of technical applications already widely available. Specialization of technique, a clear trend of the past twenty years, will continue unabated. This trend continues in spite of the fact that practitioners are applying a broader array of techniques than their counterparts thirty and more years ago.

Over the past twenty years the psychological aspects of doing massage, such as being witness to a client's emotional release, has gained attention, leading not so much to including a curriculum in psychology in massage education but to more and better training in ethics and boundaries within the healing relationship. The advent of widespread training in ethical conduct and professional boundaries is fairly recent and is now commonplace throughout the country.

The future of massage as an adjunct therapy to psychology is another trend on the increase. A number of programs that utilize massage with speech therapy for special-needs children and abuse treatments is rising from within the massage industry. This trend will continue and will grow within the public and private school systems as well as other human-resource areas of health care.

Massage is a valuable tool in the treatment of trauma, as evidenced by the growing field of emergency massage relief teams. The aftermath of any disaster brings a lot of assistance for the victims, but relief and rescue workers have little support for their efforts. Following the tragedies of September 11th, 2001, massage practitioners volunteered their time, energy, money, and products to relieve workers at the crash sites and at other locations where post-traumatic stress was being felt. Practitioners gave massages in New York near Ground Zero; in athletic stadiums around the city, where relief workers took meals and slept; and at morgues where workers brought the bodies that had been retrieved. They were on the job at the Pentagon and at the crash site in Pennsylvania. They also worked on citizens in Oklahoma City, where many people who had suffered through the Murrah Federal Building bombing only a few years ago found themselves deeply troubled after September 11th, as if the tragedy they had lived through had happened all over again.

Massage will continue to be a part of the relief efforts for large-scale disasters, and the future will bring massage increasingly to the local level as practitioners develop stronger relationships with the emergency agencies in their communities. Massage emergency relief efforts is a relatively new concept in the industry, but with more practitioners being trained and experienced working in emergency conditions and being encouraged to build ongoing relationships with local emergency organizations, we will see many advances in this area in the near future. We might see formal relationships with the military, fire departments, civil emergency organizations, and even operations overseas that contain professional elements of a massage emergency team.

The impact of state regulation on the education of massage practitioners continues to be felt in those states with a massage law. In the twenty states without regulation, competition between schools in and out of the state is a strong influence on curriculum; in those states that are regulated statewide, most of the influence on curriculum is derived from the state examination that students need to pass in order to get their credential to practice massage. That test, the NCTMB exam, has been adopted by twenty of the thirty states that are regulated, and serves as their examination of choice. Those states with statewide regulation that do not use the NCBTMB exam utilize their own testing instruments.

It is my opinion that the NCTMB has had more of an impact on schools throughout the country in terms of curriculum than any other factor over the past ten years. The NCTMB has forced hundreds of schools, in regulated and nonregulated states, to teach to the test. This is not very different from the situation that existed before there was a national certification examination for massage, because even then schools were oriented to teaching their students what they needed to pass the state exam. I operated a massage school during the early 1980s in Washington state, and even then the state exam was an important guide to the curriculum. However, today the NCTMB exam used by regulated states has broadened school curriculum to the point that it is, in my opinion, a watered-down version of what the exam was twenty years ago. There is now more diversity of technique and less hydrotherapy and hygiene. An orientation to career tracks, such as working in a spa, a hospital, or a chiropractic office, are beginning to be emphasized, while in-depth business training is slowly declining.

Even though the NCTMB is an entry-level examination it is purported to be a professional credential, and many employers are now requiring those they hire to be nationally certified. Touted by the AMTA as being a voluntary exam when it was being developed, the NCTMB exam quickly became nonvoluntary. The NCTMB exam is not a competency-based test; it is a multiple-choice exam of approximately 150 questions. More than 98 percent of those who take the exam pass it. The NCTMB certification does not confer anything other than the fact that one can pass a general test of objective knowledge, but it is the first time in the history of massage that a standard test is being administered in a large number of states. The exam, as promoted by the AMTA when it was first initiated, does not provide for reciprocity between the states either, except in a few cases and those are not any more cases than existed before the exam was established.

The AMTA has set a course to establish statewide regulation in all fifty of the United States and they spend a lot of money in their lobbying efforts, but a new player has come across the AMTA's path that promises to up the ante in the battle between those who want statewide regulation and those who do not. The Freedom to Practice Act passed by the Minnesota legislature in 2000 is serving as an initiative piece of legislation for a growing number of other states. This type of legislation protects practitioners from overly broad definitions of what constitutes medical practice, while also giving the public the freedom to make choices for the health care they want. These kinds of laws, varying in each state, allow healing arts practitioners of many kinds, including massage, who are not in a licensed or registered state to conduct their business with the public without the need for a control board.

Trends in government regulation and the efforts of trade factions for and against regulation show movement into a new phase as more and more practitioners stand up against the formerly secret and unilateral initiatives of certain groups. The Internet is providing a new forum for discussing and organizing efforts on both sides of the argument. We will see efforts at standardizing existing government regulations, and more states will adopt these standards. Future trends will see massage associations and other organizations putting themselves in the public eye; more public relations campaigns will be planned and launched, and public awareness about massage will increase. As the growing body of knowledge from other health and science fields is integrated into the profession, massage practitioners and organizations promoting specific techniques will expand their wisdom and their capacities for transmitting informed touch. Research into the efficacy and applications of massage therapy will continue to increase and the quality of these projects will improve. Future research will develop from these early models but will be far more complex, sophisticated, relevant, and useful.

As massage continues to move into distant corners of human culture, it will find continued success at helping to establish and maintain bonds between family members, society, and possibly even nation-states. The Massage for Peace in Schools program, created by Swedish massage practitioner Solveig Berggren, has advanced touch therapies into some parts of the Swedish school system such that elementary students are taught to massage each other. A massage school in Sweden has developed an initia-

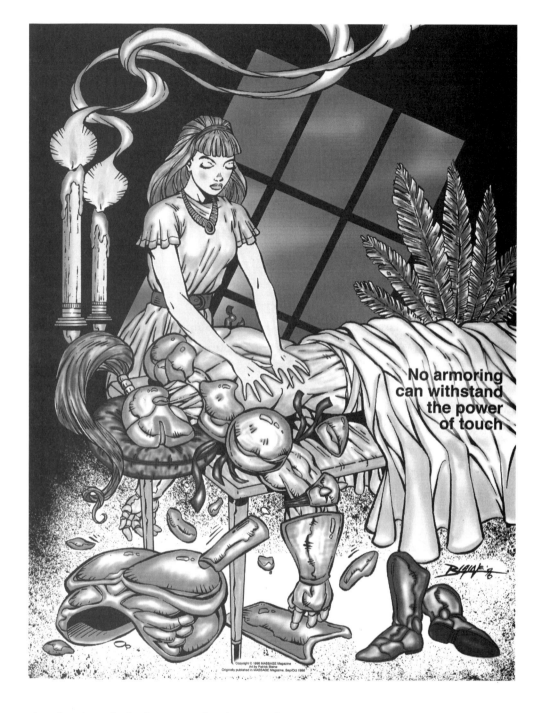

No armoring can withstand the power of touch

Copyright © 1996 MASSAGE Magazine
Art by Patrick Blaine
Originally published in MASSAGE Magazine, Sep/Oct 1996

An ancient form of the healing arts, massage continues in its long and worldwide tradition of melting the armor that builds up from our past and present actions. That armor may change its character and source as life goes on, but humans will always have need of its softening if we are to traverse the distance before us. Ilustration by Patrick Blaine, courtesy of *Massage Magazine.*

tive the aim of which is to make the use of massage a national agenda for the entire Swedish culture.

In the United States there are several programs that have their roots in the work of Peggy Farlow and her Touch to T.E.A.C.H. program. Touch to T.E.A.C.H. is an anagram for Trust, Emotional Security and Empowerment, Attachment and Attending, Communication and Connection, and Healthier Families through Healing Touch. Peggy has had considerable success incorporating her program into school districts, medical establishments, parent organizations, and various caregiver groups. In New

Zealand, Eva Scherer has created a program for children called Touch, Love, Health, which is taught through the Auckland YMCA. Finally, a program in Minneapolis utilizes touch therapy as part of its rehabilitation process for victims of torture and domestic violence.

The ancient shaman successfully utilized various forms of touch in his or her negotiations with the evil spirit or evil deed that possessed the patient. Through coaxing, jostling, cajoling and physical manipulations the shaman discovered ways to remedy the patient from the ill effects of the evil inside. When we see massage being provided free of charge in the halls of a state legislature and the subsequent passing of a bill related to massage (which has happened many times in the United States), it isn't too much of a stretch to imagine massage being used as a means of softening up the opposition in other types of negotiations.

It is a widely known fact that between the client and practitioner a relationship is created that is built upon trust. Similar to the concerns surrounding the power differential that can take place within a counseling relationship, massage practitioners are acknowledging the boundaries of their role as practitioners. Advising a client to do some homework or purchase a lotion, a book, or some other self-help tool is possible because of the relationship created in the session room. I believe the relationship that emerges from the connection of two humans in the privacy of the massage session room will one day be brought to its fullest potential in the arena of business, cultural, and political negotiations as well.

Massage as a part of the larger alternative and complementary field of health care is also very promising. Massage is the number three alternative therapy chosen most by American consumers (chiropractic being the first and biofeedback the second). Billions of dollars are spent by consumers each year for these and other alternative therapies, all out of pocket and not reimbursed by health insurance. Many a vision for a future business venture will be founded on this information about consumer use and spending.

It is my hope that a new appreciation and growing interest will evolve in the twenty-first century toward our past in the field of massage—a past full of ideas, personalities, and knowledge. Learning about the history of massage comprises the first step toward realizing its future. Knowing where we've come from can help us better understand where we might be going. To paraphrase Disraeli, by learning about our past we are less likely to repeat our previous mistakes. Losing sight of our past fosters near-sightedness that obscures our vision of the continuum of which we are a part, disrespect to those who have come before us, and an incredible loss of knowledge and wisdom.

Massage has been kicked around, gone underground, and risen to unprecedented heights, only to fall again into disuse and disarray. Yet massage has survived since before humans built shelters for themselves, devised exercise programs, or developed science and the arts. From its fundamental roots in touch behavior, massage has survived because it is a basic human need, it feels good, and it is an immediate and healthy approach to relieving pain and suffering. But most importantly, it brings humans together into contact with one another—it is a relationship connection like no other. The application of a pair of healing hands to another person is the ultimate expression of caring and giving, while receiving that touch is an ultimate expression of trust and self-compassion. Massage is a profound way to deliver love and nurturing to a suffering world.

The past century has been the busiest and most successful for massage therapy around much of the world. The next century of massage begins with the new hands-on healing arts careers of those now entering the trade. Sculpting the future of massage is a noble and exciting venture, and many of you are now forming the contours of that destiny. Some will make noteworthy contributions, but most will be satisfied to contribute to the next chapter of the history of massage—and to the healing of the world's people—one session and one person at a time. I wish each of you an adventure of discovery in the wonderful world of massage and the bliss found from doing work you love.

In touch,
Robert Noah Calvert
Valleyford, Washington
February 2002

Endnotes

Introduction

1. Joseph Rohrer, *Rohrer's Scientific Body Massage and Swedish Movements,* 1925, self-published, New York, 11.

Chapter One

1. Gertrude Beard and Elizabeth Wood, *Massage: Principles and Techniques* (Philadelphia and London: W. B. Saunders, 1964).

2. Herman L. Kamenetz, M.D., "History of Massage" in *Manipulation, Traction and Massage*, ed. Joseph P. Rogoff (Baltimore: Williams & Wilkins, 1980).

3. Robert Montraville Green, M.D., *A Translation of Galen's Hygiene (De Sanitate Tuenda)* (Springfield, Ill.: Charles C. Thomas, 1951).

4. Kamenetz, "History of Massage." Herman L. Kamenetz, M.D., was chief of physical medicine and rehabilitation at Veterans Hospital, Rocky Hill, Connecticut, and clinical instructor in medicine at Yale University School of Medicine in New Haven, Connecticut. Kamenetz is the author of a chapter entitled "History of Massage" in the fifth volume of the Physical Medicine Library series *Massage, Manipulation and Traction,* edited by Sidney Licht, M.D. (New Haven, Conn.: Elizabeth Licht, 1960).

5. Gunilla Knutson, *Gunilla Knutson's Book of Massage* (New York: Bell Publishing, 1972).

6. Douglas Graham, M.D., *Manual Therapeutics, A Treatise on Massage: Its history, mode of application and effects,* 3rd ed. (Philadelphia and London: J. B. Lippincott, 1902).

7. Kamenetz, "History of Massage."

8. Ibid.

9. Ibid.

10. William Murrell, *Massage as a Mode of Treatment* (London: H. K. Lewis, 1886).

11. Cornelius E. De Puy, M.D., "Richard P. Van Why, Father of Massage Therapy in the United States," *Massage Therapy Journal* 30, no. 3 (summer 1991).

12. *Thomas's Medical Dictionary,* 13th ed., s.v. "massage."

13. George H. Taylor, M.D., *Massage: Principles and Practice of Remedial Treatment by Imparted Motion* (New York: John B. Alden, 1887).

14. Ibid.

15. Graham, *Manual Therapeutics.*

16. John Harvey Kellogg, M.D., *The Art of Massage: Its Physiological Effects and Therapeutic Applications* (Battle Creek, Mich.: Modern Medicine Publishing, 1895).

17. Ibid.

18. Axel V. Grafstrom, M.D., *A Text-book of Mechano-Therapy (Massage and Medical Gymnastics),* 2nd ed. (Philadelphia: W. B. Saunders & Co., 1904).

19. Emil G. Kleen, M.D., *Massage and Medical Gymnastics,* trans. Mina L. Dobbie, M.D., 2nd ed. (London: J. & A. Churchill, 1921).

20. *Stedman's Medical Dictionary, Illustrated: A Practical Medical Dictionary,* 13th ed., s.v. "massage."

21. Gertrude Beard, *Massage: Principles and Techniques,* 2nd ed. (Philadelphia: W. B. Saunders Company, 1952).

22. George Downing, *The Massage Book* (New York, Berkeley: Random House and Bookworks, 1972).

23. Ruth E. Williams, *The Road to Radiant Health* (Kennewick, Wash.: self-published, 1977).

24. Frances M. Tappan, *Healing Massage Techniques,* 2nd ed. (East Norwalk, Conn.: Appleton & Lange, 1980).

25. Albert Schatz, Ph.D., professor emeritus, Temple University, in correspondence with the author, 1999.

26. Time-Life, *Massage: Total Relaxation* (Alexandria, Va.: Time-Life Books, 1987).

27. Sandy Fritz, *Mosby's Fundamentals of Therapeutic Massage* (St. Louis: Mosby Lifeline, 1995).

28. Albert Schatz, Ph.D., personal correspondence.

29. The American Massage Therapy Association, *Massage Therapy Journal,* summer, 1999. The definition given here was developed in 1995.

30. Connecticut Department of Public Health, Massage Therapy Licensure (1998).

31. Florida Department of Health, Division of Medical Quality Assurance, Board of Massage Therapy (1997).

32. Oregon Board of Massage Therapists (1998).

33. Iowa Board of Examiners for Massage Therapy (1998).

Chapter Two

1. Felix Marti-Ibanez, M.D., ed., *The Epic of Medicine* (New York: Clarkson N. Potter and M. D. Publications, 1959).

2. Ibid.

3. Adolphus P. Elkin, *Aboriginal Men of High Degree: Initiation and Sorcery in the World's Oldest Tradition* (Rochester, Vt.: Inner Traditions International, 1994).

4. Jacqueleyn Benton, "Massage in the African Tradition," *Massage Magazine* 31, (May/ June 1991).

5. Marti-Ibanez, ed., *The Epic of Medicine.*

6. Ibid.

7. Garcilaso Inca de la Vega, *Commentarios Reales de los Incas*, 1609. Translated by commission of the author.

8. Douglas Guthrie, M.D., *A History of Medicine* (Philadelphia: J. B. Lippincott Co., 1946).

9. Fikret Yegul, *Baths and Bathing in Classical Antiquity* (New York: The Architectural History Foundation, M.I.T Press, 1992).

10. Elisabeth Brooke, *Medicine Women: A Pictorial History of Women Healers* (Wheaton, Ill.: Quest Books, The Theosophical Publishing House, and Godsfield Press, 1997).

11. Ibid.

12. Ibid.

13. Mircea Eliade, *Shamanism: Archaic Techniques of Ecstasy*, Bollingen Series LXXVI, trans. Willard R. Trask (Princeton: Princeton University Press, 1974).

14. Graham, *Manual Therapeutics.*

15. Kamenetz, "History of Massage."

16. Kellogg, *The Art of Massage,* 1895.

17. Graham, *Manual Therapeutics.*

18. Charles Nordhoff, *Northern California, Oregon and the Sandwich Islands* (New York: Harper & Brothers, 1874).

19. Paul A. Lawrence, *Lomi-Lomi Hawaiian Massage* (San Anselmo, Calif.: PAL Press, 1981).

20. Emil G. Kleen, M.D., *Handbook of Massage,* trans. Edward M. Hartwell, M.D. (Philadelphia: P. Plakiston, Son & Co., 1892).

21. Walter Johnson, *The Anatriptic Art* (London: Simpkin, Marshall & Co., 1866).

22. Alan Villiers, "Tribute to Captain Cook: The Man Who Mapped the Pacific. The Voyages and Historic Discoveries of Captain James Cook," in *National Geographic* 140, no. 3, September, 1971.

23. Cornelio H. Evangelista and Virgil J. Mayor Apostol, *The Healing Hands of Hilot: Filipino Therapeutic Massage* (National City, Calif.: self-published, 1998).

24. Ibid.

25. Ibid.

26. Zhenya Kurashova Wine, *Russian School of Massage Therapy, The Kurashova Method* (Self-published, n.d.)

Chapter Three

1. Marti-Ibanez, ed., *The Epic of Medicine*.

2. Kamenetz, "History of Massage."

3. Ibid.

4. Walter Libby, M.D., *The History of Medicine* (Boston and New York: Houghton Mifflin, 1922).

5. Kamenetz, "History of Massage."

6. Libby, *The History of Medicine*.

7. Sir William Osler, *The Evolution of Modern Medicine* (New Haven, Conn.: Yale University Press, 1921).

8. Cited by Sir Osler in James Henry Breasted, *A History of the Ancient Egyptians* (New York: Scribner, 1908).

9. Brooke, *Medicine Women*.

10. Selim Hassan, Ph.D., *Excavations at Giza I* (Oxford: Egyptian University, 1932).

11. Marti-Ibanez, ed., *The Epic of Medicine*.

12. Russell T. Trall, M.D., *The Hydropathic Encyclopedia* (New York: Fowlers & Wells, 1853.)

13. Ibid.

14. Graham, *Manual Therapeutics*.

15. Barbara Metz, *Ancient Egypt* (Washington, D.C.: National Geographic Society, 1978).

16. Ibid.

17. Graham, *Manual Therapeutics*.

18. Marti-Ibanez, ed., *The Epic of Medicine*.

19. Ibid.

20. Morris Berman, *The Reenchantment of the World* (New York: Bantam, 1984).

21. J. J. M. de Groot, *The Religious System of China,* vol. 6 (Leyden, Mass.: E. J. Brill, 1910).

22. Ted J. Kaptchuk, *The Web That Has No Weaver* (Portland: NTC Publishing Group, 1983).

23. Ibid.

24. Kleen, *Handbook of Massage*.

25. Kellogg, *The Art of Massage*, 1895.

26. Kamenetz, "History of Massage."

27. Ibid.

28. Sensei Masunaga, *Zen Shiatsu* (Tokyo: Kodansha Publishing, 1977).

29. Zhang Tao, M.D., interview in *Massage Magazine* 33 (Sept/Oct 1991).

30. Sun Chengnan, ed., *Chinese Bodywork: A Complete Manual of Chinese Therapeutic Massage,* trans. Wang Qiliang (Berkeley: Pacific View Press, 1993).

31. Zhang Enqun, ed., *Chinese Massage: A Practical English–Chinese Library of Traditional Chinese Medicine* (Shanghai: Shanghai College of Traditional Chinese Medicine, 1988).

32. Kamenetz, "History of Massage."

33. Ibid.

34. Honora Lee Wolfe, "Tuina Massage in the People's Republic of China" in *Massage Magazine* 1, no. 4 (1986).

35. Yegul, *Baths and Bathing.*

36. John Bowle, ed., *The Concise Encyclopedia of World History* (New York: Hawthorne Books, 1958).

37. Marti-Ibanez, ed., *The Epic of Medicine.*

38. Guthrie, *A History of Medicine.*

39. George H. Taylor, M.D., *Health by Exercise: Showing What Exercises to Take* (New York: American Book Exchange, 1885).

40. Ibid.

41. Harish Johari, *Ayurvedic Massage* (Rochester, Vt.: Healing Arts Press, 1996).

42. Minnie Goodnow, R.N., *Nursing History,* Practice of Medicine, vol. 2, 7th ed. (Philadelphia and London: W. B. Saunders, 1943).

Chapter Four

1. Francis Adams, trans., *The Genuine Works of Hippocrates,* vol. 2 (New York: William Wood and Co., 1886).

2. Ibid.

3. Libby, *The History of Medicine.*

4. Graham, *Manual Therapeutics.*

5. Guthrie, *A History of Medicine.*

6. Johnson, *The Anatriptic Art.* Italics in text here by Johnson.

7. Adams, trans., *The Genuine Works of Hippocrates.*

8. Ibid.

9. Graham, *Manual Therapeutics.*

10. Ibid.

11. Beard and Wood, *Massage.*

12. Jurgen Thorwald, ed., *Science and Secrets of Early Medicine,* Richard and Clara Winston, trans. (New York: Harcourt, Brace & World, 1962).

13. Adams, trans. *The Genuine Works of Hippocrates.*

14. Ibid.

15. Johnson, *The Anatriptic Art.*

16. Ibid.

17. H. L. Crosby, trans., *Dio Chrysostom, Discourses* (Cambridge, Mass.: Harvard University Press, 1946).

18. Yegul, *Baths and Bathing.*

19. Ibid.

20. Ibid.

21. Ibid.

22. Johnson, *The Anatriptic Art.*

23. Bowle, ed., *The Concise Encyclopedia of World History.*

24. Guthrie, *A History of Medicine.*

25. Ibid.

26. Graham, *Manual Therapeutics.*

27. Osler, *The Evolution of Modern Medicine.*

28. Ibid.

29. Kamenetz, "History of Massage."

30. Kellogg, *The Art of Massage*, 1895.

31. Kleen, *Massage and Medical Gymnastics.*

32. Kamenetz, "History of Massage."

33. Guthrie, *A History of Medicine.*

34. Kamenetz, "History of Massage."

35. Ibid.

36. Johnson, *The Anatriptic Art.*

37. Green, *A Translation of Galen's Hygiene.*

38. Ibid.

39. Ibid.

40. William Sanger, M.D., *The History of Prostitution* (New York: Medical Publishing Co., 1927).

41. Guthrie, *A History of Medicine.*

42. Yegul, *Baths and Bathing.*

43. Ibid.

44. Ibid.

45. W. Adlington and S. Gaselee, trans., *The Golden Ass* by Apuleius (Cambridge, Mass.: Harvard University Press, 2000).

46. Yegul, *Baths and Bathing.*

47. Guthrie, *A History of Medicine.*

48. Graham, *Manual Therapeutics.*

49. Ibid.

50. Yegul, *Baths and Bathing.*

51. Graham, *Manual Therapeutics.*

52. Kamenetz, "History of Massage."

53. Ibid.

54. Ibid.

Chapter Five

1. Guthrie, *A History of Medicine.*

2. Ibid.

3. Zach Thomas, *Healing Touch, The Church's Forgotten Language* (Louisville: Westminter/ John Knox Press, 1994).

4. Ibid.

5. Graham, *Manual Therapeutics.*

6. Brooke, *Medicine Women.*

7. Ibid.

8. Ibid.

9. Yegul, *Baths and Bathing.*   ·

10. Avicenna, *Canon Medicinae.* Translated by commission of the author.

11. Ibid.

12. Johnson, *The Anatriptic Art.*

13. Kamenetz, "History of Massage."

14. Ibid.

15. Graham, *Manual Therapeutics.*

16. Ibid.

17. Ibid.

18. Ibid.

19. Kamenetz, "History of Massage."

20. Kellogg, *The Art of Massage,* 1895.

21. Ibid.

22. Brooke, *Medicine Women.*

23. Kamenetz, "History of Massage."

24. Brooke, *Medicine Women*.

25. Ibid.

26. Author conversations with Oregon midwife Sherry Lauer.

27. Montague Summers, *The History of Witchcraft and Demonology* (London: Kegan Paul, 1926).

28. Guthrie, *A History of Medicine*.

29. John V. Basmajian, ed., *Therapeutic Exercise*, 3rd ed. (Malabar, Fla.: Robert E. Drieger Publishing, 1978).

30. Kleen, *Handbook of Massage*.

31. Ibid.

32. George H. Taylor, M.D., *An Exposition of the Swedish Movement-Cure* (New York: Fowler and Wells, 1860).

33. Basmajian, *Therapeutic Exercise*.

34. Kamenetz, "History of Massage."

35. Ibid.

36. Basmajian, *Therapeutic Exercise*.

37. Jean Jacques Rousseau, quoted by Kamenentz in "History of Massage."

38. Ibid.

Chapter Six

1. George Taylor, M.D., *Health by Exercise: The Movement-Cure* (New York: Fowler & Wells, 1888).

2. Taylor, *An Exposition of the Swedish Movement-Cure*.

3. Ibid.

4. Ibid.

5. Taylor, *Health by Exercise: Showing What Exercises to Take*.

6. Taylor, *Health by Exercise: The Movement-Cure*.

7. Ibid.

8. Matthias Roth, M.D., *The Prevention and Cure of Disease by Movements* (London: John Churchill, 1851). From the introduction by Dr. Neumann.

9. Taylor, M.D., *Health by Exercise: The Movement-Cure*.

10. Kamenetz, "History of Massage."

11. Ibid.

12. Roth, *The Prevention and Cure of Disease by Movements*.

13. Ibid.

14. Ibid.

15. Ibid.

16. Ibid.

17. Ibid.

18. Ibid.

19. Taylor, *Health by Exercise: Showing What Exercises to Take.*

20. Kellogg, *The Art of Massage,* 1895.

21. Graham, *Manual Therapeutics.*

22. Kleen, *Handbook of Massage.*

23. John Harvey Kellogg, M.D., *The Art of Massage,* 4th ed. (Battle Creek, Mich.: Modern Medicine Publishing, 1929).

24. Kleen, *Massage and Medical Gymnastics.*

25. Matthias Roth, M.D., trans., *The Gymnastic Free Exercises of P. H. Ling* (London: Groombridge & Sons, 1853).

26. Roth, *The Prevention and Cure of Disease by Movements.*

27. T. J. Hartelius, M.D., *Swedish Movements or Medical Gymnastics* (Battle Creek, Mich: Modern Medicine Publishing, 1896).

28. Kellogg, *The Art of Massage,* 1895.

29. Grafstrom, *A Text-book of Mechano-Therapy.*

30. Graham, *Manual Therapeutics.*

31. Roth, *The Prevention and Cure of Disease by Movements.*

32. Patricia Benjamin, Ph.D., "Seeds of a Profession," *Massage Therapy Journal* (summer 1986).

33. Roth, *The Prevention and Cure of Disease by Movements.*

34. Ibid.

35. Ibid.

36. Kleen, *Massage and Medical Gymnastics.*

37. Esther C. Swanson, Ph.D., from the School of Swedish Massage course instruction book, 1957.

38. Beard and Wood, *Massage: Principles and Techniques,* 1964.

39. Patricia Benjamin, "Notations to the General Principles of Gymnastics by Pehr Henrik Ling," Lars Agren and Patricia Benjamin, trans., *Journal of the American Massage Therapy Association* 2, no. 1 (winter 1987).

40. Kamenetz, "History of Massage."

41. Kleen, *Handbook of Massage.*

42. Taylor, *Health by Exercise: Showing What Exercises to Take.*

43. Kleen, *Handbook of Massage.*

44. Kamenetz, "History of Massage."

45. Kurre W. Ostrom, *Massage and the Original Swedish Movements* 8th ed. (Philadelphia: P. Blakiston's Son, 1912).

46. Kleen, *Handbook of Massage.*

47. Kellogg, *The Art of Massage,* 1895.

48. Ibid.

Chapter Seven

1. Marti-Ibanez, ed., *The Epic of Medicine.*

2. Taylor, *Massage.*

3. Kleen, *Handbook of Massage.*

4. Wine, *Russian School of Massage Therapy.*

5. Ibid.

6. Leonard A. Goldstone, "Massage as an Orthodox Medical Treatment Past and Future," *Complimentary Therapies in Nursing & Midwifery* 6 (2000).

7. John Harvey Kellogg, M.D., *The Home Hand-book of Domestic Hygiene and Rational Medicine* (London: International Tract Society, 1899).

8. Johnson, *The Anatriptic Art.*

9. Ibid.

10. Ibid.

11. Ibid.

12. Murrell, *Massage as a Mode of Treatment.*

13. Ibid.

14. Ibid.

15. *Lancet,* 1852.

16. Kleen, *Handbook of Massage.*

17. Ibid.

18. Ibid.

19. Kleen, *Massage and Medical Gymnastics.*

20. Gustav Schutz, writing in his translation from the original Swedish into German of Kleen's 1892 book, *Handbook of Massage,* (Philadelphia: P. Blakiston, Son & Co.)

21. Grafstrom, *A Text-book of Mechano-Therapy.*

22. Richard Haehl, M.D., *Massage: Its History, Technique and Therapeutic Uses* (Philadelphia: Hahnemann Medical College, 1898).

23. Ibid.

24. Ibid.

25. Hartvig Nissen, Ph.D., *A Manual of Instruction for Giving Swedish Movement and Masssage Treatment* (Philadelphia and London: F. A. Davis, 1889).

26. Graham, *Manual Therapeutics.*

27. Kamenetz, "History of Massage."

28. Graham, *Manual Therapeutics.*

29. Ibid.

30. Ibid.

31. Benjamin, "Seeds of a Profession."

32. Kellogg, *The Art of Massage,* 1895.

33. Frank Foster, M.D., ed., *Reference-Book of Practical Therapeutics by Various Authors,* vol. 1 (New York: D. Appleton, 1897).

34. Ibid.

35. Ibid.

36. Karnitsky, *International Medical Annual* (n.p.: 1882).

37. Haehl, *Massage.*

38. Ibid.

39. Ibid.

40. Ibid.

41. W. R. Latson, M.D., *Common Disorders with Rational Methods of Treatment including Diet, Exercise, Massotherapy, Baths, Etc.* (New York: L.N. Fowler & Co., 1904).

42. Pye Henry Chavasse, *Advice to a Mother on the Management of Her Children and on the Treatment of the Moment of Some of Their More Pressing Illnesses and Accidents,* 9th ed. (Philadelphia: J. B. Lippincott., and London: Churchill & Sons, 1868).

43. Ibid.

44. *The People's Medical Advisor,* 19th ed. (Buffalo, N.Y.: World's Dispensary Printing Office and Bindery, 1880). Founded by Dr. R. V. Pierce, a U.S. congressman, the World's Dispensary Medical Association was an affiliation of medical doctors conducting their practices out of two offices. The main office was located in Buffalo, New York, and the other in London, England. The facility, established about 1875, was named the World's Dispensary and Surgical Institute.

45. Ibid.

46. Ibid.

47. Adams, trans., *The Genuine Works of Hippocrates.*

48. Kellogg, *The Art of Massage,* 1929.

49. Ibid.

50. Murrell, *Massage as a Mode of Treatment.*

51. Ibid.

52. Ibid.

53. Taylor, *Massage.*

54. Graham, *Manual Therapeutics.*

55. Kleen, *Handbook of Massage.*

56. Ibid.

57. Ibid.

58. Ibid.

59. Roth, *The Prevention and Cure of Disease by Movements.*

60. Taylor, *Massage.*

61. Kleen, *Handbook of Massage.*

62. William T. Smith, M.D., *The Human Body and Its Health* (New York: American Book Company, 1884).

63. Graham, *Manual Therapeutics.*

64. Goodnow, *Nursing History.*

65. Ibid.

66. Ibid.

67. Guthrie, *A History of Medicine.*

68. Thomas, *Healing Touch.*

69. Ibid.

70. Ibid.

71. Goodnow, *Nursing History.*

72. Thomas, *Healing Touch.*

73. Florence Nightingale, *Notes on Nursing: What it is, and What it is not* (London: n.p., 1859).

74. L. A. Maule, "Training Schools and Other Nursing Institutions" in Cassell's *The Art and Science of Nursing* 1 (London: Waverley, 1907).

75. Louisa L. Despard, *Text-book of Massage and Remedial Gymnastics,* 3rd ed. (London: Oxford University Press, 1932).

76. Robert Ziegenspeck, M.D., *Massage Treatment in Diseases of Women,* trans. F. H. Westerschulte. Published by the translator, 1909.

77. Nellie Elizabeth Macafee, R.N., *Massage, An Elementary Text-Book for Nurses* (Pittsburgh: Reed & Witting, 1920).

78. Mary McMillan, *Massage and Therapeutic Exercise* (Philadelphia and London: W. B. Saunders, 1921).

79. C. M. Sampson, M.D., *Physiotherapy Technic: A Manual of Applied Physics* (St. Louis: Mosby, 1923).

80. Maude Rawlins, *A Textbook of Massage for Nurses and Beginners* St. Louis, Mosby, 1933).

81. Kathryn L. Jensen, R.N., *Fundamentals in Massage for Students of Nursing* (New York: MacMillan, 1932).

82. Ibid.

83. Ibid.

Chapter Eight

1. Douglas Graham, M.D., "Massage: Its Mode of Application and Effects" in *Popular Science Monthly* 50, no. 6 (1882).

2. *The Medical Advance* 27, no. 6 (December 1891).

3. Souvenir brochure, Mayfield Sanitarium, St. Louis, 1899.

4. *Modern Medicine* 1, no. 1 (1932).

5. *Physical Culture* 89, no. 9 (1945).

6. The Lindlahr Sanitarium promotional brochure, Elmhurst, Illinois, 1891.

7. *Hygeia: The Health Magazine* 8, no. 10 (1930).

8. Dr. Strong's Sanitarium promotional brochure, Saratoga Springs, New York, 1899.

9. *Radiant Health* (Chicago: The Lindlahr Sanitarium, 1897).

10. Craig Healing Springs promotional brochure, Craig County, Virginia, 1921.

11. *Radiant Health.*

12. Ibid.

13. Cited in *The Battle Creek Idea* 1, no. 4 (1994).

14. The Battle Creek Sanitarium and Hospital Training School for Nurses promotional brochure for the class of 1908–1909.

15. Jadi Campbell, *Touch Translated: A World of Massage* (unpublished manuscript, 2001).

16. *The Kneipp Cure* (New York: The Kneipp Cure Publishing Co., 1896).

17. Pat Zacharias and Vivian Baulch, article posted on the Internet, May 1999, at www.detnews.com/history/baths.htm.

18. Robert King, "The Legend of Bathhouse John" in *Massage Therapy Journal* 32, no. 4 (fall 1993).

19. Ibid.

20. Sanger, *The History of Prostitution.*

21. Ibid.

22. George Scott, *The History of Prostitution* (London: Senate [Random House] 1968).

23. Ibid.

24. Harold Cross, M.D., *The Lust Market* (London: Torchstream Books, n.d.).

Chapter Nine

1. Smithsonian Institute Freer Gallery of Art display placard.

2. Kamenetz, "History of Massage."

3. Quoted in Johnson, *The Anatriptic Art.*

4. Kamenetz, "History of Massage."

5. Graham, *Manual Therapeutics.*

6. Kamenetz, "History of Massage."

7. Murrell, *Massage as a Mode of Treatment.*

8. Johnson, *The Anatriptic Art.*

9. Kellogg, *The Home Hand-book of Domestic Hygiene and Rational Medicine.*

10. Latson, *Common Disorders with Rational Methods of Treatment.*

11. Carl Rosen, *The Face, Hair and Scalp* (Chicago: Monarch, 1906).

12. Promotional text printed on the inside flap of the box containing the electric massage roller.

13. Latson, *Common Disorders with Rational Methods of Treatment.*

14. Ibid.

15. Albert Turner, ed., *Womanly Beauty in Form and Features* (New York: The Health-Culture Co., 1903).

16. Taylor, *Massage.*

17. Nissen, *A Manual of Instruction for Giving Swedish Movement and Massage Treatment.*

18. Rachel Maines, "Vibratory Massage in Electrotherapeutics" in *Electric Quarterly: A Quarterly Publication of the Bakken Library of Electricity In Life* 8, no. 1 (winter 1986).

19. Rachel Maines, *The Technology of Orgasm* (Baltimore and London: Johns Hopkins University Press, 1999).

20. Maines, "Vibratory Massage."

21. Kellogg, *The Art of Massage,* 1895.

22. Taylor, *Massage.*

23. Kellogg, *The Art of Massage,* 1929.

24. Kleen, *Handbook of Massage.*

25. Johnson, *The Anatriptic Art.*

26. James B. Mennell, M.D., *Physical Treatment by Movement, Manipulation and Massage,* 5th ed. (Philadelphia and Toronto: The Blakiston Co., 1947).

27. Kleen, *Handbook of Massage.*

28. Graham, *Manual Therapeutics.*

Chapter Ten

1. Adams, trans., *The Genuine Works of Hippocrates.*

2. Green, *A Translation of Galen's Hygiene.*

3. Ibid.

4. Katsusuki Serizawa, M.D., *Massage, The Oriental Method* (Tokyo: Japan Publications, 1972).

5. Tao, interview in *Massage Magazine.*

6. Taylor, *Massage.*

7. Latson, *Common Disorders with Rational Methods of Treatment.*

8. Graham, *Manual Therapeutics.*

9. Douglas Graham, M.D., "The Treatment of Sprains by Massage" in *New York Medical Record* (August 11, 1877).

10. Grafstrom, *A Text-book of Mechano-Therapy.*

11. Ibid.

12. Graham, *Manual Therapeutics.*

13. Ibid.

14. Ibid.

15. Ziegenspeck, *Massage Treatment in Diseases of Women.*

16. Ibid.

17. Kellogg, *The Art of Massage,* 1895.

18. Ibid.

19. Ibid.

20. George Abbott, *Technique of Hydrotherapy and Swedish Massage* (Mountain View, Calif.: Pacific Press, 1912).

21. McMillan, *Massage and Therapeutic Exercise.*

22. Taylor, *Health by Exercise: Showing What Exercises to Take.*

23. Taylor, *Health by Exercise: The Movement-Cure.*

24. Roth, *The Prevention and Cure of Disease by Movements.*

25. Nissen, *A Manual of Instruction for Giving Swedish Movement and Masssage Treatment.*

26. Kleen, *Handbook of Massage.*

27. Ibid.

28. Haehl, *Massage.*

29. Ibid.

30. Ibid.

31. Ibid.

Chapter Eleven

1. Graham, *Manual Therapeutics.*

2. Kamenetz, "History of Massage."

3. Goldstone, "Massage as an Orthodox Medical Treatment Past and Future."

4. De Puy, "Richard Van Why, Father of Massage Therapy in the United States."

5. *Massage Magazine* surveys 1985–2001.

6. Thomas, *Healing Touch.*

7. Graham, *Manual Therapeutics.*

8. A. Hughes, "Nursing as a Vocation" in Cassell's *The Art and Science of Nursing* 1 (London: Waverley, 1907).

9. Leonard Goldstone, "From Orthodox to Complimentary: The Fall and Rise of Massage, with Specific Reference to Orthopaedic and Rheumatology Nursing" in *Journal of Orthopaedic Nursing* 3 (1999).

10. Ibid.

11. Wine, *Russian School of Massage Therapy.*

12. Carl Dubitsky, *Bodywork Shiatsu* (Rochester, Vt.: Healing Arts Press, 1997).

13. Bonnie Horrigan, "Therapeutic Touch and a Healing Way" (interview with Janet Quinn, R.N., Ph.D.) in *Alternative Therapies in Health and Medicine* 2, no. 4 (July, 1996).

14. David Eisenberg, M.D., "Trends in Alternative Medicine Use in the United States 1990–1997" in *Journal of the American Medical Association* (Nov. 11, 1999).

Bibliography

Abbott, George. *Technique of Hydrotherapy and Swedish Massage.* Mountain View, Calif.: Pacific Press, 1912.

Adams, Francis, trans. *The Genuine Works of Hippocrates,* vol. 2. New York: William Wood and Co., 1886.

Adlington, W. , and S. Gaselee, trans. *The Golden Ass* by Apuleius. Cambridge, Mass.: Harvard University Press, 2000.

Avicenna. *Canon Medicinae.* Translated by commission of the author.

Basmajian, John V., ed. *Therapeutic Exercise,* 3rd ed. Malabar, Fla.: Robert E. Drieger Publishing, 1978.

Bassermann, Lujo. *The Oldest Profession, A History of Prostitution.* Translated by James Cleugh. New York: Dorset Press, 1993.

The Battle Creek Idea, vol. 1, no. 4, 1994.

The Battle Creek Sanitarium and Hospital Training School for Nurses promotional brochure for the class of 1908–1909. Published by The Battle Creek Sanitarium.

Beard, Gertrude. *Massage: Principles and Techniques,* 2nd ed. Philadelphia: W. B. Saunders Company, 1952.

Beard, Gertrude, and Elizabeth Wood. *Massage: Principles and Techniques,* Philadelphia and London, W. B. Saunders Co., Publishers, 1964.

Benjamin, Patricia, Ph.D. "Notations to the General Principles of Gymnastics by Pehr Henrik Ling," *Massage Therapy Journal,* vol. 2, no. 1, Winter 1987. Translated from the Swedish by Lars Agren and Patricia Benjamin, Ph.D.

Benjamin, Patricia, Ph.D. "Seeds of a Profession," *Massage Therapy Journal.* Summer 1986.

Benton, Jacqueleyn. "Massage in the African Tradition," *Massage Magazine* 31, May/June 1991.

Berman, Morris. *The Reenchantment of the World.* New York: Bantam, 1984.

Bohm, Max. *Massage: Its Principles and Technic.* Philadelphia: W. B. Saunders Co., 1913.

Bowle, John, ed. *The Concise Encyclopedia of World History.* New York: Hawthorne Books, 1958.

Breasted, James Henry. *A History of the Ancient Egyptians.* New York: Scribner, 1908.

Brooke, Elisabeth. *Medicine Women: A Pictorial History of Women Healers.* Wheaton, Ill.: Quest Books, The Theosophical Publishing House, and Godsfield Press, 1997.

Bullough, Vern, and Bonnie Bullough. *Women and Prostitution, A Social History.* New York: Prometheus Books, 1987.

Byers, Dwight C. *Better Health with Foot Reflexology.* Saint Petersburg, Fla.: Ingham Publishing, 1983.

Calder, Ritchie. *Medicine and Man.* New York: The New American Library, 1958.

Caldwell, John C. *Massage Girl and Other Sketches of Thailand.* New York: The John Day Co., 1968.

Campbell, Jadi. "Indonesia's Therapists Struggle," *Massage Magazine* 85, May/June 2000.

Campbell, Jadi. *Touch Translated: A World of Massage.* Unpublished manuscript, 2001.

Carter, Mildred. *Helping Yourself with Foot Reflexology.* West Nyack, N.Y.: Parker Publishing, 1969.

Cayce, Edgar. *Edgar Cayce's Massage, Hydrotherapy and Healing Oils.* Virginia Beach, Va.: Inner Vision Publishing, 1989.

Chavasse, Pye Henry. *Advice to a Mother on the Management of Her Children and on the Treatment of the Moment of Some of Their More Pressing Illnesses and Accidents,* 9th ed. Philadelphia: J. B. Lippincott., and London: Churchill & Sons, 1868.

Chengnan, Sun, ed. *Chinese Bodywork: A Complete Manual of Chinese Therapeutic Massage.* Translated by Wang Qiliang. Berkeley, Calif., Pacific View Press, 1993.

Clendening, Logan, M.D. *Source Book of Medical History.* New York: Dover Publications, 1960.

Cline, Kyle. *Chinese Pediatric Massage.* Portland, Ore.: Institute for Traditional Medicine, 1993.

The College of Swedish Massage, Home-Study Course in Massage and Hydro-Therapy 1939.

Colton, Buel P. *Elementary Physiology and Hygiene,* Boston: D. C. Heath & Co., 1908.

Crosby, H. L., trans. *Dio Chrysostom, Discourses.* Cambridge, Mass.: Harvard University Press, 1946.

Cross, Harold, M.D. *The Lust Market.* London: Torchstream Books, n.d.

de Groot, J. J. M. *Religious System of China,* vol. 6. Leyden, Mass.: E. J. Brill, 1910.

De Puy, Cornelius E., M.D. "Richard P. Van Why, Father of Massage Therapy in the United States," *Massage Therapy Journal.* Summer 1991.

Despard, Louisa L. *Text-book of Massage and Remedial Gymnastics,* 3rd ed. London: Oxford University Press, 1932.

Dewees, William P., M.D. *Baudelocque's Midwifery.* Translated by Heath, 3rd ed. Philadelphia: Thomas Desilver, 1823.

Diehl, Harold S., M.D. *Healthful Living.* New York: McGraw-Hill, 1941.

Downing, George. *Massage … Meditation.* New York: Random House, 1974.

———. *The Massage Book.* New York: Random House and Berkeley: The Bookworks, 1972.

Dr. Strong's Sanitarium promotional brochure, Saratoga Springs, New York, 1899.

Dubitsky, Carl. *Bodywork Shiatsu.* Rochester, Vt.: Healing Arts Press, 1997.

Eames, E. G. *Scientific Massage for Athletes.* London: Athletic Publications, unknown date (circa 1920).

Early English Voyagers. London: Thomas Nelson and Sons, 1889.

Eisenberg, David, M.D. "Trends in Alternative Medicine Use in the United States 1990–1997" in *JAMA* 11 November 1999.

Eliade, Mircea. *Shamanism: Archaic Techniques of Ecstasy.* Bollingen Series LXXVI, translated from the French by Willard R. Trask. Princeton: Princeton University Press, 1974.

Elkin, Adolphus P. *Aboriginal Men of High Degree: Initiation and Sorcery in the World's Oldest Tradition.* Rochester, Vt.: Inner Traditions International, 1994.

Enqun, Zhang, ed. *Chinese Massage: A Practical English–Chinese Library of Traditional Chinese Medicine.* Shanghai: Shanghai College of Traditional Chinese Medicine, 1988.

Evangelista, Cornelio H., and Virgil J. Mayor Apostol. *The Healing Hands of Hilot: Filipino Therapeutic Massage.* National City, Calif.: self-published, 1998.

Fay, Joseph H. *Scientific Massage for Athletes.* London: Ewart, Seymour & Co., Ltd, unknown date (circa 1920).

Florida Department of Health, Division of Medical Quality Assurance, Board of Massage Therapy (1997).

Foster, Frank, M.D., ed. *Reference-Book of Practical Therapeutics by Various Authors,* vol. 1. New York: D. Appleton, 1897.

Freeman, Morton S. *The Story Behind the Word.* Philadelphia: ISI Press, 1985.

Fritz, Sandy. *Mosby's Fundamentals of Therapeutic Massage.* St. Louis: Mosby Lifeline, 1995.

Goldberg, Audrey Githa. *Body Massage for the Beauty Therapist.* 2nd ed. Oxford: Heinemann Professional Publishing, 1989.

Goldstone, Leonard A. "Massage as an Orthodox Medical Treatment Past and Future," *Complimentary Therapies in Nursing & Midwifery* 6 (2000).

———. "From Orthodox to Complimentary: The Fall and Rise of Massage, with Specific Reference to Orthopaedic and Rheumatology Nursing" in *Journal of Orthopaedic Nursing* 3, 1999.

Goodall-Copestake, Beatrice M. *The Theory and Practice of Massage and Medical Gymnastics.* London: H. K. Lewis & Co., 1917.

Goodnow, Minnie, R.N. *Nursing History,* Practice of Medicine, vol. 2, 7th ed. Philadelphia and London: W. B. Saunders, 1943.

Grafstrom, Axel V., M.D. *A Text-book of Mechano-Therapy (Massage and Medical Gymnastics),* 2nd ed. Philadelphia: W. B. Saunders, 1904.

Graham, Douglas, M.D., *Manual Therapeutics.* Philadelphia: J. B. Lippincott, 1890.

———. *Manual Therapeutics, A Treatise on Massage: Its history, mode of application and effects,* 3rd ed. Philadelphia and London: J. B. Lippincott, 1902.

———. "Massage: Its Mode of Application and Effects" in *Popular Science Monthly* 50, no. 6 (1882).

———. "The Treatment of Sprains by Massage" in *New York Medical Record,* August 11, 1877.

Green, Robert Montraville, M.D. *A Translation of Galen's Hygiene (De Sanitate Tuenda).* Springfield, Ill.: Charles C. Thomas, 1951.

Grossinger, Richard. *Planet Medicine.* Berkeley: North Atlantic Books, 1990.

Guthrie, Douglas, M.D. *A History of Medicine.* Philadelphia: J. B. Lippincott, 1946.

Haehl, Richard, M.D. *Massage: Its History, Technique and Therapeutic Uses.* Philadelphia: Hahnemann Medical College, 1898.

Haggard, Howard W., M.D. *Devils, Drugs and Doctors.* New York: Blue Ribbon Books, 1929.

Harner, Michael. *The Way of the Shaman.* San Francisco: Harper & Row, 1980.

Hartelius, T. J., M.D. *Swedish Movements or Medical Gymnastics.* Battle Creek, Mich.: Modern Medicine Publishing, 1896.

Harvey, William. *The Circulation of the Blood.* Translated by K. J. Franklin. London: Everyman's Library, 1966.

Hassan, Selim, Ph.D. *Excavations at Giza I.* Oxford: Egyptian University, 1932.

Hertzler, Arthur E., M.D. *The Horse and Buggy Doctor.* New York: Harper & Brothers, 1938.

Hoadley, Joe E., M.D. *The Homestead Doctor.* Story, Wyo.: self-published, 1995.

Houston, F. M. *Contact Healing,* 2nd ed. Long Beach, Calif.: self-published, 1959.

Hughes A., "Nursing as a Vocation" in Cassell's *The Art and Science of Nursing,* vol. 1. London: Waverley, 1907.

Hygeia: The Health Magazine, vol. 8, no. 10. October 1930.

Jansen, W. *Sportmassage en Trainingsoefeningen.* Rotterdam: Van Ditmar's Press, 1925.

Jaschok, Maria. *Concubines and Bondservants.* London and New Jersey: Zed Books, 1988.

Jensen, Albrecht. *Massage … Exercise Combined.* New York, self-published, 1920.

Jensen, Kathryn L., R.N. *Fundamentals in Massage for Students of Nursing.* New York: MacMillan, 1932.

Johari, Harish. *Ayurvedic Massage.* Rochester, Vt.: Healing Arts Press, 1996.

Johnson, Walter. *The Anatriptic Art.* London: Simpkin, Marshall & Co., 1866.

Kamenetz, Herman L. "History of Massage" in *Manipulation, Traction and Massage,* edited by Joseph P. Rogoff. Baltimore, Md.: William and Wilkins, 1980.

Kaptchuk, Ted J. *The Web That Has No Weaver.* Portland: NTC Publishing Group, 1983.

Karnitsky, M.D., International Medical Annual (n.p. 1882).

Kellogg, John Harvey, M.D. *The Art of Massage.* Battle Creek, Mich.: Modern Medicine Publishing, 1929.

———.*The Home Hand-book of Domestic Hygiene and Rational Medicine.* London: International Tract Society, 1899.

———. *The Art of Massage: Its Physiological Effects and Therapeutic Applications.* Battle Creek, Mich.: Modern Medicine Publishing, 1895.

Kessel, Joseph. *The Magic of Touch.* London: Rupert Hart-Davis, 1961.

King, Robert. "The Legend of Bathhouse John" in *Massage Therapy Journal,* vol. 32, no. 4, fall 1993.

Kleen, Emil G., M.D. *Massage and Medical Gymnastics.* Translated by Mina L. Dobbie, M.D., 2nd ed. London: J. & A. Churchill, 1921.

———. *Handbook of Massage.* Translated by Edward M. Hartwell, M.D. Philadelphia: P. Plakiston, Son & Co., 1892.

The Kneipp Cure. New York: The Kneipp Cure Publishing Co., 1896.

Knutson, Gunilla. *Gunilla Knutson's Book of Massage.* New York: Bell Publishing, 1972.

Krohn, William O., M.D. *First Book in Physiology and Hygiene.* New York: D. Appleton and Co., 1908.

Lace, Mary V. *Massage and Medical Gymnastics.* London: J. & A. Churchill, 1936.

Lamberg-Karlovsky, C. C., and Jeremy A. Sabloff. *Ancient Civilizations.* Prospect Heights, Ill.: Waveland Press, 1979.

Latson, W. R., M.D. *Common Disorders with Rational Methods of Treatment including Diet, Exercise, Massotherapy, Baths, Etc.* New York, London: L.N. Fowler & Co., 1904.

Lawrence, Paul A. *Lomi-Lomi Hawaiian Massage.* San Anselmo, Calif.: PAL Press, 1981.

Lee, Eldon. *Scalpels and Buggywhips.* Surrey, B.C., Canada: Heritage House Publishing, 1997.

Lee, Nor Ming, and Gregory Whincup, trans. *Chinese Massage Therapy.* Compiled at the Anhui Medical School Hospital. Boulder, Colo.: Shambhala Publications, 1983.

Libby, Walter, M.D. *The History of Medicine.* Boston and New York: Houghton Mifflin, 1922.

The Lindlahr Sanitarium promotional brochure, Elmhurst, Illinois, 1891.

Macafee, Nellie Elizabeth, R.N. *Massage, An Elementary Text-Book for Nurses.* Pittsburgh: Reed & Witting, 1920.

Maines, Rachel. *The Technology of Orgasm.* Baltimore and London: Johns Hopkins University Press, 1999.

———. "Vibratory Massage in Electrotherapeutics" in *Electric Quarterly: A Quarterly Publication of the Bakken Library of Electricity in Life,* vol. 8, no. 1, winter 1986.

Majno, Guido. *The Healing Hand: Man and Wound in the Ancient World.* Cambridge, Mass.: Harvard University Press, 1982.

Marti-Ibanez, Felix, M.D., ed. *The Epic of Medicine.* New York: Clarkson N. Potter and M. D. Publications, 1959.

Masseur, A Qualified. *Massage for the Million.* London: Thorsons Publishers, 1946.

Masunaga, Sensei. *Zen Shiatsu*. Tokyo: Kodansha Publishing, 1977.

Maule, L. A. "Training Schools and Other Nursing Institutions" in Cassell's *The Art and Science of Nursing*, vol. 1. London: Waverley, 1907.

McMillan, Mary. *Massage and Therapeutic Exercise*. Philadelphia and London: W. B. Saunders, 1921.

The Medical Advance, vol. 27, no. 6, December 1891.

Mennell, James B., M.D. *Physical Treatment by Movement, Manipulation and Massage,* 5th ed. Philadelphia and Toronto: The Blakiston Co., 1947.

Metz, Barbara. *Ancient Egypt*. Washington D.C.: National Geographic Society, 1978.

Miller, Roberta DeLong. *Psychic Massage*. New York: Harper Colophon Books, 1975.

Mitchell, Donald G. *English Lands, Letters and Kings*. New York: Charles Scribner's Sons, 1889.

Modern Medicine, vol. 1, no. 1. October 1932.

Montague, Ashley. *Touching, The Human Significance of the Skin*. New York: Harper & Row, 1971.

Moor, Fred B., M.D., et al. *Manual of Hydrotherapy and Massage*. Boise, Id.: Pacific Press Publishing, 1964.

Murrell, William. *Massage as a Mode of Treatment*. London: H. K. Lewis, 1886.

Mussen, Paul, and Nancy Eisenberg-Berg, *Roots of Caring, Sharing and Helping*. San Francisco: W. H. Freeman and Co., 1977.

Ni, Maoshing, Ph.D. *The Yellow Emperor's Classic of Medicine*. Boston: Shambhala, 1995.

Nichols, Frank C. *Theory and Practice of Body Massage*. Chicago: Nelson-Hall Company, 1958.

Nightingale, Florence. *Notes on Nursing: What it is, and What it is not*. London: n.p., 1859. Reprinted by J.B. Lippincott Co., London, 1946.

Nissen, Hartvig, Ph.D. *A Manual of Instruction for Giving Swedish Movement and Masssage Treatment*. Philadelphia and London: F. A. Davis, 1889.

Nordhoff, Charles. *Northern California, Oregon and the Sandwich Islands*. New York: Harper & Brothers, 1874.

Osler, Sir William. *The Evolution of Modern Medicine*. New Haven, Conn.: Yale University Press, 1921.

Ostrom, Kurre W. *Massage and the Original Swedish Movements,* 7th ed. Philadelphia: P. Blakiston's Son, 1912.

Palmer, Margaret D. *Lesson on Massage,* 5th ed. London: Bailliere, Tindal and Cox, 1918.

The People's Medical Advisor, 19th ed. Buffalo, N.Y.: World's Dispensary Printing Office and Bindery, 1880.

Physical Culture, vol. 89, no. 9. June 1945.

Popular Science Monthly, vol. 40, no. 6. October 1882.

Radiant Health. Chicago: Lindlahr Sanitarium, promotional pamphlet, 1897.

Rama, Gloria, and Bright Light. *Our Method of Gentle Massage*. New York: Rayma Publications, 1948.

Rawlins, Maude. *A Textbook of Massage for Nurses and Beginners*. St. Louis: Mosby, 1933.

Richard, David. *Anoint Yourself with Oil*. Bloomingdale, Ill.: Vital Health Publishing, 1997.

Robbins, R. H., M.D. *Textbook of Anatomy and Physiology for Nurses and Masseuses*. London: The Scientific Press, 1928.

Rodman, Julius Scammon. *The Kahuna Sorcerers of Hawaii*. New York: Exposition Press, 1979.

Rohrer, Joseph. *Rohrer's Scientific Body Massage and Swedish Movements*. New York: self-published, 1925.

Rosen, Carl. *The Face, Hair and Scalp.* Chicago: Monarch, 1906.

Rossiaud, Jacques. *Medieval Prostitution.* Translated by Lydia G. Cochrane. New York: Barnes & Noble Books, 1996.

Roth, Matthias, M.D., trans. *The Gymnastic Free Exercises of P. H. Ling.* London: Groombridge & Sons, 1853.

————. *The Prevention and Cure of Disease by Movements.* London: John Churchill, 1851.

————. *Gymnastic Exercises Without Apparatus, according to Ling's System for the Due Development and Strengthening of the Human Body.* 5th ed. London: A. N. Myers & Co., 1876.

Sampson, C. M., M.D. *Physiotherapy Technic: A Manual of Applied Physics.* St. Louis: Mosby, 1923.

Sanger, William, M.D. *The History of Prostitution.* New York: Medical Publishing Co., 1927.

Schutz, Gustav. Writing in his translation from the original Swedish into German of Kleen's 1892 book, *Handbook of Massage.* Philadelphia: P. Blakiston, Son & Co.

Scott, George. *The History of Prostitution,* 3rd ed. London: Random House, 1968.

Serizawa, Katsusuki, M.D. *Massage, The Oriental Method.* Tokyo: Japan Publications, 1972.

Shires, Ida C., and Dorothy Wood. *Advanced Methods of Massage and Medical Gymnastics.* (n.p. 1931).

Sills, Jennifer. *Massage Parlor.* New York: Ace Books, 1973.

Smellie, W., M.D. *Midwifery.* Boston: J. Norman, 1786.

Smith, Bonnie G. *The Gender of History.* Cambridge, Mass.: Harvard University Press, 1998.

Smith, William T., M.D. *The Human Body and Its Health.* New York: American Book Company, 1884.

Standardized Textbook of Barbering. Chicago: Associated Master Barbers of America, 1931.

Stedman, Thomas L., M.D. *Stedman's Medical Dictionary, Illustrated: A Practical Medical Dictionary,* 13th ed. Baltimore: William Wood & Co., 1936.

Summers, Montague. *The History of Witchcraft and Demonology.* London: Kegan Paul, 1926.

Tao, Zhang, M.D. Interview in *Massage Magazine* 33. Sept/Oct 1991.

Tappan, Frances M. *Healing Massage Techniques,* 2nd ed. East Norwalk, Conn.: Appleton & Lange, 1980.

————. *Massage Techniques, A Case Method Approach.* New York: Macmillan, 1961.

Taylor, George, M.D. *Health by Exercise: The Movement-Cure.* New York: Fowler & Wells, 1888.

————. *Massage: Principles and Practice of Remedial Treatment by Imparted Motion.* New York: John B. Alden, 1887.

————. *Health by Exercise: Showing What Exercises to Take.* New York: American Book Exchange, 1885.

————. *An Exposition of the Swedish Movement-Cure.* New York: Fowler and Wells, 1860.

Thomas, Zach. *Healing Touch, The Church's Forgotten Language.* Louisville: Westminter/John Knox Press, 1994.

Thorwald, Jurgen, ed. *Science and Secrets of Early Medicine.* Richard and Clara Winston, trans. New York: Harcourt, Brace & World, 1962.

Tidy, Noel M. *Massage and Remedial Exercises in Medical and Surgical Conditions,* 7th ed. London: John Wright and Sons, 1947.

Time-Life. *Massage: Total Relaxation.* Alexandria, Va.: Time-Life Books, 1987.

Trall, R. T., M.D. *The Hydropathic Encyclopedia.* New York: Fowlers & Wells, 1853.

Turner, Albert, ed. *Womanly Beauty of Form and Feature.* New York: The Health-Culture Co., 1903.

Tyrrell, Charles A., M.D. *The Royal Road to Health or the Secret of Health Without Drugs*, 7th ed. New York: self-published, 1911.

Uilamakamakane, Kili Luika, and Likeke Helemano Smith. *The Art of Hawaiian Lomilomi Massage*. Captain Cook, Hawaii: Hawaiian Islands Publishing, 1982.

Van Why, Richard P. "A Brief History and Exhortation Concerning Massage Therapy in America," *Massage Therapy Journal*, vol. 31, no. 1, winter 1992.

Villiers, Alan. "Tribute to Captain Cook: The Man Who Mapped the Pacific. The Voyages and Historic Discoveries of Captain James Cook," in *National Geographic* 140, no. 3. September, 1971.

Vogel, Morris J. *The Invention of the Modern Hospital*. Chicago: The University of Chicago Press, 1980.

Wallnofer, Heinrich, and Anna Von Rottauscher. *Chinese Folk Medicine*. Translated by Marion Palmedo. New York: Crown Publishers, 1965.

Williams, Ruth E. *The Road to Radiant Health*. Kennewick, Wash.: self-published, 1977.

Wine, Zhenya Kurashova. *Russian School of Massage Therapy, The Kurashova Method*. Self-published, n.d.

Wolfe, Honora Lee. "Tuina Massage in the People's Republic of China" in *Massage Magazine* 1, no. 4, 1986.

Wood, Elizabeth C. *Beard's Massage Principles and Techniques*, 2nd ed. Philadelphia, London, Toronto: W. B. Saunders Co., 1974.

Yegul, Fikret. *Baths and Bathing in Classical Antiquity*. New York: The Architectural History and Foundation, MIT Press, 1992.

Zacharias, Pat, and Vivian Baulch. Article posted on the Internet, May 1999, at www.detnews.com/history/baths.htm.

Zhen, Cao Xi. *The Massotherapy of Traditional Chinese Medicine*. Translated by Ding Chang Hao. Hong Kong: Hai Feng Publishing, 1985.

Ziegenspeck, Robert, M.D. *Massage Treatment in Diseases of Women*. Translated by F. H. Westerschulte. Published by the translator, 1909.

Zinn, Howard. *A People's History of the United States*, 2nd ed. New York: HarperPerennial, 1995.

INDEX

266

BOOKS OF RELATED INTEREST

THAI YOGA MASSAGE
A Dynamic Therapy for Physical Well-Being and Spiritual Energy
by Kam Thye Chow

BODY ROLLING
An Experiential Approach to Complete Muscle Release
by Yamuna Zake

THE REFLEXOLOGY MANUAL
An Easy-to-Use Illustrated Guide to the Healing Zones of the Hands and Feet
by Pauline Wills

AMMA THERAPY
A Complete Texbook of Oriental Bodywork and Medical Principles
by Tina Sohn and Robert Sohn

INFORMED TOUCH
A Clinician's Guide to the Evaluation and Treatment of Myofascial Disorders
by Donna Finando, L.Ac., L.M.T., & Steven Finando, Ph.D., L.Ac.

TRADITIONAL REIKI FOR OUR TIMES
Practical Methods for Personal and Planetary Healing
by Amy Z. Rowland

REIKI ENERGY MEDICINE
Bringing Healing Touch into Home, Hospital, and Hospice
by Libby Barnett and Maggie Chambers with Susan Davidson

THE HANDBOOK OF CHINESE MASSAGE
Tui Na Techniques to Awaken Body and Mind
by Maria Mercati

Inner Traditions • Bear & Company
P.O. Box 388
Rochester, VT 05767
1-800-246-8648
www.InnerTraditions.com

Or contact your local bookseller